Renal Nursing

This book is dedicated to my family

For Baillière Tindall

Senior Commissioning Editor: Ninette Premdas
Project Development Manager: Karen Gilmour
Project Manager: Joannah Duncan
Designer: Judith Wright

Renal Nursing

SECOND EDITION

Edited by

Nicola Thomas
RGN BSc(Hons) MA
Senior Lecturer
St Bartholomew School of Nursing and Midwifery
City University
London, UK
Past President of EDTNA/ERCA

The first edition of *Renal Nursing* was edited by

Toni Smith MBE
RGN
(Retired) Formerly Senior Nurse Manager
Department of Nephrology
Leicester General Hospital Trust
Leicester, UK

Foreword by

Corinne Jeffrey
Chair
Royal College of Nursing
Nephrology Nursing Forum
UK

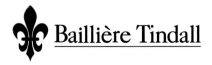 Baillière Tindall

BAILLIÈRE TINDALL
An imprint of Elsevier Science Limited

First edition 1997
Second edition 2002

ISBN 0 7020 2642 5

British Library Cataloguing in Publication Data
A catalogue record for this book is available from the British Library

Library of Congress Cataloging in Publication Data
A catalog record for this book is available from the Library of Congress

Note
Medical knowledge is constantly changing. As new information becomes
available, changes in treatment, procedures, equipment and the use of
drugs become necessary. The editor and contributors and the publishers
have taken care to ensure that the information given in this text is accurate
and up to date. However, readers are strongly advised to confirm that the
information, especially with regard to drug usage, complies with the latest
legislation and standards of practice.

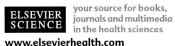 your source for books,
journals and multimedia
in the health sciences
www.elsevierhealth.com

The
publisher's
policy is to use
**paper manufactured
from sustainable forests**

Printed in China by RDC Group Limited

Contents

Contributors

Tim Armstrong Formerly Charge Nurse, Oxford Kidney Centre, Oxford, UK

Juliet Auer Renal Patient Support Manager, Oxford Kidney Centre, Oxford, UK

Gemma Bircher Dietetic Manager (Nephrology), Leicester General Hospital Trust, Leicester, UK

Charlotte A Chalmers Lecturer, Faculty of Health and Life Sciences, Napier University, Borders General Hospital NHS Trust, Melrose, UK

Jean-Yves De Vos Head Nurse, Dialysis Unit, Werken Glorieux, Ronse, Belgium

Patricia M Franklin Senior Clinical Nurse Specialist and Psychologist in Transplantation, Oxford Transplant Centre, Churchill Hospital, Oxford, UK

Jane Hattersley (Retired) Formerly Research Sister, Department of Nephrology, Leicester General Hospital Trust, Leicester, UK

Judith A Hurst Lecturer in Adult Nursing and Specializing in Renal Care, School of Nursing and Midwifery, City University, London, UK

Althea Mahon Nurse Consultant – Peritoneal Dialysis (community), Barts and the London NHS Trust, St Bartholomew's Hospital, London, UK

Toni Smith (Retired) Formerly Senior Nurse Manager, Department of Nephrology, Leicester General Hospital Trust, Leicester, UK

Nicola Thomas Senior Lecturer, St Bartholomew School of Nursing and Midwifery, City University, London, UK, Past President of EDTNA/ERCA

Marianne Vennegoor Dietitian, SRD, Consultant Specialist Renal Dietitian, formerly of the Department of Renal Medicine, Guy's and St Thomas' Hospital Trust, London, UK

Geraldine Ward Previously Paediatric Chronic Renal Failure Sister, Guy's and St Thomas' Hospital Trust, London, UK

Victoria Warmington Formerly Community PD Specialist Nurse, Wandsworth Community Health Trust, London, UK

Janet Wild Clinical Education Manager, Baxter Healthcare Ltd, Renal Division, Newbury, UK

Foreword

This second edition of *Renal Nursing* aims to give more up-to-date guidance to nurses caring for those with renal failure. It has been re-edited to include aspects of care that have previously not been addressed, such as the important area of pre-dialysis.

Renal Nursing is written by specialist professionals who have extensive experience and knowledge of practice within this field of nursing. The text has been produced for all nursing staff, including care assistants and support workers, who work in nephrology, dialysis and transplantation. It also provides a valuable educational resource for nurses undertaking further study in renal nursing as well as National Vocational Qualifications.

There is a lack of good evidence-based literature for nephrology nurses and this book aims to bridge the gap. It has been adapted to increase the level of knowledge, thus improving the standard of care being provided; and can be used as a reference or a resource to inform health care professionals of the developments in renal nursing.

Renal Nursing will be well received by health care professionals in the UK and throughout the world.

Corinne Jeffrey

Preface

I was delighted to edit the second edition of this successful book for nurses working in nephrology, dialysis and transplantation.

The text has been completely updated and is now fully referenced. At the beginning of each chapter there are learning outcomes and a number of chapters have useful case studies that can be used as the basis for ward or class discussions.

There are new chapters on predialysis care, clinical standards and nursing audit, plus future trends in renal nursing: all topical and pertinent issues in today's changing health care arena.

This book is mostly for those who are new to the renal specialty. Nurses who are studying on preregistration courses and practitioners who are commencing a postregistration course in renal nursing will find it particularly helpful. It also serves as a good foundation for nurses who wish to refresh their knowledge in a part of the renal field in which they are currently not practising, or for other members of the multiprofessional team who are commencing a career in renal care. The book has been written in a style that promotes renal nursing for what it is: a dynamic, varied and rewarding specialty.

Each chapter has been written by an expert in his or her field. Recognition must also go to those authors who wrote chapters for the first edition, but were unable to contribute to this edition. They are Sue Wharton, Phil Saunders, Eleanor Meldrum, Marie-Claire Richards, Maggie Hicklin and Marcelle De Sousa. I would like to thank particularly the editor of the first edition, Toni Smith, who identified the need for this book and had the drive to get it published.

Renal nurses in the 21st century face a constant challenge to keep up to date with new technologies and to use resources effectively. At the same time they must reflect on and evaluate nursing practice. However, what must always be central to their practice are those for whom they are caring, who have to cope with constant physical and psychosocial challenges. Whilst editing this book I have been mindful of the many people with renal failure I have met during my career as a nephrology nurse. Over the years I have heard their pleas for health care professionals to emphasis what *can* be done rather than what cannot. The word 'restriction' should not be part of a renal nurse's vocabulary: why not fluid or dietary *allowance*? So I have endeavoured to use a language that promotes the patient-centred care philosophy, and hope that this book will encourage renal nurses to care for their patients with understanding, compassion and sensitivity.

London 2002   *Nicola Thomas*

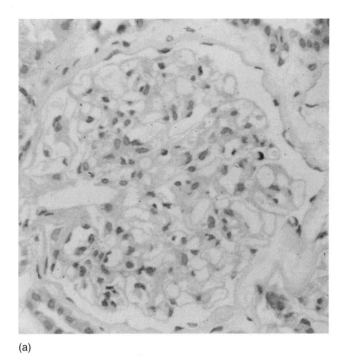

(a)

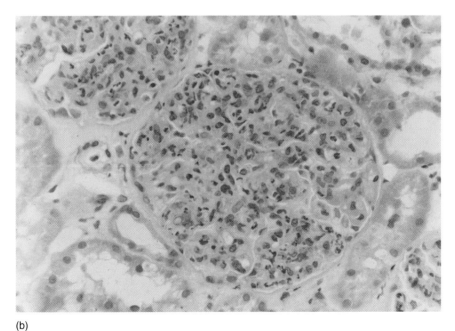

(b)

Plate 1 Renal histology from biopsy specimen (light micrographs). (a) A normal glomerulus. (b) A glomerulus from a patient with a diffuse proliferative (poststreptococcal) glomerulonephritis. Note how 'full' the glomerulus appears with a great increase in the number of cells due to inflammation (See Ch. 2.).

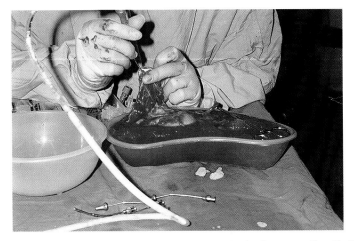

Plate 2 Kidney undergoing perfusion (in ice) immediately after harvesting. (See Ch. 11.)

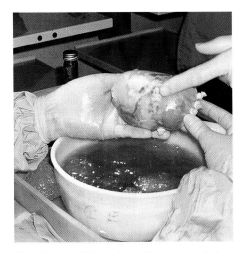

Plate 3 Cooled kidney in surgical glove, ready for transplantation. (See Ch. 11.)

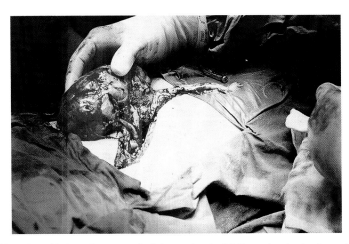

Plate 4 Transplanted kidney after removal of clamps showing 'pinking up' and urine formation. (See Ch. 11.)

The history of dialysis and transplantation

Toni Smith   Nicola Thomas

■ **CONTENTS**

■ **LEARNING OUTCOMES FOR THIS CHAPTER**

- To understand the evolution of haemodialysis (HD), peritoneal dialysis (PD) and transplantation
- To appreciate the difficulties that healthcare professionals have had to overcome in the development of the nephrology specialty
- To evaluate the changing focus of renal care in the 20th century
- To identify the challenges for nephrology nursing in the future.

INTRODUCTION

The introduction of dialysis as a life-saving treatment for kidney failure was not the result of any large-scale research programme, rather it emerged from the activities of a few pioneering individuals who were able to utilise ideas, materials and methods from a range of developing technologies.

HD as a routine treatment for renal failure was initiated in the 1960s, followed by continuous ambulatory peritoneal dialysis (CAPD) in the late 1970s. The recognition of the need for immunosuppression in transplantation in the 1960s enabled it to become the preferred treatment for many patients.

HAEMODIALYSIS

The beginning

It was the Romans who first used a form of dialysis therapy by giving hot baths to patients to remove urea. The action of the hot water made the patient sweat profusely and this, together with the toxins diffusing through the skin into the bath water, would temporarily relieve symptoms. However, the Romans did not understand why the treatment worked. The effect was to leave the patient fatigued but, as the only hope, this treatment was still used on occasions into the 1950s.

The first time that the term 'dialysis' was used was in 1854 by Thomas Graham (Fig. 1.1), a Scottish chemist (Graham, 1854). He used dialysis to

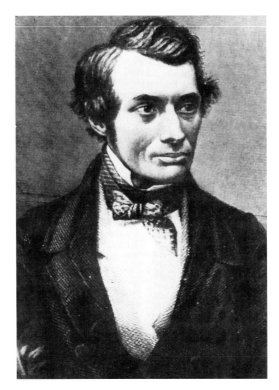

Figure 1.1 Thomas Graham 1805–1869. (Engraving by C. Cook after photograph by Claudet.)

describe the transport of solutes through an ox bladder, and this was the catalyst for other researchers working in a similar field to focus on the membrane.

Membranes were made from a variety of substances, including parchment and collodion (Eggerth 1921). Collodion is a syrupy liquid that dries to form a porous film, and allows the passage of small-molecular-weight substances, whilst being impermeable to substances with a molecular weight greater than 5 kDa. In 1889, BW Richardson referred to the use of collodion membranes in the dialysis of blood. So, by this method, living animals were dialysed in experimental conditions (Richardson 1889), but the limiting factor that prevented the treatment being used in humans at this time was the lack of suitable materials.

Pre-1920

It was not until 1913 that the first article on the technique of HD, named the 'artificial kidney', was reported. Experimental dialysis was performed on animals, by using variances in the composition of dialysis fluid (Abel et al, 1914). Substances could be added to the solution to avoid their net removal. The main aim of the experiments was the removal of salicylates. The removal of fluid and toxins accumulated due to kidney disease was not, at this time, considered.

In 1914, Hess & McGuigan were experimenting with dialysis in a pharmacology laboratory in Chicago. As a result they were able to transfer sugar from tissue to blood and from the blood across a collodion membrane. The design of the dialyser minimised the length of tubing from the patient, and a high blood flow was achieved by connection to the carotid artery in an effort to minimise the necessity to use an anticoagulant. A single U-shaped collodion tube was inserted into a glass cylinder with a rubber stopper at one end. The blood flow both to and from the dialyser was at one end, with a port for adjusting the pressure inside the tube. These experiments were still only performed on animals. The only anticoagulant available was in the form of an extract obtained from crushed leech heads, called hirudin. This was far from satisfactory, even though leeches were plentiful and readily available from the corner shop for around $25 per 1000.

The 1920s

The first dialysis performed on a human was carried out by the German physician, Georg Haas, in Giessen in the latter half of the 1920s. He performed six treatments in six patients. Hand-made collodion membranes were used, and clotting was prevented by using hirudin and, later, a crude form of heparin. Haas used multiple dialysers to increase the surface area of blood exposed to the dialysis fluid. This necessitated as many as six dialysers arranged in parallel and he found that the arterial pressure of the blood was insufficient to propel the blood through the entire extracorporeal circuit. He therefore introduced a pump into the circuit (Fig. 1.2). Haas was aware of the lack of support given to him by the hospital and his colleagues and by the late 1920s he gave up and the work was stopped. Georg Haas died in 1971, aged 85 years, and was honoured as the pioneer of dialysis.

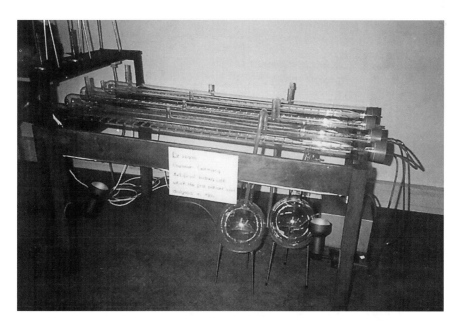

Figure 1.2 The equipment used by Georg Haas.

In spite of these treatments carried out from the 1920s to the 1940s, those with uraemia suffering from poor appetite and vomiting could be offered nothing more than bed-rest, and a bland salt-free diet composed mainly of vegetables, carbohydrate and fat to reduce protein metabolism. Dialysis was not considered a realistic option and the conservative therapy was only offered as a palliative measure.

Heinrich Necheles was the founder of the contemporary dialyser. In 1923, he experimented with the sandwiching of membranes, thus giving an increased surface area without the necessity for multiple dialysers. The membrane used was the peritoneum of a sheep, and because the membrane was prone to expansion, support sheets were placed between the layers of membrane, thus allowing a large surface area of membrane to come into contact with the dialysis fluid. Other features introduced by Necheles were a heater, the priming of the pathway for the blood, and a filter to prevent clots returning to the patient.

The 1930s

The 1920s and 1930s saw great advances in synthetic polymer chemistry, resulting in the availability of cellulose acetate which could be used as a membrane for HD. It was in 1937 that the first synthetic membrane was used by the American scientist William Thalhimer. The material, cellophane—a form of cellulose acetate, which was used extensively in the sausage industry—had potential which was not recognised for some years. In the mid-1930s came the purification of heparin (Thalhimer et al, 1938) which could be used as an anticoagulant and together these two advances gave rise to the next stage of development, which took place in 1943 in occupied Holland.

The 1940s and 1950s

Willem Kolff, a physician working in Groningen in Nazi-occupied Holland, had his attention drawn to the work of a colleague who was concentrating plasma by using cellulose acetate as a membrane and immersing it in a weak solution of sugar. Kolff noticed that toxins in the blood were altered by this method (Kolff 1950). He built a rotating drum dialyser (Figs 1.3 and 1.4) which provided sufficient surface area for his first attempt at human dialysis (Kolff & Berk 1944). His machine consisted of 30 m of cellophane tube that was wound round a large cylinder. The cylinder was placed in a tank containing a weak solution of salts—the dialysate. The patient's blood was passed through the cellophane tube, the walls acting as a semipermeable membrane. Blood flow was achieved by the addition of a circuit containing a burette which, when filled with blood, could be raised high enough to allow the blood to flow into the dialyser. The burette was then lowered, allowing the blood to drain back, and raised again to allow the blood to return to the patient. The slats in the construction of the cylinder were of wood due to the shortage at this time of materials such as aluminium—in retrospect, this was fortunate since the toxicity of aluminium is now appreciated. Six hours were required for the treatment, and it is interesting to note that with this method, similar efficiency of dialysis could be achieved as is possible with the dialysers in use today: a clearance of 170 ml min^{-1} urea could be achieved.

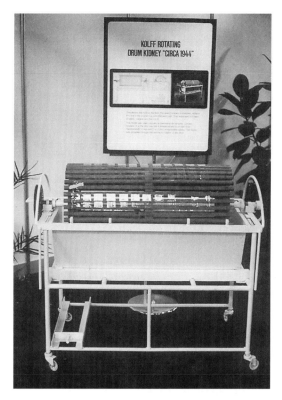

Figure 1.3 The Kolff rotating drum.

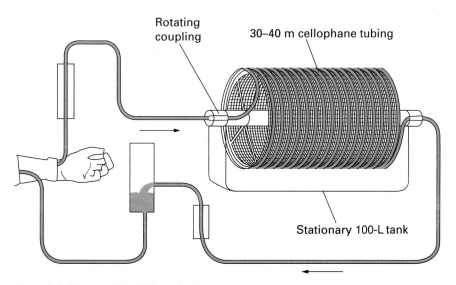

Rotating
coupling

30–40 m cellophane tubing

Stationary 100-L tank

Figure 1.4 Diagram of the Kolff rotating drum system.

Fluid could only be removed by increasing the osmotic pressure of the dialysate fluid by the addition of sugar, as an increase in pressure on the membrane would result in rupture (Kolff 1965).

The whole procedure was very time-consuming and labour-intensive, as the process required attention at all times, to raise and lower the burette and observe the membrane for rupture, which happened frequently. Repairs to the membrane were carried out by inserting a glass tube at the point of rupture.

Kolff's first clinical experience was gained on a 29-year-old woman with chronic nephritis. The blood urea was kept stable for 26 days, but after 12 sessions of dialysis, her blood urea began to increase, and she subsequently died.

After the war, in 1945, Kolff's technique was widely used, particularly in Sweden and the USA. The treatment was initially for acute renal failure when kidney function could be expected to return to normal following a short period of dialysis treatment. It was widely used in the Korean war in 1952 to treat trauma-induced renal failure. The group, led by Paul Teschan, trained to use the rotating drum dialyser and saved many lives by lowering the high potassium levels of the victims (Teschan 1955).

Some of the earliest research carried out on fluid removal from the blood using negative pressure was conducted by MR Malinow and W Korzon at Michael Reese Hospital in Chicago in 1946 (Malinow & Korzon 1947). The device used was the earliest version of a dialyser with multiple blood paths and negative pressure capacity. It had parallel sections of cellulose acetate tubing and, by adding layers of tubing, the surface area of the device could be increased. The diffusion properties of this device were not considered, as it was intended for removal of water only from the blood. The device required a low priming volume and the circuit included a blood pump.

In the 1940s, interest in dialysis as a treatment for renal failure had spread throughout Europe and across to Canada as the need was becoming widely recognised by the medical profession. After obtaining drawings of the Kolff dialyser, Russell Palmer and a colleague, from Vancouver in Canada, built a replica and dialysed their first patients in September 1947 (Palmer & Rutherford 1949).

Kolff was invited to take his artificial kidney to New York where he trained physicians in the operation of the life-saving device. There was resistance from hospital staff at the Mount Sinai Hospital, who only permitted the treatment to be administered in the surgical suite after normal surgical schedules were completed for the day. The first patient scheduled for treatment was a victim of mercuric chloride poisoning, but treatment was cancelled when a spontaneous diuresis occurred.

The first successful dialysis in Mount Sinai Hospital was in January 1948, in a female admitted to hospital having inserted mercury tablets into her vagina to induce an abortion (Fishman et al 1948). Eight hours after the first dialysis using the Kolff machine, the patient passed urine. The treatment had been a success. Victims of drug overdose were then regularly treated by use of the rotating drum dialyser until 1950.

To expand the use, the rotating drum would have to be modified to become easier to use. Kolff enlisted the help of Dr Carl Walter, who worked at the Peter Brent Brigham Hospital. Together with Edward Olson, an associate engineer from Fenwal, they set about designing and building a new version of the Kolff device. Stainless steel was used for the drum, and refinements included a hose for filling the pan with the 100 L of dialysate fluid, which was heated, and a hood to cover the drum. A tensioning device was used on the cellophane membrane as it had a tendency to stretch during use. The split connection for the patient's tubing was introduced, and this allowed the patient's tubing to remain stationary whilst the drum rotated. This was made leakproof, and a Lucite hood was added to overcome heat loss from the extracorporeal blood. These improvements paved the way for wider acceptance of the use of dialysis treatment (Merrill et al 1950).

When the Kolff–Brigham kidney was used, the heparin dose ranged from 6000 to 9000 units, and was infused prior to the start of the treatment. The dialyser was primed with blood, and the blood flow to the dialyser was limited to 200 mL at a time to prevent hypotension. To assist blood flow a pump was inserted in the venous circuit rather than the arterial side, to minimise the probability of pressure build-up in the membrane, which would cause a rupture.

This version of the Kolff–Brigham dialysis machine was used in 1948, and in all, over 40 machines were built and exported all over the world. Orders for spare parts were still being received as late as 1974, from South America and behind the Iron Curtain.

The 1950s

The Allis–Chalmers Corporation was one of the first companies to produce dialysis machines commercially. They were prompted into the manufacture when an employee developed renal failure. There was no machine available and so the firm turned its attention to producing a version of the Kolff rotating drum. The resulting machine was commercially available for $5600 and included all the sophistication available at the time. Allis–Chalmers produced 14 of these machines and sold them all over the USA into the early 1950s.

In October 1956, the Kolff system became commercially available, so the unavailability of equipment could no longer be used as an excuse for non-treatment of patients. Centres purchased the complete delivery system for around $1200 and the disposables necessary for the treatment were around $60. The system was still mainly used for reversible acute renal failure drug overdose, and poisoning (Fig. 1.5).

The development of the dialyser

Jack Leonards and Leonard Skeggs produced a plate dialyser which would permit a reduction in the priming volume, and allow negative pressure to be used to remove fluid from the patient's system (Skeggs et al 1949). A modification to this design included a manifold system which allowed variation of the surface area without altering the blood distribution. Larger dialysers followed, which necessitated the introduction of a blood pump.

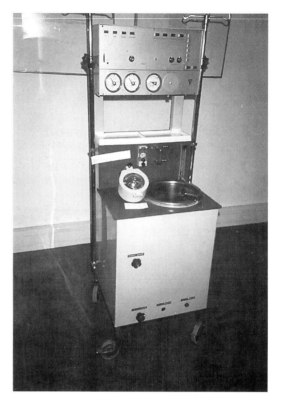

Figure 1.5 A typical dialysis machine from the 1950s: Fresenius.

In the late 1950s Fredrik Kiil of Norway developed a parallel plate dialyser, with a large surface area (1 m²) requiring a low priming volume (Fig. 1.6). A new cellulose membrane, Cuprophan, was used and this allowed the passage of larger molecules than other materials which were available at that time. The Kiil dialyser could be used without a pump. Kiil dialysed the patients using their own arterial pressure. This dialyser was widely used because the disposables were relatively inexpensive when compared with other dialysers at that time.

A crude version of the capillary-flow dialyser, the parallel dialyser using a new blood pump, and a more advanced version of the Alwall kidney was developed (MacNeill 1949). However, it was John Guarino who incorporated the important feature of a closed system, a visible blood pathway.

To reduce the size of the dialyser without reducing the surface area, William Y Inouye and Joseph Engelberg produced a plastic mesh sleeve to protect the membrane. This reduced the risk of the dialysis fluid coming into contact with the blood. Because this was a closed system, the effluent could be measured to determine the fluid loss of the patient. It is the true predecessor of the positive-and negative-pressure dialysers used today.

The first commercially available dialyser was manufactured by Baxter and based on the Kolff kidney. It provided a urea clearance of approxi-

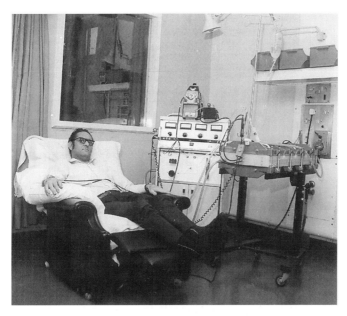

Figure 1.6 The Kiil dialyser.

mately 140 ml min^{-1}, equivalent to today's models, and was based on the coil design. The priming volume was 1200–1800 mL and this was drained into a container at the end of treatment, refrigerated and used for priming for the next treatment. It was commercially available in 1956 at $59.00.

The forerunner of today's capillary-flow dialyser was produced by Richard Stewart in 1960. The criteria for design of this hollow-fibre dialyser were low priming volume and minimal resistance to flow. The improved design contained 11 000 fibres which provided a surface area of 1 m^2.

Future designs for the dialyser will focus on refining the solute and water removal capabilities, as well as reducing the size and priming requirements of the device, thus allowing an even higher level of precise individual care.

The emergence of home haemodialysis

It was Scribner's shunt which provided vascular access, thus leading to the first dialysis unit to be established for chronic patients at the University of Washington Hospital. Belding Scribner also developed a central dialysate delivery system for multiple use and set this up in the chronic care centre, which had 12 beds. These beds were quickly taken and his plan for expansion was rejected. The only alternative was to send the patients home, and so the patient and family were trained to perform the dialysis and care for the shunts. Home dialysis was strongly promoted by Scribner (Fig. 1.7).

Stanley Shaldon reported in 1961 that a patient dialysing at the Royal Free Hospital in London was able to self-care by setting up his own

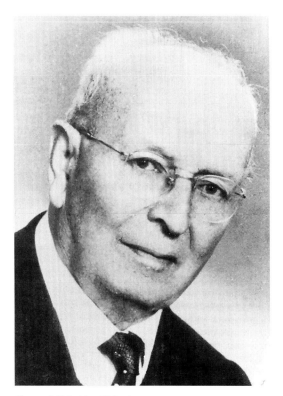

Figure 1.7 Belding H Scribner.

machine, initiating and terminating dialysis; so home HD in the UK was made possible. The shunt was formed in the leg for vascular access, to allow the patient to have both hands free for the procedures. Hence Shaldon was able to report the results of his first patient to be placed on overnight home HD in November 1964. With careful patient selection, the venture was a success. Scribner started to train patients for home at this time, and his first patient was a teenager assisted by her mother. Home dialysis was selected for this patient, so that she would not miss her high-school education. The average time on dialysis was 14 h twice weekly. To allow freedom for the patient, overnight dialysis was widely practised. At first, emphasis was on selection of the suitable patient and family, even to the extent of a stable family relationship, before the patient could be considered for home training (Baillod et al 1965).

From these beginnings, large home HD programmes developed in the USA and in the UK, thus allowing expansion of the dialysis population without increasing hospital facilities. Many patients could now be considered for home treatment, often with surprisingly good results, as the dialysis could be moulded to the requirements of the individual, rather than the patients conforming to a set pattern. However, with the development in the late 1970s and early 1980s of CAPD as the first choice for home treatment, the use of home HD has steadily dwindled.

Vascular access for haemodialysis

It was Sir Christopher Wren, of architectural fame, who in 1657 successfully introduced drugs into the vascular system of a dog. In 1663, Sir Robert Boyle injected successfully into humans. Prison inmates were the subjects and the cannula used was fashioned from a quill. For HD to become a widely accepted form of treatment for renal failure, a way to provide long-term access to the patient's vascular system had to be found and until this problem was solved, long-term treatment could not be considered. In order for good access to be established, a tube or cannula had to be inserted into an artery or vein, thus giving rise to good blood flow from the patient. The repeated access for each treatment quickly led to exhaustion of blood vessels for cannulation. The need for a system whereby a sufficiently large blood flow could be established for dialysis, without destroying a length of blood vessel every time dialysis was required, was imperative.

Teschan, in the 11th Evacuation Hospital in Korea, was responsible in the 1950s for developing a method of heparin lock for continuous access to blood vessels. The cannulae were made from Tygon tubing and stopcocks, and the blood was prevented from clotting by irrigation with heparinised saline. It was not a loop design, as the arterial and venous segments were not joined together.

In 1960 in the USA, George Quinton, an engineer, and Belding Scribner, a physician, made use of two new synthetic polymers—Teflon and Silastic—and, using the tubing to form the connection between a vein and an artery, were able to re-route the blood outside the body (usually in the leg). This was known as the arteriovenous (AV) shunt. The tubing was disconnected at a union joint in the centre, and each tube then connected to the lines of the dialysis machine. At the end of treatment, the two ends were then reconnected, establishing a blood flow from the artery to the vein outside the body. In this way, repeat dialysis was made possible without further trauma to the vascular system.

This external shunt, whilst successful, had drawbacks. It was a potential source of infection, often thrombosed and had a restrictive effect on the activity of the patient. This form of access is still occasionally used for acute treatment, although the patient's potential requirements for chronic treatment must be considered when the choice of vessels is made, so that vessels to be used in the formation of an AV fistula are not scarred. In 1966, Michael Brescia and James Cimino developed the subcutaneous radial artery-to-cephalic vein AV fistula (Cimino & Brescia 1962), with Cimino's colleague Kenneth Appel performing the surgery.

The AV fistula required less anticoagulation, had reduced infection risk and gave access to the blood stream without danger of shunt disconnection. Subsequently, a number of synthetic materials have been introduced to create internal AV fistulae (grafts). These are useful when the patient's veins are not suitable to form a conventional AV fistula, such as in severe obesity, with loss of superficial veins due to repeated cannulation or in the elderly or those with diabetes.

Venous access by cannulation of the jugular, subclavian or femoral veins has now largely replaced the shunt for emergency dialysis.

The present

Monitoring and total control of the patient's therapy became more important as dialysis became widespread, and so equipment development continued. Sophisticated machines incorporated temperature monitoring, positive-pressure gauges and flow meters. Negative-pressure monitoring followed, as did a wide range of dialysers with varying surface areas, ultrafiltration capabilities and clearance values. Automatic mixing and delivery of the dialysate and water supply to the machine greatly increased the margin of safety for the procedure, and made the dialysis therapy much easier to manage. The patient system that has evolved provides a machine that monitors all parameters of dialysis through the use of microprocessors, allowing the practitioner to programme a patient's requirements (factors such as blood flow, duration of dialysis and fluid removal) so that the resulting treatment is a prescription for the individual's needs. Average dialysis time is reduced to 4 h three times weekly, or less if a high-flux (high-performance) dialyser is used.

The early 1970s saw the number of patients increase due to the increased awareness brought about by the availability of treatment. Free-standing units for the sole use of kidney dialysis came into being, leading to dialysis becoming a full-time business. Committees for patient selection were disbanded, and the problems concerned with inadequate financial resources came to the fore. Now that the 21st century, have been set for treatment quality. Attempts continue to reduce treatment duration, to enhance the patient's quality of life. Good nutrition has also emerged as playing a vital role in reducing dialysis morbidity and mortality. Dialysis facilities are demanded within easy reach of patients' homes, and this expectation has led to the emergence of small satellite units, managed and monitored by larger units, as a popular alternative to home HD treatment. In 2000, there were 82 satellite dialysis units in the UK (Kidney Alliance 2001).

PERITONEAL DIALYSIS

CAPD as a form of therapy for renal failure has been brought about by a climax of the innovative efforts and the tenacity of many pioneers over the past 2 centuries. It was probably the early Egyptian morticians who first recognised the peritoneum and peritoneal cavity as they embalmed the remains of their influential compatriots for eternity. The peritoneal cavity was described in 3000 BC in the Ebers papyrus as a cavity in which the viscera were somehow suspended. In Greek times, Galen, a physician, made detailed observations of the abdomen whilst treating the injuries of gladiators.

The earliest reference to what may be interpreted as PD was in the 1740s when Christopher Warrick reported to the Royal Society in London that a 50-year-old woman suffering from ascites was treated by infusing Bristol water and claret wine into the abdomen through a leather pipe (Warrick 1744). The patient reacted violently to the procedure, and it was stopped after three treatments. The patient is reported to have recovered, and was able to walk 7 miles (approximately 13 km) a day without difficulty. A modification of this was subsequently tried by Stephen Hale of Teddington in England: two trocars were used—one on each side of the abdomen—allowing the fluid to flow in and out of the peritoneal cavity during an operation to remove ascites (Hale 1744).

Subsequent experiments on the peritoneum (Wegner 1877) determined the rate of absorption of various solutions, the capacity for fluid removal (Starling & Tubby, 1894) and evidence that protein could pass through the peritoneum. It was also noted that the fluid in the peritoneal cavity contained the same amount of urea that is found in the blood, indicating that urea could be removed by PD (Rosenberg 1916). This was followed by Tracy Putnam suggesting that the peritoneum might be used to correct physiological problems, when he observed that under certain circumstances fluids in the peritoneal cavity can equilibrate with the plasma and that the rate of diffusion was dependent on the size of the molecules. Research also suggested at this time that the clearance of solutes was proportional to their molecular size and solution pH, and that a high flow rate maximised the transfer of solutes, which also depended on peritoneal surface area and blood flow (Putman 1923).

George Ganter was looking for a method of dialysis that did not require the use of an anticoagulant (Ganter 1923). He prepared a dialysate solution containing normal values of electrolytes and added dextrose for fluid removal. Bottles were boiled for sterilisation and filled with the solution, which was then infused into the patient's abdomen through a hollow needle.

The first treatment was carried out on a woman who was suffering acute renal failure following childbirth. Between 1 and 3 L of fluid was infused at a time, and the dwell time was 30 min to 3 h. The blood chemistry was reduced to within acceptable limits. The patient was sent home, but unfortunately she died, as it was not realised that it was necessary to continue the treatment in order to keep the patient alive.

Ganter recognised the importance of good access to the peritoneum, as it was noted that it was easier to instil the fluid than it was to attain a good return volume. He was also aware of the complication of infection, and indeed it was the most frequent complication that he encountered. Ganter identified four principles, which are still regarded as important today:

- There must be adequate access to the peritoneum.
- Sterile solutions are needed to reduce infection.
- Glucose content of the dialysate must be altered to remove greater volumes of fluid.
- Dwell times and fluid volume infused must be varied to determine the efficiency of the dialysis.

There are reports of 101 patients treated with PD in the 1920s (Abbott & Shea 1946; Odel et al 1950). Of these, 63 had reversible causes, 32 irreversible and in two the diagnosis was unknown. There was recovery in 32 of 63 cases of reversible renal failure. Deaths were due to uraemia, pulmonary oedema and peritonitis.

Stephen Rosenak, working in Europe, developed a metal catheter for peritoneal access, but was discouraged by the results because of the high incidence of peritonitis. In Holland, PSM Kop, who was an associate of Kolff during the mid-1940s, created a system of PD by using materials for the components that could easily be sterilised: porcelain containers for the fluid, latex rubber for the tubing, and a glass catheter to infuse the fluid into the patient's abdomen. Kop treated 21 patients and met with success in 10.

Morton Maxwell, in Los Angeles, in the latter part of the 1950s, had been involved with HD, and it was his opinion that HD was too complicated for regular use. Aware of the problems with infection, he designed a system for PD with as few connections as possible. Together with a local manufacturer, he formulated a peritoneal solution, and customised a container and plastic tubing set and a single polyethylene catheter. The procedure used was to instil 2 L of fluid into the peritoneum, leave it to dwell for 30 min, and return the fluid into the original bottles. This would be repeated until the blood chemistry was normal. This technique was carried out successfully on many patients and the highly regarded results were published in 1959. This became known as the Maxwell technique (Maxwell et al 1959). This simple form of dialysis recognised that it was no longer necessary to have expensive equipment with highly specialised staff in a large hospital to initiate dialysis. All that was required was an understanding of the procedure and available supplies.

The catheter

Up to the 1970s, PD was used primarily for patients who were not good candidates for HD, or who were seeking a gentler form of treatment. Continuous flow using two catheters (Legrain & Merrill 1953) was still sometimes used, but the single-catheter technique was favoured because of lower infections rates.

The polyethylene catheter was chosen by Paul Doolan (Doolan et al 1959) at the Naval Hospital in San Francisco when he developed a procedure for the treatment to use under battlefield conditions in the Korean war. Because of the flexibility of the catheter, it was considered for long-term treatment. A young physician called Richard Ruben decided to try this procedure, known as the Doolan technique (Ruben et al unpublished work), on a female patient who improved dramatically, but deteriorated after a few days without treatment. The patient was therefore dialysed repeatedly at weekends, and allowed home during the week, with the catheter remaining in place. This was the first reported chronic treatment using a permanent indwelling catheter.

Catheters were made from tubing available on the hospital ward and included gallbladder trocars, rubber catheters, whistle-tip catheters and stainless-steel sump drains. However, as with the polyethylene plastic tubes, the main trouble was kinking and blockage. Maxwell described a nylon catheter with perforations at the curved distal end and this was the catheter which became commercially available. Advances in the manufacture of the silicone peritoneal catheter by Palmer (Palmer et al 1964) and Gutch (Gutch 1964) included the introduction of perforations at the distal end and later Tenckhoff included the design of a shorter catheter, a straight catheter and a curled catheter. He also added the Dacron cuff, either single or double, to help to seal the openings through the peritoneum (Tenckhoff & Schechter 1968). He was also responsible for the introduction of the trocar that gave easy placement of the catheter. Dimitrios Oreopoulos, a Greek physician, was introduced to PD in Belfast, Northern Ireland, during his training and he noted the difficulties encountered with the catheters there. He had been shown a simple technique for inserting the catheter by Norman Dean from New York City, which allowed the access to be used over and over again.

Peritoneal dialysis at home

In 1960, Scribner and Boen (Boen 1959) set up a PD programme that would allow patients to be treated at home. An automated unit was developed which could operate unattended overnight. The system used 40-L containers that were filled and sterilised at the University of Washington. The bottles were then delivered to the patient's home, and returned after use. The machine was able to measure the fluid in and out of the patient by a solenoid device. An indwelling tube was permanently implanted into the patient's abdomen, through which a tube was inserted for each dialysis treatment. The system was open, and therefore was vulnerable to peritonitis. A new method was then used, whereby a new catheter was inserted into the abdomen for each treatment, and removed after the treatment ended. This was still carried out in the home, when a physician would attend the patient at home for insertion of the catheter, leaving once the treatment had begun. The carer was trained to discontinue the treatment and remove the catheter. The wound was covered by a dressing, and the patient would be free of dialysis until the next week. This treatment was carried out by Tenckhoff et al (1965) in a patient for 3 years, requiring 380 catheter punctures.

The large 40-L bottles of dialysate were difficult to handle and delivery to the home and sterilisation were not easy. Tenckhoff, at the University of Washington, installed a water still into the patient's home, thus providing a sterile water supply. The water was mixed with sterile concentrate to provide the correct solution, but this method was not satisfactory as it remained cumbersome and dangerous due to the high pressure in the still. Various refinements were tried using this method, including a reverse osmosis unit, and this was widely used later for HD treatment.

Lasker, in 1961, realised the potential of this type of treatment and concentrated on the idea of a simple version by instilling 2 L of fluid by a gravity-fed system. This proved to be cheaper to maintain but was labour-intensive. Later that year, he was approached by Ira Gottscho, a businessman who had lost a daughter through kidney problems, and together they designed the first peritoneal cycler machine. The refinements included the ability to measure the fluid in and out, and the ability to warm the fluid before the fill cycle. Patients were sent home using the automated cycler treatment as early as 1970, even though there was a bias for HD at that time.

In 1969, Oreopoulos accepted a position at the Toronto Western Hospital and, together with Stanley Fenton, decided to use the Tenckhoff catheter for long-term treatment. Because of a lack of space and facilities at the hospital, it was necessary to send the patients home on intermittent PD. He reviewed the Lasker cycler machine and ordered a supply, and by 1974 was managing over 70 patients on this treatment at home. Similar programmes were managed in Georgetown University and also in the Austin Diagnostic Clinic in the USA.

The beginning of continuous ambulatory peritoneal dialysis

It was in 1975, following an unsuccessful attempt to haemodialyse a patient at the Austin Diagnostic Clinic, that an engineer, Robert Popovich, and Jack Moncrief became involved in working out the kinetics of 'long-dwell equilibrated dialysis' for this patient. It was determined that five exchanges each of 2 L per day would achieve the appropriate blood chemistry, and that the removal of 1–2 L of fluid from the patient was needed per day. Thus came the evolution of CAPD (Popovich et al 1976).

The treatment was so successful that the Austin group were given a grant to allow them to continue dialysing patients with CAPD. Strangely, their first description and account of this clinical experience was rejected by the American Society for Artificial Internal Organs. At this time the treatment was called 'a portable/wearable equilibrium dialysis technique'. The stated advantages compared to HD included:

- good steady-state biochemical control
- more liberal diet and fluid intake
- improvement in anaemia.

The main problems were protein loss (Popovich et al 1978) and infection. It was recognised that the source of infection was almost certainly related to the use of the bottles. Oreopoulos found that collapsible polyvinylchloride (PVC) containers for the solution were available in Canada. Once the fluid was instilled, the bag could then be rolled up and concealed under the clothing. The fluid could be returned into the bag during draining by gravity, without a disconnection taking place (Oreopoulos et al 1978). New spike connections were produced for access to the bag of fluid, and a Luer connection for fitting to the catheter; together with tubing devised for HD, greatly reduced the chances of infection. The patients treated on an intermittent basis (by intermittent peritoneal dialysis or IPD) were rapidly converted to CAPD and evaluation of the new treatment was rapid, due to the large numbers being treated. Following approval by the US Food and Drug Administration, many centres were then able to develop CAPD programmes.

The first complete CAPD system was released on to the market in 1979, giving a choice of three strengths of dextrose solution. Included in this system were an administration line, and sterile items packed together to form a preparation kit, to be used at each bag change in an attempt to keep infection at bay. The regime proposed by Robert Popovich and Jack Moncrief entailed four exchanges over a 24-h period, three dwell times of approximately 4 h in the daytime, and one dwell overnight of 8 h. This regime is the one mainly used today.

The systems are continually being improved, with connectors moving from spike to Luer to eliminate as far as possible the accidental disconnection of the bag from the line. A titanium connector was found to be the superior form of adaptor for connection of the transfer set to the catheter, and probably led to a reduced infection rate for peritonitis. A disadvantage of this technique is the flow of fresh fluid down the transfer set along the area of disconnection, thus encouraging any bacteria from the disconnection to be instilled into the abdomen. The development of the Y-system (flush before fill) in the mid-1980s in Italy resulted in a further decrease in peritonitis.

Automated peritoneal dialysis

Automated PD in the form of continuous cyclic peritoneal dialysis (CCPD) was further developed by Diaz-Buxo in the early 1980s to enable patients who were unable to perform exchanges in the day to be treated with PD overnight (Fig. 1.8).

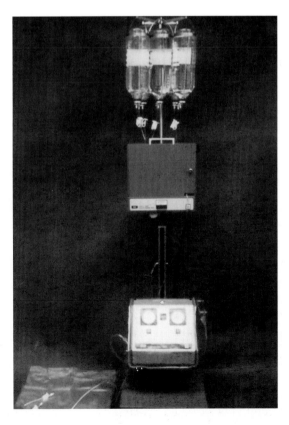

Figure 1.8 The American Medical Products (AMP)
continuous cyclic peritoneal dialysis (CCPD) machine 1980.

Advances in peritoneal dialysis for special needs

Recent advances in CAPD treatment include a dialysate which not only provides dialysis, but which contains 1.1% amino acid, to be administered to malnourished patients. This may be particularly useful for the elderly on CAPD, in whom poor nutrition is a well-recognised complication.

Those with diabetes were initially not considered for dialysis, because of the complications of the disease. Carl Kjellstrand, at the University of Minnesota, suggested that insulin could be administered to those with diabetes by adding it to the PD fluid (Crossley & Kjellstrand 1971). However, when this suggestion was first put forward, it was not adopted because the 30-min dwell did not give time for the drug to be absorbed into the patient. It became viable later, when the long dwell dialysis was initiated, and this gave the advantage of slow absorption, resulting in a steady state of blood sugar in the normal range, thus alleviating the need for painful injections (Flynn & Nanson 1979).

The realisation that patients are individuals, bringing their own problems associated with training, brought many exchange aid devices on to the market to assist the patient in the exchange procedure. These exchange devices were mainly used to assist such disabilities as blindness, arthritis (particularly of the hands) and patients prone to repeated episodes of peritonitis (Fig. 1.9).

The future

PD is a first choice of treatment for end-stage renal disease in many countries and, because of the lack of facilities for in-centre HD, will remain so. In the UK in 1998, 36% of all patients on dialysis were on PD therapies (Ansell & Feest 2000). However the relative prevalence of PD in the UK has been declining since its peak in the early 1990s, possibly because of the

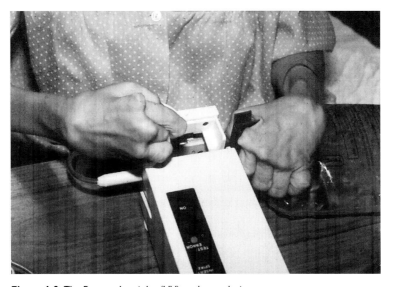

Figure 1.9 The Baxter ultraviolet (UV) exchange device.

availability of satellite haemodialysis and a high level of PD technique failure.

TRANSPLANTATION

In the beginning

Kidney transplantation as a therapeutic and practical option for renal replacement therapy (RRT) was first reported in published literature at the turn of the 20th century. The first steps were small and so insignificant that they were overlooked or condemned.

The first known attempts at renal transplantation on humans were made without immunosuppression between 1906 and 1923 using pig, sheep, goat and subhuman primate donors (Elkington 1964). These first efforts were conducted in France and Germany but others followed. None of the kidneys functioned for long, if indeed at all, and the recipients all died within a period of a few hours to 9 days later.

Of all the workers at this time, the contribution made by Alixis Carrel (1873–1944) remains the most famous. His early work in Lyons, France and in Chicago involved the transplantation of an artery from one dog to another. This work later became invaluable in the transplantation of organs. In 1906, Carrel and Guthrie, working in the Hull Laboratory in Chicago, reported the successful transplantation of both kidneys in cats and later a double nephrectomy on dogs, reimplanting only one of the kidneys. He found that the secretion of urine remained normal and the animal remained in good health, despite having only one kidney (Carrel 1908). Carrel was awarded the Nobel Prize in 1912 for his work on vascular and related surgery.

While at this stage there was no clear understanding of the problem, some principles were clearly learned. Vascular suture techniques were reviewed and the possibility of using pelvic implantation sites was investigated and practised. No further renal heterotransplantations (animal to human) were tried until 1963 when experiments using kidneys from chimpanzee (Reemtsma et al 1964) and baboon were tried, with eventual death of the patients. This ended all trials using animal donation.

The first human-to-human kidney transplant was reported in 1936, by the Russian Voronoy, when he implanted a kidney from a cadaver donor of B-positive blood type into a recipient of O-positive blood type, a mismatch that would not be attempted today. The donor had died 6 h before the operation and the recipient died 6 h later without making any urine. The following 20 years saw further efforts in kidney transplantation, all without effective immunosuppression (Groth 1972). The extraperitoneal technique developed by French surgeons Dubost and Servelle became today's standard procedure.

The first successes

The first examples of survival success of a renal transplant can probably be attributed to Hume. Hume placed the transplanted kidney into the thigh of the patient, with function for 5 months. Then at the Peter Bent Brigham Hospital in Boston, USA, in December 1954, the first successful identical-twin transplant was performed by the surgeon Joseph E Murray in collaboration with the nephrologist John P Merrill (Hume et al 1955). The recipient survived for more than 2 decades. The idea of using identical twins had been proposed when it was noted by David C Miller of the Public Health Service Hospital, Boston, that skin grafts between identical twins were not rejected (Brown 1937). The application of this information resulted in rigorous matching, including skin grafting, prior to effective immunosuppression.

Over the period between 1951 and 1976 there were 29 transplants performed between identical twins, and the survival rate for 20 years was 50%. Studies of two successfully transplanted patients, who were given kidneys from their non-identical twins, were also reported (Merrill et al 1960). The first survived 20 years (died of heart disease) and the second, 26 years (died of carcinoma of the bladder). Immunosuppression used in these cases was irradiation.

Immunosuppression

It was Sir Peter Medawar who appreciated that rejection is an immunological phenomenon (Medawar 1944), and this led to research into weakening the immune system of the recipients to reduce the rejection. In animals, corticosteriods, total body irradiation and cytotoxic drug therapy were used. Experiments in animals were still far from successful, as were similar techniques when used in humans. It was concluded that the required degree of immunosuppression would lead to destruction of the immune system and finally result in terminal infections.

A few patients were transplanted between 1960 and 1961 in Paris and Boston, using drug regimes involving 6-mercaptopurine or azathioprine with or without irradiation. They all died within 18 months. Postmortem examination of failed kidney grafts showed marked changes in the renal histology, which at first were thought unlikely to be due to immunological rejection, but later it was convincingly shown that this was indeed the underlying process.

In the early days of kidney transplantation, the kidney was removed from either a living related donor or a cadaver donor and immediately transferred to the donor after first flushing the kidney with cold electrolyte solution such as Hartman's solution. In 1967, Belzer and his colleagues developed a technique for continuous perfusion of the kidney using oxygenated cryoprecipitated plasma, which allowed the kidney to be kept up to 72 h before transplantation. This machine perfusion required constant supervision, and it was found that flushing the kidney with an electrolyte solution and storage at 0°C in ice saline allowed the kidney to be preserved for up to 24 h or more (Marshall et al 1988). This was a major development in transplantation techniques.

During the 1950s it was recognised that many of the survivors of the Hiroshima atomic bomb in 1945 suffered impairment to their immune system. It was concluded that radiation could therefore induce immunosuppression, and clinical total body irradiation was used to prolong the survival of renal transplants in Boston in 1958. This did improve the survival of some transplants; however, the overall outcomes were poor. There was clearly a need for a more effective form of immunosuppression than irradiation.

A breakthrough in immunosuppressive therapy occurred in 1962 in the University of Colorado, when it was discovered that the combination of azathioprine and prednisone allowed the prevention and, in some cases, reversal, of rejection (Starzl et al 1963). Transplantation could at last expand. A conference sponsored by the National Research Council and National Academy of Sciences in 1963 in Washington resulted in the first registry report, which enabled the tracing of all the early non-twin kidney recipients. In 1970 work commenced on the development of ciclosporin by Sandoz in Basle, Switzerland, following recognition of the potential (Borel et al 1976). Clinical trials carried out in Cambridge, UK (Calne et al 1979), showed that outcomes on renal transplantation were greatly improved, both with graft and with patient survival. Ciclosporin revolutionised immunosuppression treatment for transplant patients, even though it is itself nephrotoxic and its use needs close monitoring.

Tissue typing is a complex procedure and, as yet, is far from perfect. The use of the united networks for organ sharing has increased the efforts of matching donor and recipient, and data available from these sources show a significant gain in survival of well-matched versus mismatched cadaver kidneys. Cross-matching remains as important today as it was 25 years ago at its conception. None of the immunosuppressive measures available today can prevent the immediate destruction of the transplanted organ by humoral antibodies in the hyperacute rejection phase. This was recognised as early as 1965 (Kissmeyer-Neilsen et al 1966), and it may be that this phenomenon holds the key to the future of successful heterotransplantation.

Blood transfusions

It was observed in the late 1960s that patients who had received multiple blood transfusions before organ transplantation did not have a poorer graft survival than those who had not been transfused. In 1974, Opelz & Terasaki observed that patients who had received no transfusions whatsoever were more likely to reject the transplant. It became evident, therefore, that a small number of blood transfusions resulted in an improved organ survival and so the transfusion policies for non-transfused recipients were changed throughout the world. This 'transfusion effect' is of much less importance with the ciclosporin era.

Present

Renal transplantation has been a dramatic success over the past 30 years, with patient survival rates not less than 97% after 6 months transplantation for both living related and cadaver transplants. Although short-term survival for the graft is good—around 90% expectation of survival of the graft at 1 year)—cadaveric graft survival at 5 years of around 60% is less impressive, with a substantial minority losing their renal graft after 10 years.

The future

There is no doubt that renal transplantation is the treatment of choice for many patients requiring RRT giving, in general, a better quality of life than dialysis. However, organs are in short supply, the numbers of transplants having diminished slightly over the last 10 years (United Kingdom Transplant Support Service Authority 1999). A change in the law may result in more kidneys becoming available for transplantation, by allowing easier access to donors or removing the need for relatives' consent, but until a significant breakthrough is achieved there will continue to be a waiting list for transplantation and it will be necessary to continue to improve the techniques of dialysis.

SUMMARY

The Kidney Alliance (an umbrella body representing all organisations involved in renal services) suggested in 2001 that acceptance rates for RRT are rising, but there remain geographical inequalities. Some areas in the UK do not have autonomous renal services or satellite dialysis units. Acceptance rates in some areas are lower than in other European countries (Fig. 1.10). Therefore, both hospital and community-based services need to be expanded to enable patients to have a choice of treatment, and the standard of dialysis therapy offered to patients should be monitored.

Since acceptance rates exceed death rates, the numbers receiving RRT will not plateau for at least 10 years and, since transplant rates are static, the numbers on dialysis will continue to increase. Another challenge is the difficulty in recruiting and retaining nursing staff skilled in dialysis care.

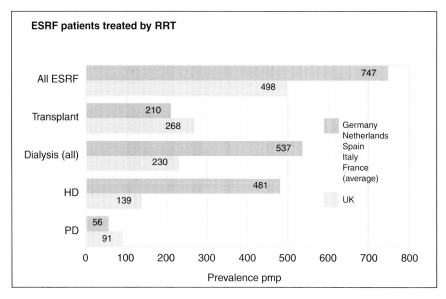

Figure 1.10 End-stage renal failure (ESRF) patients treated by renal replacement therapy. HD, haemodialysis; PD, peritoneal dialysis; pmp, per million population. (From Kidney Alliance 2001, with permission.)

Dialysis has come a long way from the small beginnings of the hot baths in Rome. Refinements and improvements continue, most recently with the emergence of erythropoietin in the late 1980s to correct the major complication of anaemia in these patients.

Improvements in access for both HD and PD will emerge. The challenge of adequate dialysis for all who need treatment remains.

Transplantation is still not available for all those who are eligible, and changes in the law may help with availability of donor organs.

The multidisciplinary teams will continue to strive to give patients the best possible quality of treatments until a revolutionary breakthrough in prevention of renal failure happens.

REFERENCES

Abbott WE, Shea P. Treatment of temporary renal insufficiency (uraemia) by peritoneal lavage. Am J Med Sci 1946; 211:312.

Abel JJ, Rowntree LG, Turner BB. The removal of diffusable substances from the circulating blood of living animals by dialysis. J Pharmacol Exp Ther 1914; 5:275–316.

Ansell D, Feest T (eds). Third annual report of the UK Renal Registry. Bristol: UK Renal Registry, 2000.

Baillod RA, Comty C, Ilahi M et al. Proceedings of the European Dialysis and Transplant Association 2. Amsterdam: Excerpta Medica, 1965: 99.

Boen ST. Peritoneal dialysis. Amsterdam: Van Gorcum, 1959: 26.

Borel JF, Feurer C, Gubler HU et al. Biological effects of cyclosporin A. A new antilymphocytic agent. Agents Actions, 1976; 6:468–475.

Brown JB Homografting of the skin. With report of success in identical twins. Surgery 1937; 1:558–563.

Calne, RY, Rolles K, White DJG et al. Cyclosporin A initially as the only immunosuppressant in 34 recipients of cadaveric organs: 32 kidneys, 2 pancreases, and 2 livers. Lancet 1979; 1:1033–1036.

Carrel, A. Results of the transplantation of blood vessels, organs and limbs. JAMA 1908, 51:1662–1667. Reprinted in JAMA 1983; 250:994–953.

Cimino, JE, Brescia MJ. Simple venepuncture for haemodialysis. N Engl J Med 1962; 267:608–609.

Crossley K. Kjellstrand CM. Intraperitoneal insulin for control of blood sugar in diabetic patients during peritoneal dialysis. Br Med J 1971; 1:269–290.

Doolan PD, Murphy WP Jr, Wiggins RA et al. An evaluation of intermittent peritoneal lavage. Am J Med 1959; 26:831–844.

Eggerth AH. The preparation and standardization of collodion membranes. J Biol Chem 1921; 48(1):203–221.

Elkington JR. Moral problems in the use of borrowed organs artificial and transplanted. Ann Intern Med 1964; 60:309–313.

Fishman AP, Kroop IG, Leiter HE et al. Management of anuria in acute mercurial intoxication. NY State J Med 1948; 48:2393–2396.

Flynn CT, Nanson, JA. Intraperitoneal insulin with CAPD—an artificial pancreas. Trans Am Soc Artif Intern Organs 1979; 25:114–117.

Ganter G. About the elimination of poisonous substances from the blood by dialysis. Munch Med Wochenschr 1923; 70:1478–1480.

Graham T. The Bakerian lecture—on osmotic force. Phil Trans R Soc Lond 1854; 144:177–228.

Groth CG. Landmarks in clinical renal transplantation. Surg Gynecol Obstet 1972 134:323–328.

Gutch CF. Peritoneal dialysis. Trans Am Soc Artif Intern Organs 1964; 10:406–407.

Hale S. A method of conveying liquors into the abdomen during the operation of tapping. Phil Trans R Soc 1744; 43:20–21.

Hess CLV McGuigan H. The condition of the sugar in the blood. J Pharmacol Exp Ther 1914; 6:45–55.

Hume DM, Merrill JP, Miller BF et al. Experience with renal homotransplantation in the human. Report of nine cases. J Clin Invest 1955; 34:327–382.

Kidney Alliance. End-stage renal failure—a framework for Planning and Service Delivery. Kidney Alliance: 2001.

Kissmeyer-Neilsen F, Olsen S, Peterson VP et al. Hyperacute rejection of kidney allografts, associated with pre-existing humoral antibodies against donor cells. Lancet 1966; 2:662–665.

Kolff WJ. Artificial kidney—treatment of acute and chronic uraemia. Cleveland Clin Q 1950; 17:216–228.

Kolff WJ. First clinical experience with the artificial kidney. Ann Intern Med 1965; 62:608–619.

Kolff WJ, Berk HT. The artificial kidney: a dialyser with a great area. Acta Med Scand 1944; 117:121–134.

Legrain M Merrill JP. Short term continuous transperitoneal dialysis. N Engl J Med 1953; 248:125–129.

MacNeill AE. Some possible uses of blood dialysers. Surgeons practice meeting. New England Surgical Society Sept 23 1949. Bretton Woods, NH: Proceedings of the New England Surgical Society, 1949:3.

Malinow MR, Korzon W. Experimental method for obtaining an ultrafiltrate of the blood. J Lab Clin Med 1947; 31:461–471.

Marshall VC, Jablonski P Scott DF. Renal preservation. In: Morris PJ, ed. Kidney transplantation: principles and practice. 3rd edn. Philadelphia: WB Saunders, 1988:151–182.

Maxwell MH, Rockney RE., Kleeman CR. Peritoneal dialysis, techniques and application. JAMA 1959; 170:917–924.

Medawar PB. The behaviour and fate of skin autografts and skin homografts in rabbits. J Anat 1944; 78:176–199.

Merrill JP, Thorn GW, Walter CW et al. The use of an artificial kidney. 1. Technique. J Clin Invest 1950; 29:412–424.

Merrill JP, Murray JE, Harrison JH et al. Succesful homotransplantation of the kidney between non-identical twins. N Engl J Med 1960; 262:1251–1260.

Odel HM, Ferris DO, Power H. Peritoneal lavage as an effective means of extrarenal excretion. Am J Med 1950; 9:63–77.

Opelz G, Terasaki PI. Poor kidney transplant survival in recipients with frozen-blood transfusions or no transfusions. Lancet 1974; 2:696–698.

Oreopoulos DG, Robson M, Izatt S et al. A simple and safe technique for continuous ambulatory peritoneal dialysis. Trans Am Soc Artif Organs 1978; 24:484–489.

Palmer RA, Rutherford PS. Kidney substitutes in uraemia: the use of Kolff's dialyser in two cases. Can Med Assoc J 1949; 60: 261–266.

Palmer RA, Quinton WE, Gray JF. Prolonged peritoneal dialysis for chronic renal failure. Lancet 1964; 1:700–702.

Popovich RP, Moncrief JF, Decherd JF et al. The definition of a novel portable/wearable equilibrium peritoneal dialysis technique. Abstract Trans Am Soc Artif Organs 1976; 5:64.

Popovich RP, Moncrief JW, Nolph KD et al. Continuous ambulatory peritoneal dialysis. Ann Intern Med 1978; 88:449–456.

Putman T. The living peritoneum as a dialysing membrane. Am J Physiol 1923; 63:548–555.

Reemtsma K, McCracken BH, Schlegel JU et al. Renal heterotransplantation in man. Ann Surg 1964; 160:384–410.

Richardson BW. Practical studies in animal dialysis. Asclepiad (Lond) 1923; 6:331–332.

Rosenberg M. Nitrogenous retention of substances in the blood and in other body fluids in the core of the kidneys. J Berl Klin Wochenshr 1916; 53:1314–1316.

Skeggs LT Jr, Leonards JR, Heisler CR. Artificial kidney: 11. Construction and operation of an improved continuous dialyser. Proc Soc Exp Biol Med 1949; 72(3):539–543.

Starling EH, Tubby AH. On the paths of absorption from the peritoneal cavity. J Physiol 1894 16:140.

Starzl TE, Marchioro TL, Waddell WR. The reversal of rejection in human renal homografts with subsequent development of homograft tolerance. Surg Gynecol Obstet 1963; 117:385–395.

Tenckhoff H, Schechter H. A bacteriologically safe peritoneal access device. Trans Am Soc Artif Intern Organs 1968; 14:181–186.

Tenckhoff H, Shilipetar G, Boen ST. One year experience with home peritoneal dialysis. Trans Am Soc Artif Intern Organs 1965; 11:11–14.

Teschan PE. Haemodialysis in military casualties. Trans Am Soc Artif Intern Organs 1955; 2:52–54.

Thalhimer W, Solandt DY, Best CH. Experimental exchange transfusion using purified heparin. Lancet 1938; 11:554–555.

United Kingdom Transplant Support Service Authority (UKTSSA) Transplant Activity 1998. Bristol: UKTSSA, 1991.

Warrick C. An improvement in the practice of tapping, whereby that operation instead for the relief of symptoms, became an absolute cure for ascites, exemplified in the case of Jane Roman. Phil Trans R Soc 1744; 43:12–19.

Wegner G. Surgical comments on peritoneal cavity with special emphasis on ovariotomy. Arch Klin Chir 1877; 20:53–145.

Applied anatomy and physiology and the renal disease process

Charlotte A Chalmers

2

◼ LEARNING OUTCOMES FOR THIS CHAPTER

- To understand the structure and main functions of the kidney
- To explain the basic renal processes of filtration, reabsorption and secretion
- To identify the main conditions causing chronic and end-stage renal failure
- To analyse the clinical features of these conditions and explain the principles of care management.

INTRODUCTION

This chapter provides the reader with a detailed discussion on all aspects of renal physiology, together with the relationship to important patho-physiological processes in renal disease and some brief discussion on related nursing observations. The first part of the chapter explores the normal renal anatomy and physiology and the second part deals with disease processes causing renal failure. This is not intended as a complete reference to all kidney diseases, rather to illustrate how altered renal physiology can affect the whole body, and indeed how other diseases can impact on kidney function.

STRUCTURE AND FUNCTIONS OF THE KIDNEY

The kidneys are paired organs lying behind the peritoneum, on either side of the vertebral column. The upper pole of the kidney is at the spinal level of T12 and the lower pole at approximately L3. The right kidney is a little lower due to the presence of the liver on that side. Usually, the kidneys are oriented with the concave surface facing the spine. However, due to developmental aberrations, other orientations of the kidney may occasionally exist (e.g. lying in the pelvis) but these do not usually affect function. Each kidney is approximately 11 cm long and weighs about 150 g (Fig. 2.1).

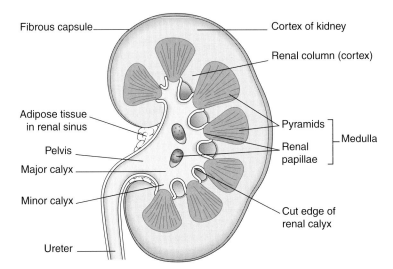

Figure 2.1 Coronal section of a kidney. (After Hinchliff SM, Montague SE, Physiology for nursing practice. London: Baillière Tindall' 1988, with permission of Baillière Tindall.)

On the concave surface of the kidney lies the hilus, from which the ureter and the main blood vessels and nerves access the kidney. The cut surface of the kidney reveals two distinct regions: a dark outer region, the cortex, and a pale inner region called the medulla. The outer cortex is covered by a fibrous capsule and the whole kidney is surrounded by a pad of fat that offers some protection against injury. Broadly speaking, the cortex contains the filtering and reabsorptive components of the nephrons, whilst the medulla contains the concentrating and diluting components of the nephrons and a system of collection ducts. These ducts funnel the urine into the pelvis at the heart of the medulla, from where it moves down the ureter into the bladder (Fig. 2.2).

The nephron

The nephron is the functional unit of the kidney and each kidney contains approximately 1 million nephrons (Fig. 2.3). The unique structure of the nephron is critically related to its complex functions and contains five components, each performing a distinct process:

• the Bowman's capsule—forming a blind-ending capsule around a knot of capillaries called the glomerulus (the site of filtration)
• the proximal convoluted tubule (the site of bulk-phase reabsorption and some secretion)
• the loop of Henle (where the concentration and dilution of urine mainly occur)
• the distal convoluted tubule (the site of 'fine-tuning' reabsorption and more secretion)
• the collecting duct (also important for the concentration of urine and for carrying urine into the renal pelvis).

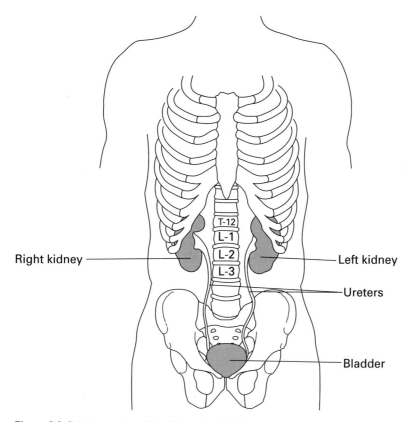

Right kidney

Left kidney

Ureters

Bladder

T-12
L-1
L-2
L-3

Figure 2.2 Relative position of the kidneys in the body.

These processes do not occur in isolation but are interdependent and intimately related to each other by the shape of the nephron. The importance of this fact will become clear when the renal processes are discussed in more detail.

There are broadly two types of nephron found in the kidney (Fig. 2.4). Approximately 85% of nephrons are cortical nephrons, which have short loops of Henle that are contained in the cortex of the kidney. The other 15% of nephrons are called juxtamedullary nephrons and they have long loops of Henle which extend deep into the medulla of the kidney. It is the long loops of Henle which enable concentration of urine; animals adapted to arid environments have long loops of Henle compared with those which have a lesser requirement to conserve water. It is the loops of Henle, together with the collecting ducts which also pass through the medulla, that give the pyramids of the medulla a striated appearance.

The main functions of the kidney are to rid the body of the end-product of metabolism and to regulate the electrolytes found in the body fluids. A more detailed list of the functions of the kidney can be found in Box 2.1. Before looking at how the kidney achieves its functions, there follows a discussion on the impressive versatility of urine.

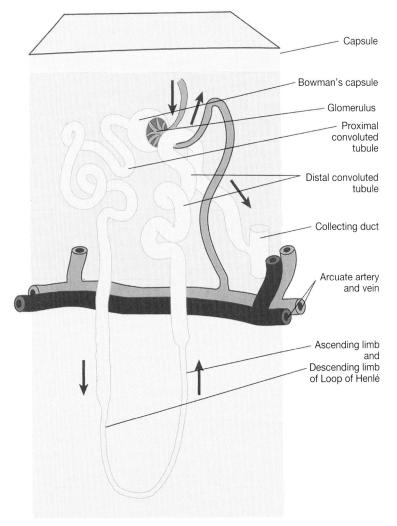

Figure 2.3 Microanatomy of nephron. (From Hinchliff SM, Montague SE, Watson R Physiology for nursing practice. London: Bailliére Tindall, 1999, with permission of Baillière Tindall.)

The versatility of urine

When the immense variability in the qualities of urine that can be produced in order to control our internal environment is considered, one cannot fail to be impressed by the complexities of the workings of the kidney. Broadly speaking, there are three parameters that can be varied in order to maintain the constancy of our bodily fluids: urinary volume, urinary concentration and urinary content.

Urinary volume

In a healthy person, the volume of urine produced per day can vary from as little as 300 mL, if no water is ingested or there is excessive water loss from the body (as in diarrhoea), up to a maximum of 23 L in cases of excessive

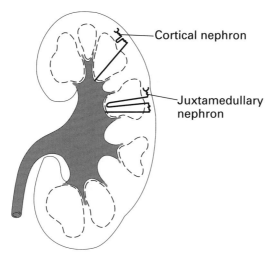

Figure 2.4 The position of the nephrons in the kidney.

■ BOX 2.1 The functions of the kidney

Excretory
- Excretion of metabolic waste products, e.g. urea and creatinine

Regulatory
Regulation of:
- Body water volume
- Body fluid osmolality
- Electrolyte balance
- Acid–base balance
- Blood pressure

Metabolic
- Activation of vitamin D
- Production of renin
- Production of erythropoietin

---

fluid ingestion. In health, urine output cannot drop below 300 mL day^{-1} because this is the absolute minimum water volume required to excrete the daily load of toxic waste products. If the amount of waste products to be removed by the kidney rises, then the minimum urine volume must also rise. However, the average urine output per day is approximately 1500 mL. The kidneys' ability to vary the volume of daily urine output over such a wide range is essential if we are to maintain a constant body fluid volume in the face of adverse factors such as excessive heat, which causes sweating; colonic infections causing diarrhoea; or excessive thirst and water ingestion, as seen in the condition psychogenic polydipsia (Table 2.1).

Table 2.1 Normal fluid inputs and outputs

Inputs (mL)		Outputs (mL)		
Water	1500	Urine[a]		1500
Food	500	Insensible loss	lungs	400
			skin[b]	400
Water of metabolism	400	Faeces[c]		100
Total	2400			2400

[a] Urinary volume is the only factor that can be regulated by the body to balance fluid inputs.
[b] This insensible loss of fluid through the skin is by simple evaporation (not sweat). Sweat is called 'sensible loss' and may reach up to 5 L h^{-1}, for example, when a person is exercising excessively.
[c] Loss of fluid with the faeces can be as high as several litres per day in the presence of severe colonic infections such as cholera.

Urinary concentration

Though the volume of urine can vary over a wide range, the amount of solutes to be excreted by the kidney each day is much less variable. Thus, in order to excrete a fairly fixed volume of solutes each day in a very variable volume of water, the kidney must have the ability to concentrate or dilute the urine. On a hot summer's day when very little fluid has been drunk, urine is dark in colour and of low volume, whereas if liberal amounts of beer have been consumed at a party, large volumes of watery urine are passed all evening. In fact this diuretic effect of beer is not wholly due to the volume imbibed, but also to the fact that the alcohol present in the beer suppresses the secretion (from the posterior pituitary gland) of antidiuretic hormone (ADH, also known as vasopressin), a hormone which would normally prevent diuresis. The hangover suffered the next day is therefore caused by dehydration.

The ability of the kidneys to excrete all the body's excess solutes in varying amounts of water by concentrating or diluting the urine is essential for maintaining a constant body osmolality (Box 2.2). The mechanism in the kidney that controls the concentration or dilution of urine is often affected early on in renal disease, making it difficult for the individual to control both body fluid volume and osmolality in response to changes in fluid inputs and outputs. This can result in the individual tipping back and forth from states of dehydration to fluid overload.

Urinary content

The range of substances that can be constituents of urine is varied and includes:

- Ions: sodium, potassium, calcium, magnesium, chloride, bicarbonate, phosphate and ammonium
- Metabolic waste: urea, creatinine and uric acid
- Drug metabolites: most metabolites of pharmacological agents are eventually excreted from the body through the kidneys; many are detoxified in the liver first

---

■ BOX 2.2 Concepts of osmosis and body osmolality

- Water can move between the different body fluid compartments across semipermeable membranes by the process of osmosis
- The more concentrated a solution, the more water will be drawn into this solution
- Any solute that can cause the movement of water across a semipermeable membrane is said to be 'osmotically active'
- The osmotic activity of substances in solution is dependent on the number of dissolved particles in the solution and not on their size or charge
- Sodium chloride (NaCl) dissociates in solution into Na^+ and Cl^- ions, so the number of osmotically active particles is almost double the number of NaCl molecules (but not exactly double, since the dissociation is not complete; the solution consists of NaCl, Na^+ and Cl^- particles)
- Osmotically active particles in solution are measured by the unit called the osmole or milliosmole (mosmol)
- Osmolality is measured in $mosmol\ kg^{-1}$ water and is a measure of the potential osmotic activity of dissolved solutes in solution
- Normal body fluid osmolality is 285 $mosmol\ kg^{-1}$ water
- The concentration (rather than the osmotic activity) of individual electrolytes is measured in mmol (millimoles) or μmol (micromoles) rather than mosmol, e.g. normal fasting blood glucose range = 3.6–5.8 $mmol\ L^{-1}$

- Other products of normal metabolism: metabolites of hormones can be detected in the urine by appropriate assays and may be a diagnostic aid, for example, the appearance of human chorionic gonadotrophin (hCG) in the urine in the early stages of pregnancy forms the basis of the pregnancy test.

Normal urine is clear in appearance, though it may vary in colour from pale to dark amber, depending on its concentration. It has no unpleasant odour, though urine that has been standing a long time may develop a strong ammonia smell. Finally, normal urine has a pH that is slightly acidic—around pH 6—though urine can have a pH in the range 4.0–8.0 in cases of severe acidosis or alkalosis respectively.

BASIC RENAL PROCESSES

Glomerular filtration

This is a process of filtration of plasma across the glomerular basement membrane from the glomerulus into the Bowman's capsule (Fig. 2.5). The glomerular filtration surface is a unique structure composed of three layers:

- the endothelial lining of the glomerular capillaries
- the basement membrane

- the epithelial cells of the Bowman's capsule, or podocytes. Filtration occurs between the slits formed by the finger-like processes of these cells (called pedicels) which surround the glomerular capillaries (Fig. 2.6).

These three layers are fused together and act as a barrier to the filtration of large-molecular-weight molecules such as proteins.

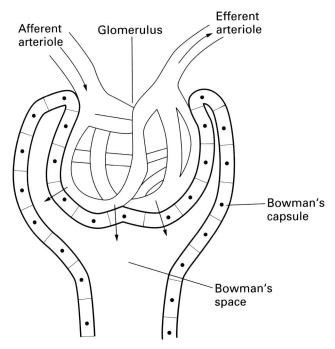

Figure 2.5 The glomerulus and Bowman's capsule.

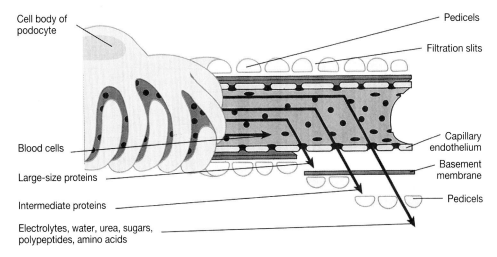

Figure 2.6 Schematic representation of the filtration barrier. (Redrawn from Creager JG. Human anatomy and physiology. CA: Wodsworth, 1983, with permission.)

Blood enters the glomerulus from a series of branches of the renal artery, ending in the afferent arteriole. Blood then leaves the glomerulus through the efferent arteriole rather than a vein. In the majority of nephrons (those situated in the cortex), the efferent arteriole from the glomerulus divides up into capillaries which cover the surfaces of the convoluted tubules. The capillaries finally empty into the venous system. In the deeper juxta-medullary nephrons the efferent arteriole from the glomerulus divides to form loops which lie parallel to the loops of Henle and so run down into the medulla. These vessels are called the vasa recta and are concerned with the process of concentration of the urine (Fig. 2.7). Blood then leaves the kidney through a series of larger converging veins, ending in the renal vein which returns the blood to the vena cava.

In effect, the nephrons contain two capillary beds, one within the glomerulus and a second which surrounds the convoluted tubules of the nephrons. This unusual arrangement of two capillary beds in tandem enables a pressure gradient to exist within the nephron, with high pressure

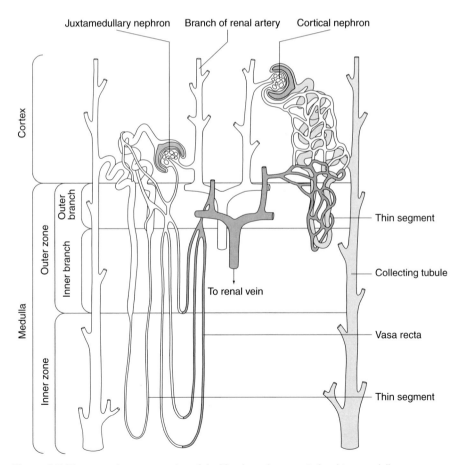

Figure 2.7 Diagrammatic representation of the blood supply to cortical and juxtamedullary nephrons. (From Lamb JF, Pitman RM. Essentials of physiology. 3rd edn. London: Blackwell Scientific, 1991, with permission.)

in the glomerulus, favouring filtration, and a relatively low pressure in the peritubular capillaries, favouring reabsorption.

The formation of a filtrate from plasma flowing through the glomerulus occurs due to Starling's forces (Fig. 2.8). These are the same forces that cause the filtration and reabsorption of tissue fluid in other capillary beds in the body, but with some important adaptations. In the glomerulus, fluid is forced across the glomerular basement membrane because of the high hydrostatic pressure of blood flowing through the afferent arteriole. This pressure is greater than the oncotic pressure opposing it. Oncotic pressure is essentially osmotic pressure, exerted by proteins in the blood. In an ordinary capillary bed, this filtrate would be almost entirely reabsorbed back into the capillary at the venule end because the hydrostatic pressure would

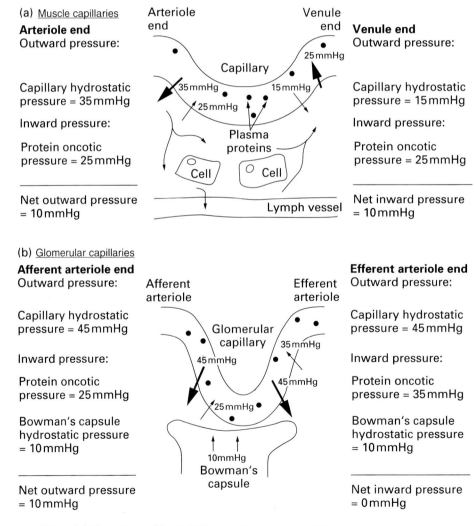

(a) Muscle capillaries

Arteriole end
Outward pressure:

Capillary hydrostatic pressure = 35 mmHg

Inward pressure:

Protein oncotic pressure = 25 mmHg

Net outward pressure = 10 mmHg

Venule end
Outward pressure:

Capillary hydrostatic pressure = 15 mmHg

Inward pressure:

Protein oncotic pressure = 25 mmHg

Net inward pressure = 10 mmHg

(b) Glomerular capillaries

Afferent arteriole end
Outward pressure:

Capillary hydrostatic pressure = 45 mmHg

Inward pressure:

Protein oncotic pressure = 25 mmHg

Bowman's capsule hydrostatic pressure = 10 mmHg

Net outward pressure = 10 mmHg

Efferent arteriole end
Outward pressure:

Capillary hydrostatic pressure = 45 mmHg

Inward pressure:

Protein oncotic pressure = 35 mmHg

Bowman's capsule hydrostatic pressure = 10 mmHg

Net inward pressure = 0 mmHg

Figure 2.8 Comparison of Starling's forces between muscle capillaries and glomerular capillaries. (a) Starling's forces operating in muscle capillaries, resulting in the formation and reabsorption of tissue fluid. (b) Starling's forces operating in glomerular capillaries, resulting in the formation of glomerular filtrate.

have fallen to below the oncotic pressure of the capillary, which would then pull the fluid back in by osmosis. However, in the glomerulus, because blood leaving enters another arteriole (the efferent arteriole) rather than a venule, a high hydrostatic pressure is maintained and oncotic pressure is insufficient to draw fluid back into the capillary. This situation is obviously desirable so that large amounts of filtrate can be made. All of the filtrate formed in the glomerulus passes into the Bowman's capsule and is often referred to as tubular urine (Fig. 2.8).

Amount and composition of glomerular filtrate

The amount of glomerular filtrate formed per minute is referred to as the glomerular filtration rate (GFR), and in the average healthy person is approximately 125 mL min^{-1}. This volume is the sum amount from all 2 million nephrons in the kidneys and thus the amount from each nephron is relatively small. A quick calculation shows that at a GFR of 125 mL min^{-1}, the total amount of filtrate formed per day is 180 L—approximately 60 times the circulating plasma volume. Obviously, the majority of this must be reabsorbed to prevent severe dehydration.

The 'average' GFR quoted is generally only average for a young adult. Children have a lower GFR than this because their nephrons are still increasing in size (all nephrons are present at birth). After the age of about 30 years the number of functioning nephrons starts to decrease because of the ageing process, thus the GFR decreases proportionately. However this only becomes significant to health when the GFR falls to around 5 mL min^{-1}—a situation that only occurs in a diseased kidney. The GFR can be calculated clinically by measuring the creatinine clearance rate. This requires a 24-h urine sample and blood sample from the patient. The principles of this test are described in Chapter 6.

The composition of the initial glomerular filtrate is that of a plasma ultrafiltration; that is, without proteins. The main determinant of what can pass through the glomerular basement membrane is molecular size, although the molecular shape and charge are also important. The passage of strongly negatively charged molecules such as albumin tends to be retarded because of the presence of fixed negative charges in the basement membrane which repel their movement. Albumin, a small protein, has a molecular weight of 69 kDa, a weight just below the cut-off point for filtration. It can therefore cross the filter, but does so only in minute quantities since it is also hindered by its negative charge. It is because of this free permeability of small molecules that the composition of the initial glomerular filtrate is the same as that of the plasma for small molecules, and will include the major ions sodium, potassium, chloride, bicarbonate, calcium and phosphate; glucose, amino acids and the toxic waste products of urea and creatinine. Any albumin filtered is reabsorbed through the proximal tubule into the renal lymph system and returned to the blood stream.

Selective reabsorption

Reabsorption is a process that involves the movement of water and dissolved substances from the tubular fluid back into the blood stream. The term 'selective' infers a regulatory function to this process, as indeed not all of the filtered substances are returned to the blood. Any substances not reabsorbed will pass with the urine into the bladder to be excreted from the body. The main sites for reabsorption in the nephron are the proximal and distal convoluted tubules.

Mechanisms of reabsorption

Broadly speaking, there are three mechanisms in the nephron for the reabsorption of water and solutes: osmosis, diffusion and active transport. Osmosis is the movement of water from an area of low concentration to a more concentrated solution across a membrane which allows water molecules through but is selectively permeable to solute molecules (a semipermeable membrane).

Diffusion occurs where a concentrated solution meets one which is less concentrated. The solute will equilibrate throughout the solvent. This may occur across a membrane so long as the membrane is permeable to the solute. Diffusion may also occur through specialised 'protein carriers' in the membrane. This is sometimes known as 'facilitated diffusion'. In these cases, the number of protein carriers in the membrane is limited, meaning that movement of the solute will be limited. This is true for tubular reabsorption of glucose (which is also linked to sodium transport). Once all the carriers are active, reabsorption of glucose has reached its maximum. If the filtered load of glucose is excessive, not all can be reabsorbed and glucose will appear in the urine, as happens in untreated diabetes mellitus.

Active transport is so named because it is an energy-requiring process. The energy source is adenosine triphosphate (ATP). Active transport can move solutes against a concentration gradient. Cells which carry out a lot of active transport will have a lot of mitochondria present (the 'power-generating' organelles of cells).

In the proximal tubule cells, where most reabsorption is by active transport, the cells are packed with mitochondria. Proximal tubule cells also have a large brush border on their luminal surface (the surface facing into the tubule) to increase their surface area for reabsorption. In contrast, cells lining the descending loop of Henle are comparatively thin, have no brush border and have relatively few mitochondria. This suggests that these cells are not very metabolically active and are adapted for reabsorption by passive diffusion. The epithelial cells of the distal tubule are similar to those of the proximal tubule but with a less well-defined brush border and fewer mitochondria. This suggests that these cells are capable of active transport of substances but in much lesser quantities than in the proximal tubule. This again illustrates how each segment of the nephron is anatomically adapted to carry out its unique functions. The different cell types lining the tubules are illustrated in Figure 2.9.

Reabsorption in the proximal convoluted tubule—the site of bulk-phase reabsorption

Approximately 65% of all reabsorption occurs in the proximal tubule (hence the term 'bulk phase') and is obligatory rather than regulatory. Most

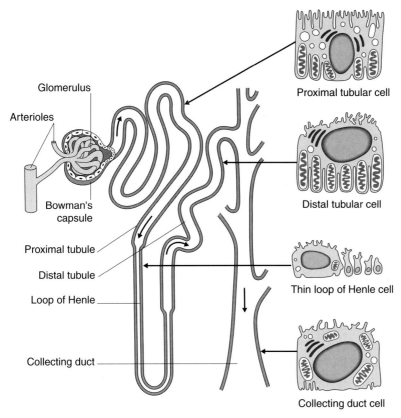

Figure 2.9 Essential features of the structure of a nephron. (After Hinchliff SM, Montague SE. Physiology for nursing practice. London: Baillière Tindall, 1988, with permission of Baillière Tindall.)

substances here are reabsorbed by active transport mechanisms, including sodium, chloride, potassium, glucose, amino acids, phosphate and bicarbonate. Urea is absorbed by passive diffusion and water is reabsorbed by osmosis. Some substances are reabsorbed almost entirely in the proximal tubule, such as glucose and amino acids, which do not appear in the urine, whereas others have only between 60 and 70% reabsorption, such as sodium, water and potassium. Approximately 50% of urea is reabsorbed here but creatinine is not reabsorbed at all. However, for all substances that are reabsorbed, the proximal tubule is the site where the bulk of this reabsorption occurs.

Reabsorption in the distal convoluted tubule—the site of fine-tuning reabsorption

This is the site where more specific regulation of substances occurs according to the needs of the body. In order for the distal tubule to be aware of precisely what the body's reabsorptive needs are, there needs to be some method of communication between the cells of the distal tubule and the rest of the body. This communication system is via a range of hormones which form part of a negative-feedback system for the homeostatic control of ions and water. For example, sodium and water reabsorption are under the control of aldosterone (secreted by the adrenal cortex) and ADH secreted by the posterior pituitary gland. Potassium reabsorption is also controlled by aldosterone, whereas calcium and phosphate are controlled by parathyroid hormone (PTH). The precise mechanisms for controlling the electrolytes outlined above will be dealt with in later sections in this chapter.

Secretion

The process of secretion occurs in both the proximal and distal tubules and involves the movement of substances from blood flowing through the peritubular capillaries, through the tubule wall cells, into the tubular fluid. In this respect, secretion is the opposite process to reabsorption. Substances that are secreted into the tubules are excreted in the urine. Though creatinine is freely filtered at the glomerulus, total creatinine excretion is increased by 20% by the process of secretion. Ions that are transported into the tubules by secretion are hydrogen, which is secreted in both the proximal and distal tubules and is important in acid–base control, and potassium, which is secreted in the distal tubule in exchange for sodium reabsorption. The hormone involved is aldosterone.

Excretion of drugs and drug metabolites

Many drugs and their metabolites are finally excreted from the body through the kidneys by the processes of glomerular filtration and secretion. Like other filtered substances, the rate of filtration of drugs will depend on their molecular size and charge: smaller molecules are filtered more rapidly than larger ones. Drugs that bind to plasma proteins are filtered very slowly because of the size of the complex. Some drugs are cleared from the blood purely by glomerular filtration and thus the rate of clearance cannot exceed the GFR of 125 mL min^{-1}, whereas other drugs are excreted by a combination of filtration and secretion, such as benzylpenicillin, which achieves a total clearance rate of 480 mL min^{-1} (Laurence & Bennett 1987).

Concentration and dilution of urine

The components of the nephron that are involved in the concentration and dilution of the urine are the loop of Henle and the collecting ducts. The concentration of urine is measured in units of osmolality (mosmol kg^{-1} water). The most dilute urine that humans can produce is approximately 60 mosmol kg^{-1} water, but this situation occurs in the pathological condition of diabetes insipidus in which the pituitary gland fails to produce ADH. The most concentrated urine that can be produced is approximately 1400 mosmol kg^{-1} water, which is greater than four times more concentrated than plasma (plasma osmolality = 285 mosmol kg^{-1} water) and requires maximum ADH secretion. The average range of urine osmolality in people with normal kidneys is between 300 and 500 mosmol kg^{-1} water.

Countercurrent mechanism of urinary concentration

The countercurrent mechanism is a complex physiological process which will not be discussed in great detail.

In order to concentrate the urine the following factors are required:

- the creation and maintenance of a local environment in the kidney that allows large quantities of water to be reabsorbed by osmosis from the collecting duct back into the blood
- a mechanism that can influence the opening and closing of water channels in the collecting ducts in order to control the exact amount of water reabsorbed.

Creation of the local environment (Fig. 2.10)

This local environment consists of an increasing hyperosmotic medullary interstitium as one moves towards the tip of the loops of Henle. In other words, the tissue spaces between the loops of Henle in the medulla of the

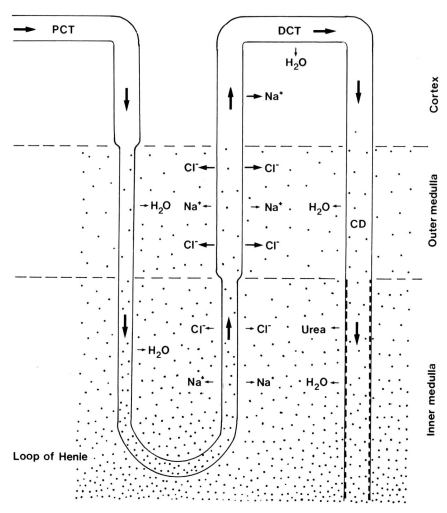

Figure 2.10 Countercurrent mechanism. Thick horizontal arrows, active transport; PCT, proximal convoluted tubule; DCT, distal convoluted tubule; thin horizontal arrows, passive transport. (From Hubbard JL, Mechan DJ. Physiology for health care students. Churchill Livingstone, Edinburgh, 1987, with permission.)

kidney must be made hyperosmotic compared to the fluid in the collecting duct. As the collecting ducts pass through the medulla on their way to the renal pelvis, water can be pulled out by osmosis, resulting in less water entering the urine.

This hyperosmotic environment is created by the active and passive transport of ions (mainly sodium and chloride) out of the tubular fluid as it passes through the loop of Henle into the medullary interstitium. The build-up of ions here gradually increases and becomes more concentrated as the loop of Henle descends into the medulla. The tip of the medulla can reach osmolalities of up to 1400 mosmol kg^{-1} water. Water does not follow the transport of ions into the medullary interstitium by osmosis because the thick ascending limb of the loop of Henle is impermeable to water. Urea also makes an important contribution to the creation of the hyperosmotic environment. Urea can diffuse passively through the walls of the tubules at most points along the nephron, but urea diffusion is greatly enhanced across the collecting tubule wall in the presence of even small amounts of ADH. Thus large amounts of urea become concentrated in the medullary interstitium.

Maintenance of the local environment: the countercurrent mechanism

It could be thought that as fast as the hyperosmotic environment is created it will be washed out by processes of diffusion and reabsorbed back into blood. However, the environment is maintained because of the unique arrangement of the looped vasa recta capillaries around the loops of Henle (Fig. 2.7 and Fig. 2.11). The vasa recta are only supplied with 1–2% of the blood entering the kidneys, so there is very little blood flow for ions to be reabsorbed back into. In addition, the vasa recta lie with their ascending and descending limbs in very close proximity. This close proximity allows for rapid exchange of water and solutes between the two limbs. So, as blood flows down the descending limb of the vasa recta, the high concentration of ions in the medullary interstitium enables ions to diffuse into the vasa recta (markedly increasing their concentration), and water to move out by osmosis, but as the blood moves into the ascending limb of the vasa recta, the high concentration of ions in the blood then enables ions to diffuse back out into the medullary interstitium (and water back into the blood), maintaining the hyperosmotic environment.

The regulation of body fluid volume and osmolality

Sodium is the main extracellular cation (positively charged ion) and is intimately related to extracellular volume. An increase in body sodium content could lead to an increase in extracellular fluid volume, leading to hypertension and oedema; and a decrease in body sodium content could lead to a decrease in extracellular fluid volume leading to hypotension and dehydration. Thus, it is vitally important that body sodium content is kept at a constant level if body fluid volume is to remain constant. Fortunately, the healthy kidney conserves sodium very efficiently in shortage, and can excrete 10–150 mmol day^{-1} when sodium is in excess.

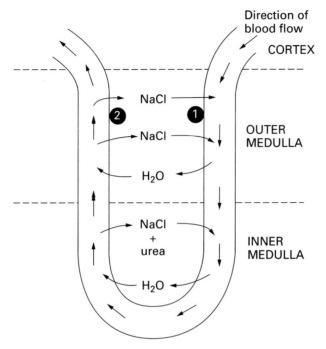

Figure 2.11 Maintenance of the hyperosmotic environment. (1) As blood flows down the descending limb of the vasa recta, the high concentration of sodium chloride and urea in the medullary interstitium causes passive diffusion of these ions into the blood, whilst water diffuses out of the blood by osmosis. (2) As blood enters the ascending limb, the high concentration of sodium chloride and urea that has accumulated in the tip of the vasa recta then diffuses back out into the interstitium, whilst water is osmotically attracted back into the blood, thus maintaining the hyperosmotic environment in the medullary interstitium. The net result of this process is that solutes circulate around in the vasa recta but are not washed out into the main circulation.

Sodium levels, and hence fluid volume, are regulated by three hormones:

- ADH
- aldosterone
- atrial natriuretic peptide.

Antidiuretic hormone

ADH is secreted from the posterior pituitary gland in response to a rise in plasma osmolality. Osmoreceptors in the hypothalamus detect small changes in the plasma osmolality and send signals to the posterior pituitary to secrete more or less ADH. Since sodium, along with its associated anion (negatively charged ion) chloride (Cl^-), contributes approximately 95% of the extracellular fluid osmolality, sodium concentration of extracellular fluid is obviously important in determining ADH secretion.

ADH receptors are found in the collecting ducts of kidney tubules and ADH acts to open water channels found here. Remember that the collecting ducts pass through the inner medulla of the kidney—a region of high osmolality. If water channels in the walls of the collecting ducts open, water will move out of the collecting duct into the medullary interstitium and

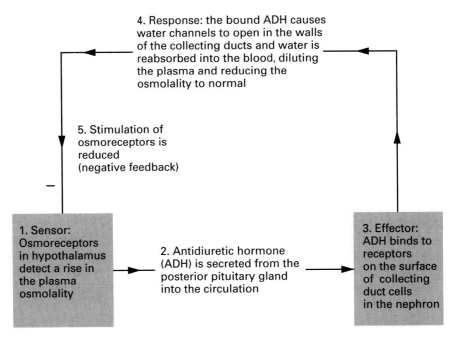

Figure 2.12 Negative-feedback loop for antidiuretic hormone (ADH) release and control of plasma osmolality.

finally into the circulation. The fall in plasma osmolality then leads to a slowing-down of ADH secretion by negative feedback (Fig. 2.12).

Aldosterone

Aldosterone is a steroid hormone secreted from the adrenal cortex. It has its effect on the distal tubule of the nephron: the more aldosterone is secreted, the more sodium is reabsorbed. Aldosterone, however, is not the sole determinant of body sodium balance, although in extreme cases of over-secretion of aldosterone, such as in Cushing's disease, hypertension may result from over-retention of sodium and water.

The secretion of aldosterone, unlike ADH, is not directly triggered by extracellular osmolality, but is regulated by a peptide, angiotensin II. The function of this peptide is described in the section on the renin–angiotensin system, below.

Atrial natriuretic peptide

This peptide is released from cardiac atrial cells in response to an increased atrial stretch. It has five known major effects:

- inhibition of aldosterone secretion by the adrenal cortex
- reduction of renin release by the kidney
- reduction of ADH release from the posterior pituitary
- vasodilation
- natriuresis and diuresis.

All of these effects result in the excretion of sodium and water through the kidney, reducing the extracellular fluid volume back to normal. Other factors which may be important in sodium regulation are renal prostaglandins, kinins and the renal nerves. Failure to regulate the extra-cellular fluid volume occurs commonly in people with renal disease and leads to hypertension.

The renin–angiotensin system

The distal convoluted tubule forms a unique contact with the glomerulus, passing in the angle between the afferent and efferent arterioles. At this point, specialised cells called the macula densa in the wall of the distal tubule make contact with cells in the endothelium of the arterioles which release a hormone called renin. (Fig. 2.13). The macula densa and the renin-releasing cells are collectively called the juxtaglomerular apparatus or complex.

The juxtaglomerular apparatus is responsible for maintaining a constant blood flow through the glomerulus and thus a constant GFR despite fluctuations in arterial pressure. This is achieved through a tubule feedback mechanism in which a fall in GFR results in a fall in the chloride ion con-centration in the distal tubule. This stimulates the macula densa cells which send 'signals' to the renin-secreting cells to release renin. Renin acts via the renin–angiotensin system (Fig. 2.14) to produce both local vasoconstriction

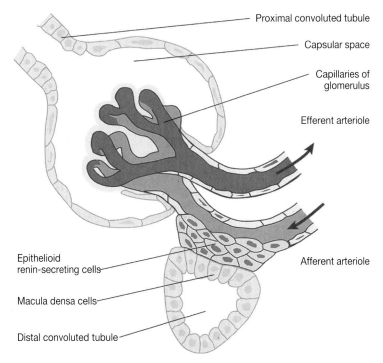

Proximal convoluted tubule

Capsular space

Capillaries of glomerulus

Efferent arteriole

Afferent arteriole

Epithelioid renin-secreting cells

Macula densa cells

Distal convoluted tubule

Figure 2.13 The juxtaglomerular apparatus showing the macula densa. (From Hinchliff SM, Montague SE, Watson R. Physiology for nursing practice. London: Baillière Tindall 1988, with permission of Baillière Tindall.)

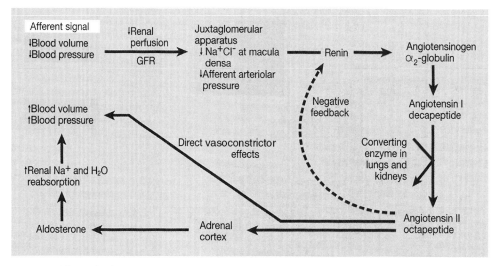

Figure 2.14 The renin-angiotensin system. GFR, glomerular filtration rate. (From Hinchliff SM, Montague SE, Watson R. Physiology for nursing practice. London: Baillière Tindall 1988, with permission of Baillière Tindall.)

of the efferent arteriole (increasing GFR) and peripheral vasoconstriction to increase arterial blood pressure. In addition, salt and water retention increase due to the effects of aldosterone.

Aldosterone and the control of body potassium content

Potassium is the main intracellular cation. Only about 2% of the total body potassium content is extracellular. Potassium ions are freely filtered at the glomerulus: 65% of reabsorption takes place in the proximal tubule. However, the renal handling of potassium ions is not as efficient as that of sodium, nor is potassium conserved so well when there is a shortage. The secretion of potassium is also linked to that of sodium and hydrogen ions. Unlike sodium regulation, where aldosterone is just one factor in the regulation of sodium content, aldosterone is the only hormone involved in the control of potassium content and thus has a very important regulatory role. Small increases in extracellular potassium concentration directly stimulate aldosterone secretion from the adrenal cortex. The effect of aldosterone in the distal tubule of the nephron is to increase the secretion of potassium into the urine. When aldosterone levels fall, the reverse occurs and less potassium is secreted. The release of aldosterone stimulated by rises in extracellular potassium concentration is strongly controlled by a negative-feedback system. Once the potassium concentration returns to normal the stimulus to secrete aldosterone is quickly switched off.

The hormone aldosterone increases sodium reabsorption in exchange for potassium or hydrogen ions. If excess potassium ions need to be secreted, then fewer hydrogen ions can be secreted and vice versa. Clinically, this phenomenon results in an association between metabolic acidosis and hyperkalaemia (or conversely, metabolic alkalosis and hypokalaemia), since in patients with acidosis the distal tubules will increase the rate of hydrogen ion secretion (to prevent a fall in plasma pH) by reducing the rate of potassium ion secretion, resulting in the retention of potassium ions in the blood, leading to hyperkalaemia.

Hypokalaemia and hyperkalaemia

Potassium is important in maintaining the membrane potential of nerve and muscle cells and hence affects their excitability. Disturbances in potassium balance show their effects in abnormal nerve and muscle function and may be life-threatening.

Changes in muscle tone and in the electrocardiogram (ECG) may indicate an altered potassium balance. The diet almost invariably contains adequate potassium, so hypokalaemia generally occurs due to excessive losses. Persistent vomiting, diarrhoea, or the use of certain prescribed diuretics are the most likely causes of low blood potassium. Dialysis using an inappropriate concentration of potassium may also result in hypokalaemia. Treatment of hypokalaemia by the administration of a potassium salt must be undertaken with care since this may result in hyperkalaemia. The uptake of potassium into cells is also dependent on the acid–base balance in the patient. Acidosis (low blood pH) causes the release of potassium from cells so acid–base disturbances must first be corrected.

Hyperkalaemia can occur as a result of decreased potassium excretion in the renal patient. Insulin promotes uptake of potassium into cells, so insulin deficiency may lead to hyperkalaemia, as can excessive tissue breakdown following trauma.

Regulation of calcium, phosphate and magnesium

Calcium and phosphate are the main mineral constituents of bone and thus the majority of calcium and phosphate in the body is found in the skeleton. However, small amounts of both these ions are found in extracellular fluid. Calcium exists in the plasma in two forms. Approximately 50% exists in the free ionised form (1.25 mmol L^{-1}), and the other 50% in a bound form, mainly bound to protein, particularly albumin (1.25 mmol L^{-1}). Usually when serum calcium levels are measured, the total calcium concentration is measured (2.5 mmol L^{-1}). This total calcium is then 'corrected' depending on the blood albumin level, since it is the ionised form of the calcium that is important in the extracellular fluid in controlling nerve and muscle conduction. Any condition which leads to a fall in the ionised calcium concentration (even if total calcium remains normal) will lead to the classic symptoms of hypocalcaemia—tetany, muscle cramps and even convulsions. In situations of hypercalcaemia, the main effects seen are pruritus, extraskeletal calcification, renal calculi, peptic ulceration and changes in mental function such as memory loss and depression.

Inorganic phosphate (i.e. those ions carrying a charge) exists in several forms—'acid' phosphate ($H_2PO_4^-$) and 'alkaline' phosphate HPO_4^- . The normal plasma range of total inorganic phosphate is 0.87–1.45 mmol L^{-1}. Phosphate is important in buffer systems to maintain the plasma pH and exists in equilibrium with calcium.

Both calcium and phosphate are freely filtered at the glomerulus. When the plasma phosphate level is below 1 mmol L^{-1}, all the filtered phosphate is reabsorbed in the early proximal tubule. However, once the plasma phosphate level rises above 1 mmol L^{-1}, the amount of phosphate excreted in the urine rises in proportion to the plasma concentration. Further excretion of phosphate in the distal tubule (by secretion) can occur in response to the rise in the circulating level of PTH. Calcium reabsorption is very similar to that of sodium, in that approximately 65% occurs in the proximal tubule, and a further 20–25% in the ascending limb of the loop of Henle, leaving around 10–12% of filtered calcium being delivered to the distal tubule. How much more calcium is reabsorbed in the distal tubule depends on the levels of circulating PTH.

Magnesium is an important intracellular cation involved in energy storage and production. In all, 55% of total body magnesium is found within bones, so it is not surprising that magnesium balance is linked to that of calcium.

PTH increases tubular reabsorption of magnesium. Under normal circumstances, gastrointestinal absorption and urinary excretion of magnesium are equal. Gastrointestinal disorders may therefore decrease magnesium uptake but this is matched by a decrease in renal excretion. Most diuretics, and alcohol, increase renal magnesium excretion.

The renal handling of calcium and phosphate—the roles of parathyroid hormone, vitamin D and calcitonin

The mechanisms by which plasma calcium and phosphate are regulated are closely interrelated. The two major regulators are PTH and vitamin D. Calcium and phosphate can enter the plasma from the gut and from the bone. Indeed almost all of the approximately 1 kg of calcium in a 70-kg person is found in the bone. Of this, a few grams exchange daily with the plasma calcium pool. Calcium and phosphate can leave the plasma by being redeposited in bone, or by renal excretion.

PTH is secreted by the parathyroid glands situated next to the thyroid. Secretion is stimulated by a decrease in plasma calcium concentration, and reduced when plasma calcium levels rise. Its effect is to raise plasma calcium concentration, mainly by increasing bone breakdown (resorption), releasing calcium ions. PTH also acts in the kidney, stimulating one step in the conversion of vitamin D to its active metabolite, 1,25-dihydroxycholecalciferol.

Vitamin D is a steroid that enters the body either through dietary intake or by the effect of sunlight on the skin. However, this is an inactive form of the vitamin called cholecalciferol. To become activated it needs to undergo two metabolic conversions, one in the liver and one in the kidney. These conversions result in the formation of 1,25-dihydroxycholecalciferol. This active form has its effect in the gut, kidney and (in the presence of PTH) on bone, raising plasma calcium levels. The actions of vitamin D are summarised in Figure 2.15.

The effects of both vitamin D and PTH are to increase the plasma calcium concentration. However, these effects are carefully controlled by a negative-feedback system which prevents the calcium level rising to high. The negative-

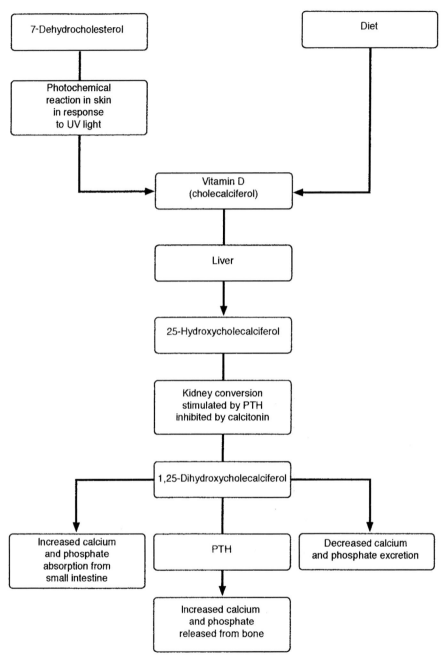

Figure 2.15 The actions of vitamin D. UV, ultraviolet; PTH, parathyroid hormone. (From Lote CJ. Principles of renal physiology. 3rd edn. Croom and Helm, London 1994, with kind permission from Kluwer Academic Publishers.)

feedback system is outlined in Figure 2.16. Only if calcium levels suddenly rise high (as after a high-calcium meal) is calcitonin stimulated to be released from the C cells of the thyroid gland, causing calcium to be redeposited in the bone. This is a rapid and relatively short-acting effect. The control of calcium and

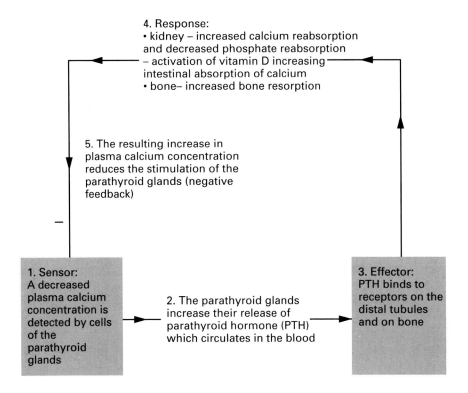

Figure 2.16 Negative-feedback loop for parathyroid hormone release and calcium and phosphate control.

phosphate levels is essential for the maintenance of normal bone. In renal disease this finely tuned negative-feedback control system is disturbed, leading to the complication of renal bone disease. Renal bone disease is discussed in Chapter 5.

Calcium ions play an important role in the regulation of nerve and muscle function and in blood clotting. Hypocalcaemia is characterised by increased excitability of muscles leading to tetany, when skeletal muscles go into spasm. Hypercalcaemia is a common finding in an individual with renal failure.

Acid–base control

Acid–base balance is about maintaining the constancy of the pH of the body's fluids. The pH scale is a logarithmic scale (range 1–14) that measures the concentration of free hydrogen ions in a fluid. In fact the scale is reciprocal, which means that as the pH becomes lower, the hydrogen ion concentration gets increasingly greater. Thus at acidic pHs (below 7), the hydrogen ion concentration of the fluid is very high relative to that at basic pHs (above 7). In fact, for each point on the scale there is a 10-fold difference in the hydrogen ion concentration. When we consider that the normal pH range of our bodily fluids is between 7.35 and 7.45, this appears very narrow but actually represents over a 20% difference in the hydrogen ion concentration! It is doubtful we would tolerate a 20% change in our sodium ion concentration with such ease.

So what are acids and bases? Simply put, acids are molecules that in the right environmental conditions will give up or donate a hydrogen ion to the solution it is in, and a base is a molecule that mops up or accepts free hydrogen ions from the solution. Thus, in order to maintain a constant hydrogen ion concentration (and hence constant pH), both acids and bases need to be present in the solution to donate or accept free hydrogen ions as required. Acids and bases working together in this way to minimise changes in pH are called buffers.

Though there are several buffering systems in the body, including haemoglobin, plasma proteins, organic and inorganic phosphates, the most important one physiologically is the bicarbonate buffering system and it is this one that will be described.

Bicarbonate buffering system

To understand the bicarbonate buffering system, the following reaction sequence needs to be understood:

$$CO_2 + H_2O \leftrightarrow H_2CO_3 \leftrightarrow H^+ + HCO_3^-$$

This equation explains how the components of the buffering system are generated in the plasma. Carbon dioxide is generated by cells as an end-product of metabolism and diffuses into the plasma. The CO_2 dissolves in water to form carbonic acid (H_2CO_3), which is the acid component of the buffering system. The carbonic acid, in turn, is in equilibrium with the hydrogen (H^+) and bicarbonate ions (HCO_3^-). This forms the basic component of the buffering system. This reaction sequence can run in either direction, thus if there is a build-up of CO_2 in the plasma then more carbonic acid will be formed and the reaction will be driven to the right in order that more bicarbonate ions can be formed to minimise changes in the pH. However, if an excess of hydrogen ions builds up (from metabolic processes) then the reaction will be driven to the left, resulting in CO_2 and water forming. The excess CO_2 can then be blown off in the lungs. Since this reaction sequence constantly runs backwards and forwards to maintain a constant pH, then it follows that pH must be dependent on the relative proportions of CO_2 to bicarbonate ions. This can be shown in the following equation:

$$pH \propto \frac{HCO_3^-}{P\text{CO}_2}$$

Both components of this equation can be controlled by the body. The bicarbonate ion concentration is carefully controlled by the kidneys, whereas the $P\text{CO}_2$ is controlled by the lungs. Thus the lungs and the kidneys are the two main organs that together control the acid–base balance of the body.

Control of bicarbonate ion concentration by the kidney

Bicarbonate ions are freely filtered in the glomerulus. When the plasma bicarbonate concentration is normal (25 mmol L^{-1}) then all of the filtered bicarbonate is reabsorbed: 90% reabsorption occurs in the proximal tubule and 10% in the distal tubule. However, if plasma bicarbonate concentration is higher than normal then this excess bicarbonate is lost in the urine.

The reabsorption of bicarbonate ions in the nephron is not a straightforward transport of ions from the tubular fluid into the plasma as with other ions but involves various chemical reactions inside the tubular wall cells. The filtered bicarbonate in the tubule undergoes the whole reaction sequence identified above for the bicarbonate buffering system so that CO_2 and water are formed. This is catalysed by the enzyme carbonic anhydrase which is found in the brush border of the proximal tubular cells. The resulting CO_2 then diffuses into the tubular cell where it undergoes the same reaction sequence, reforming the bicarbonate ion plus a hydrogen ion. The hydrogen ion is secreted into the tubule to be excreted and the bicarbonate ion diffuses into the plasma. This process is sometimes referred to as bicarbonate 'trapping' (Fig. 2.17).

This process preserves bicarbonate ions in the blood, but to excrete excess hydrogen ions, substance must take up these ions in the kidney tubule to prevent their reabsorption into the blood. This is the role of the phosphate ions HPO_4^{2-} and the ammonia ions (NH_3), both of which take up one hydrogen ion to form $H_2PO_4^-$ and NH_4^+ respectively. The process also generates HCO_3^- ions which can be reabsorbed. NH_4^+ ions cannot readily diffuse back across cell membranes, so the H^+ ions are effectively trapped in the tubule lumen.

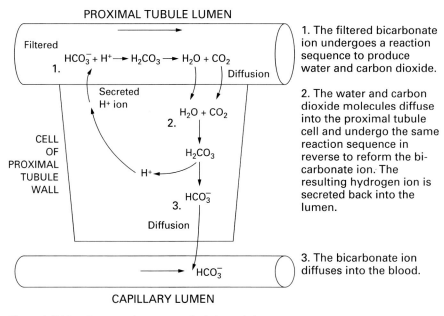

1. The filtered bicarbonate ion undergoes a reaction sequence to produce water and carbon dioxide.

2. The water and carbon dioxide molecules diffuse into the proximal tubule cell and undergo the same reaction sequence in reverse to reform the bicarbonate ion. The resulting hydrogen ion is secreted back into the lumen.

3. The bicarbonate ion diffuses into the blood.

Figure 2.17 Bicarbonate reabsorption in the kidney tubules.

Correcting acid–base fluctuations in the healthy individual

Fall in plasma pH

This is a condition called acidaemia or, more commonly, acidosis. This problem arises when there are excess hydrogen ions in the body fluids. In the absence of respiratory or renal disease, the initial response to control pH is for the excess hydrogen ions to drive the bicarbonate reaction sequence to the left to produce CO_2 and water. The lungs can then deal with this excess CO_2 by increasing the respiratory rate to 'blow off' the CO_2. This process gives a quick short-term compensation to the problem but not long-term correction. The rise in hydrogen ion concentration is then corrected by the kidneys secreting the excess hydrogen into the urine and in the process generating further bicarbonate for reabsorption into the plasma.

Rise in plasma pH

This condition is called alkalaemia or alkalosis, and arises when there is a reduction in the hydrogen ion concentration of the body fluids. The kidney plays the main role in correcting this problem by reducing the amount of hydrogen ion secretion. However, because hydrogen ion secretion and bicarbonate reabsorption are coupled together, this also results in a reduction in the plasma bicarbonate level. The plasma bicarbonate concentration is then corrected by a reduction in ventilation rate by the lungs, which leads to a build-up of CO_2, which drives the reaction sequence to the right to generate more bicarbonate ions.

Though the above compensatory and correction processes buffer the small fluctuations that occur in the acid–base balance in the healthy individual, larger fluctuations in acid–base balance tend to occur when there is either respiratory or metabolic disease. This is because the normal correction mechanisms are blocked. For example, in disorders of ventilation, a respiratory acidosis or, rarely, alkalosis may develop, whereas in disorders of metabolism (including renal disease) a metabolic acidosis or alkalosis may develop. Descriptions of these disorders are beyond this chapter, but the reader is referred to Box 2.3 for a brief outline of the causes and symptoms of the metabolic acidosis of renal failure.

Erythropoietin production by the kidney

The final important role that the kidney has is the production of the hormone erythropoietin. Erythropoietin is a glycoprotein that promotes the proliferation and differentiation of erythrocyte precursors in the bone marrow. Thus, erythropoietin is necessary for the maintenance of a normal red cell count and prevention of anaemia. The erythropoietin-producing cells of the kidney have been identified as being peritubular cells, most likely endothelial cells of the cortex and outer medulla (Lacombe et al, 1991). Erythropoietin production is stimulated by hypoxia and inhibited when the hypoxia is corrected, thus its production is controlled by the negative-feedback principle. The kidney is not the only site of erythropoietin production. Approximately 20% of erythropoietin is produced at

---

■ **BOX 2.3 Metabolic acidosis**

Causes of acidosis in renal failure

- Reduced renal excretion of acids
- Reduced renal reabsorption of bicarbonate

Markers and symptoms

- Fall in plasma pH (as hydrogen ion concentration rises)
- Fall in plasma bicarbonate concentration
- Increased anion gap (difference between the plasma concentration of cations Na^+ and K^+ and anions Cl^- and HCO_3^-)
- Possible hyperkalaemia which may lead to fatal cardiac arrhythmias
- Depressed central nervous system causing coma
- Respiratory compensation, hyperventilation (Kussmaul's breathing)
- Possible development of renal bone disease

---

extrarenal sites, thought mainly to be the liver. However, in the presence of severe renal disease, this extrarenal production of erythropoietin is insufficient to maintain the red cell count at normal levels, achieving only one-third to one-half the normal level. Anaemia is therefore a problem in most patients with chronic and end-stage renal failure, although this has now been overcome with the use of recombinant erythropoietin. See Chapter 5 for nursing management of anaemia in renal failure.

CONDITIONS CAUSING CHRONIC AND END-STAGE RENAL FAILURE

In this part of the chapter the reader is introduced to some of the common causes of chronic and end-stage renal failure and the altered physiology that results from, or may lead to, renal dysfunction. It is not intended as a complete guide to chronic renal failure, but as a starting point for understanding how important the kidneys are and how their function interacts with other body systems.

Chronic renal failure is a result of a number of pathological processes causing irreversible damage to kidney tissue. There is a mass destruction of nephrons, so that the kidneys are unable to maintain fluid and electrolyte balance and excrete waste products from the body.

Chronic renal failure is caused by a slow progressive kidney disease over a course of many years (perhaps 10–20). There may be an insidious onset of renal failure with the minimum of symptoms developing in the patient on the approach to end-stage renal failure. Unlike acute renal failure, where a full recovery of renal function can occur, in chronic renal failure the kidneys are permanently damaged and the disease is usually progressive.

The relationship between blood pressure and renal function

Despite normal fluctuations in the systemic blood pressure, the kidneys are to some extent able to autoregulate the pressure of blood entering the glomerular capillaries. This ensures that the glomerular hydrostatic pressure remains constant and GFR is maintained. In addition the kidneys are the source of the hormone renin, which has a direct effect on blood pressure via the renin–angiotensin pathway (see Fig. 2.14). If the blood pressure entering the glomerulus drops then more renin is released, resulting in a rise in systemic blood pressure.

If the filtering mechanism of the kidney is impaired by a drop in hydrostatic pressure within the glomeruli or by damage to glomerular tissue, the ability of the kidney to excrete nitrogenous waste products, and to regulate water and electrolytes may be impaired. This will ultimately result in symptoms associated with renal failure, including fluid retention which leads to hypertension.

Conversely, if blood pressure is persistently raised (hypertension), there is a risk of damage to blood vessels throughout the body, but particularly those in the brain (leading to stroke), coronary vessels and renal vessels. The renal artery, or smaller renal arteries, may become narrowed by arteriosclerosis (e.g. renal artery stenosis or renovascular disease). This will lead to impaired renal blood flow which will stimulate the release of renin, and the cycle of hypertension is worsened.

Hypertension may therefore be the cause and the result of renal failure.

Renal artery stenosis

In renal artery stenosis there is a major reduction in renal perfusion. This alteration results in increased renin secretion and activation of the renin–angiotensin system. If left untreated, accelerated hypertension will develop, resulting in further pathological changes and damage to the kidneys. The changes that take place in arterial stenosis include:

- Atherosclerosis: lipids and fibrous tissue lining the main renal artery and its larger branches.
- Hyaline arteriolar sclerosis: thickening vessel walls due to the deposition of hyaline material, narrowing the lumen. Occurs naturally after 50 years of age, but is also seen earlier in diabetics.
- Thickening of small arteries: increase of fibrous tissue in the media of arteries, narrowing the lumen. Obstruction to the renal blood flow can also be caused by:
- Vasculitis: necrosis and inflammation of the vessel walls because of immunological changes.
- Embolism: the kidney is a common site of embolism from circulating cardiac thrombi.
- Thrombosis: intravascular coagulation in the arterioles and glomerular capillaries of the kidney, which will result in renal tissue infarction (Figs 2.18–2.21).

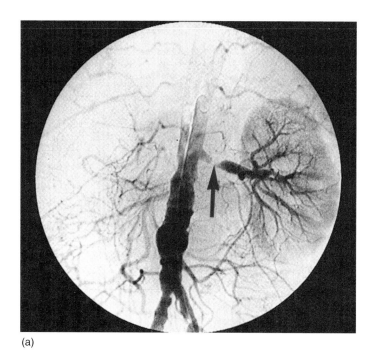

(a)

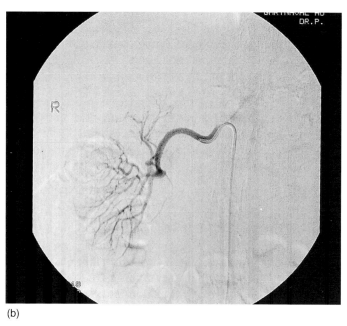

(b)

Figure 2.18 Renal arteriograms. (a) Digital subtraction arteriogram following injection of contrast material into the aorta, showing renal artery stenosis. The right renal artery is absent. The left renal artery is stenosed (arrow), but contrast medium has passed the stenosis and the developing nephrogram can be seen. The abdominal aorta is severely irregular and atheromatous. (b) In another patient, a catheter has been passed beyond a stenosis at the ostium of the right renal artery in preparation for balloon dilatation/stenting. (From Davison AM, Cumming AD, Swainson CP et al. Diseases of the kidney and urinary system. In: Haslett CC, Chilvers ER, Hunter JAA et al (eds) Davidson's principles and practice of medicine. 18th edn. Edinburgh: Churchill Livingstone, 1999:417–470, with permission.)

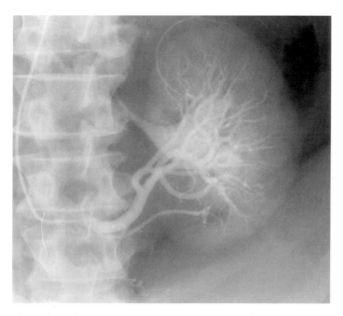

Figure 2.19 Conventional angiogram showing a normal right renal artery. Contrast material has been injected into the renal artery by means of a catheter, seen just to the left of the vertebral column.

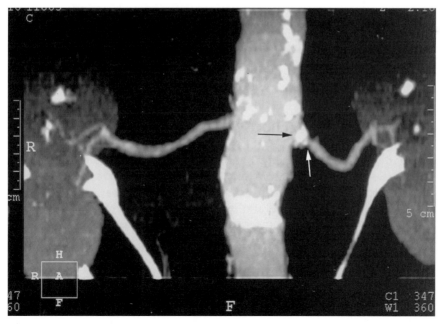

Figure 2.20 Computed tomography scan showing left renal artery stenosis. The black arrow points to a calcified plaque at the origin of the artery with narrowing of the artery distal to the plaque (white arrow). Heavy calcification is seen in the aorta (bright patches).

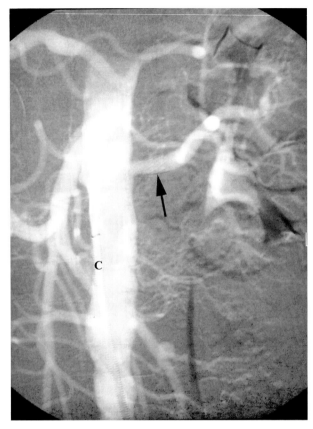

Figure 2.21 Digital subtraction angiogram of the same patient shown in Figure 2.20 following treatment by insertion of a metallic stent (black arrow) to improve the blood flow to the left kidney. C, catheter.

Disease progression and prognosis

It is estimated that renal artery stenosis accounts for 25% of end-stage renal failure in dialysis patients aged over 60 years (Scoble 1999).

Hypertension resulting from renal artery stenosis may be treated by drugs to reduce blood pressure or by lipid-lowering treatment. The stenosis itself can be treated by angioplasty of the renal artery with intra-arterial balloon catheters, by insertion of a stent or by surgical bypass of the narrowed vessel (McLaughlin et al 2000).

Nephrosclerosis

Hypertension can cause nephrosclerosis and is a major precipitating factor of renal disease. Hypertension that is not treated leads to sclerosis of the renal arterioles and the blood supply to glomeruli, tubules and interstitium gradually decreases. Scar tissue develops in the kidney, resulting in loss of renal function and eventually chronic renal failure.

Blood pressure control

The control of hypertension is the treatment of priority in patients with chronic renal failure in preventing the progression of renal failure and cardiovascular complications. Health education pertaining to cessation of smoking and alcohol, healthy eating and regular exercise for weight control is just as important in patients with chronic renal failure as in other patients with hypertension.

Nephrotic syndrome

The nephrotic syndrome is not a disease, but a collection of symptoms. It is characterised by:

- heavy proteinuria (greater than 3.5 g in 24 h)
- a reduction in plasma proteins
- severe and generalised oedema.

The nephrotic syndrome may develop in a patient with a primary renal disease of unknown cause (idiopathic nephrotic syndrome) or it may be associated with other conditions in which kidney involvement is secondary, such as amyloidosis or diabetes mellitus (Fig. 2.22).

Pathology

The nephrotic syndrome is the result of glomerular damage increasing the glomerular basement membrane permeability, allowing large amounts of small albumin molecules to pass through into the urine. It should be

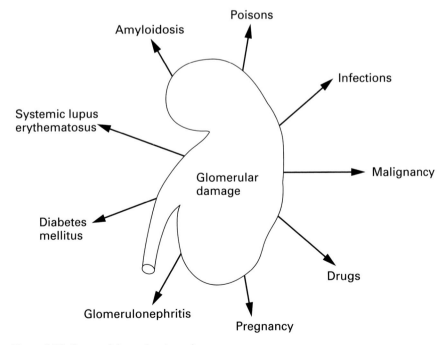

Figure 2.22 Causes of the nephrotic syndrome.

remembered that the size of the albumin molecule is just at the cut-off point in size of particle which may pass through the glomerular filter (see Fig. 2.6). As the disease progresses, larger-molecular-weight proteins leak through the glomerular basement membrane and GFRs may also reduce as the glomerular damage increases.

As the protein continues to be excreted, the serum albumin decreases (hypoalbuminaemia). This in turn leads to a low plasma oncotic pressure and diffusion of fluid into the tissue spaces causing generalised oedema (see Fig. 2.8a).

A reduction in the circulating blood volume stimulates the release of renin from the kidney, resulting in more aldosterone being released from the adrenal cortex, which is responsible for the retention of sodium and water. Retained fluid also passes out of the capillaries into the tissue, causing more oedema (Fig. 2.23).

In the early stages of the nephrotic syndrome, the protein leak may be the only disorder of renal function, but with some glomerular lesions, the disease progresses and nephrons are destroyed. This will lead to end-stage renal failure and the patient will require dialysis.

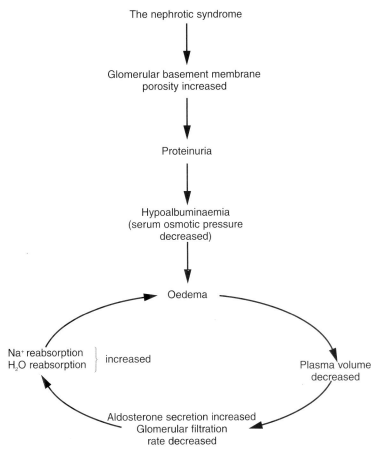

Figure 2.23 Oedema formation in the nephrotic syndrome.

CLINICAL FEATURES AND MANAGEMENT OF CARE

Oedema

In the early stages of the nephrotic syndrome, swollen eyes at the start of the day and swollen feet and ankles at the end of the day may be observed. As the disease progresses, or as a result of poor symptom control, the oedema becomes more generalised, causing pleural and peritoneal effusions resulting in breathlessness and congestion of the gastrointestinal tract.

Fluid removal will be the treatment of priority for patients, but diuretic therapy needs to be administered carefully as profound hypoalbuminaemia may cause a reduced circulating blood volume, triggering a hypotensive response in some patients following the administration of large doses of intravenous diuretics. Infusions of small volumes of intravenous salt-poor albumin prior to the administration of diuretics will increase plasma volume and restore a diuretic response in the patient. In the majority of patients the albumin is excreted after 24–48 h.

All patients with severe oedema and receiving aggressive diuretics should be weighed daily and have 4-hourly lying and standing blood pressure recordings to observe for deficits caused by a reduced plasma volume.

Proteinuria

Urine has a frothy appearance due to the high protein content (losses greater than 3.5 g in 24 h) and as a consequence hypoalbuminaemia develops. The loss of immunoglobulins increases the risk of infection. Hyperlipidaemia is also a clinical sign of the nephrotic syndrome, as a result of the liver synthesising more cholesterol and lipids. This makes the plasma milky in appearance.

Muscle wasting

The loss of skeletal muscles becomes apparent when the generalised oedema has subsided. Muscle wasting is a result of protein mobilisation into the blood to counteract protein lost in the urine.

Weight loss and malnutrition

Chronic nausea, vomiting and poor appetite may result from congestion in the gastrointestinal tract due to oedema. Weight loss also results from proteinuria and muscle wasting.

A dietetic referral should be made, and the patient encouraged to take a high-calorie diet with a protein allowance compensating for the protein loss.

Tiredness and lethargy

These symptoms may be attributed to a combination of reduced calorie intake, to muscle wasting and to the generalised oedema which may increase body weight by up to 10 kg.

Patients should be encouraged to take plenty of rest.

Intravascular clotting

There is a risk of spontaneous intravascular clotting in a patient with nephrotic syndrome due to the increase in circulating clotting proteins along with venous stasis in the legs and a reduction in plasma volume.

During episodes of hospitalisation and immobility, prophylactic anticoagulants may be used (for example, subcutaneous heparin). The use of antiembolic stockings increases venous return and reduces venous stasis.

Care for those with nephrotic syndrome can be very challenging for the renal care team. Fogo (2000) explored the significance and consequences of proteinuria in nephrotic syndrome and this paper is useful for further reading on the management of this disease.

Common causes of end-stage renal failure

The most common causes of end-stage renal failure in the UK are diabetes mellitus (approximately 20% of all new patients), glomerulonephritis, pyelonephritis, polycystic kidney, renal vascular disease and hypertension (Ansell & Feest, 2000).

Diabetic nephropathy

Diabetic nephropathy is the term used to describe damage to the kidney structure and function that occurs as a result of the long-term complications of diabetes mellitus.

Pathology

Patients initially develop microalbuminuria, i.e. 30–300 mg 24 h^{-1}. This may not occur for up to 10 years after diagnosis of type 1 diabetes mellitus, but diabetes mellitus may go undetected for so long that microalbuminuria is present at diagnosis. After 1–5 years, proteinuria becomes clinical, even to nephrotic levels (>3.5 g day^{-1}). With good glycaemic and blood pressure control, the disease may not progress towards inevitable end-stage renal failure, but in practice there is little evidence that the incidence of diabetic nephropathy is declining (Steffes 1997). Up to 75% of patients who develop proteinuria progress to end-stage renal failure (Goldberg, 1999). Ritz et al (1999) have highlighted that the incidence of those with end-stage renal failure and diabetes mellitus has increased progressively in the past decade, and have argued that the challenge for the future will be better patient management in the earlier phases of nephropathy.

The kidneys may be of normal size or slightly larger than normal and the glomerular lesions that occur are:

- pyelonephritis, the most common lesion found in those with diabetes mellitus, causing chronic renal failure and a result of autonomic neuropathy in the bladder
- diffuse intercapillary glomerulosclerosis, causing thickening and sclerosis of the basement membrane of the glomerular capillary and proliferation of the mesangial cells
- the glomerulus becoming increasingly replaced and destroyed by the deposition of nodules of a glycoprotein material—nodular glomerulosclerosis (or Kimmelstiel–Wilson nodules)

- arteriosclerosis develops in the arteries supplying the glomerulus due to hyaline deposits in the afferent and efferent arterioles, causing ischaemia and accelerating the disease process
- papillary necrosis.

Renal failure and glucose control

The kidneys have an important role in the metabolism of insulin and, as the GFR decreases in renal failure, so does the delivery of insulin to the proximal tubule cells where it is metabolised. Consequently, the circulating half-life of insulin increases with higher levels in the body after any given dose. Insulin requirements or oral hypoglycaemic agents should therefore be decreased so that hypoglycaemia does not occur.

Good glucose and blood pressure control are vital to prevent the progression of renal disease—the American Diabetes Association (2001) has published a position statement on diabetic nephropathy which has useful care recommendations.

Glomerulonephritis

The term glomerulonephritis covers a group of conditions in which inflammation in the glomerulus occurs, either as a primary disease, or as part of a systemic illness. It is therefore important to consider the possibility of an underlying systemic condition if glomerulonephritis is diagnosed. See Couser (1999) for further reading.

Glomerular disease occurs when the structure or function of the glomerular capillary network has been damaged as a result of antigen–antibody reactions in the glomeruli.

There are contributions from lymphocytes, macrophages, antibodies, immune complexes and inflammatory mediators. The glomerular cells may proliferate, basement membrane thicken or exudates of leukocytes and platelets build up in the glomerulus. These tissue reactions result in changes in the filtration properties of the glomerulus, leading to proteinuria, haematuria, impaired excretory renal function and hypertension.

Any age group may be affected, though some types are particularly common in children. The estimated incidence of glomerulonephritis in the UK is 17–60/million population.

See Plate 1 for histopathology and Box 2.4 for histopathology and clinical manifestations.

Treatment

In some cases, an underlying cause of the autoimmune response can be identified and eradicated. For example, drugs, tumours or infectious agents (e.g. streptococci) may result in glomerulonephritis which may resolve on removal of the tumour or drug. Treatment for glomerulonephritis tends to involve anti–inflammatory and/or immunosuppressive drugs. In rare conditions with rapid deterioration of renal function, plasma exchange may be used.

The prognosis depends to a large extent on the particular subtype of glomerulonephritis, identified by the pattern of glomerular injury involved.

■ **BOX 2.4 Glomerular disease**

Glomerulonephritis is the term used to describe a variety of disorders that principally affect the glomeruli in the kidney. Such glomerulopathies may arise as primary disorders of the glomerulus, or as part of a systemic disorder such as systemic lupus erythematosus (SLE) or diabetes mellitus.

Histopathology

Glomerular damage may be manifest as one or more of the following tissue reactions:

- Cellular proliferation—leading to an increase in the number of cells in the glomerular tufts.
- Leukocyte infiltration of inflammatory cells—mainly neutrophils and monocytes.
- Basement membrane thickening—as occurs in diabetes mellitus, or this may be a response caused by precipitated immune complexes.
- Hyalinisation and sclerosis—hyalinisation is the accumulation of homogeneous, amorphous substance in the glomerular tuft composed of mesangial matrix, basement membrane and plasma protein. Sclerosis is the total obliteration of structural detail in the glomerular tuft and is the end-result of glomerular damage.

Clinical manifestations

Clinical presentation of glomerular disease may range from an acute onset of disease with a reversible outcome, to a chronic insidious onset that eventually leads to renal failure after several decades. A number of syndromes of glomerular disease are defined:

- Proteinuria—occurs if the glomerular basement membranes are damaged so that they leak protein.
- Nephrotic syndrome—occurs if the basement membranes are damaged more severely and increase the protein leak to greater than 3.5 g protein 24 h^{-1}. This in turn induces a low serum albumin and generalised oedema. Hyperlipidaemia usually also occurs.
- Haematuria—occurs if capillary walls are disrupted, allowing red cells to pass into the urine. This may be microscopic or macroscopic. However, most forms of haematuria are non-glomerular in origin.
- Nephritic syndrome—occurs when basement membrane damage and red blood cell leakage are present together, leading to proteinuria and haematuria, accompanied by generalised oedema and mild hypertension.
- Renal failure (acute or chronic)—occurs when damage to the glomeruli is severe enough to impair the normal filtering function of the glomerulus, resulting in an accumulation in the blood of substances such as urea, creatinine and potassium.

continued

> ■ **BOX 2.4 Glomerular disease** (*continued*)
>
> ## *Specific nursing observations*
>
> | Parameter | Rationale |
> | --- | --- |
> | Temperature | Patients with nephrotic syndrome are prone to infection which exacerbates the disease if not detected and treated promptly |
> | Blood pressure | Hyper- or hypotension may be present, dependent on the patient's fluid and cardiac status. One should also monitor for a postural drop |
> | Respiration | Rapid, shallow breaths may indicate pulmonary oedema. Severely acidotic patients may develop Kussmaul's respirations (deep, sighing hyperventilation) |
> | Daily weight | Serial measurements of the patient's weight (at the same time each day) give the clearest indication of changes in fluid status |
> | Urinalysis | The urine should be tested for protein and blood as indicators of glomerular disease. Urinary volume should also be monitored, and the urine sent for culture if infection is suspected |
> | Skin | The skin should be observed for: oedema, dehydration, pruritus, flaking and dryness, pressure sores and rashes. A skin rash may indicate a systemic disease such as SLE, vasculitis or Henoch–Schönlein purpura. |

Subtypes of glomerulonephritis

- Minimal-change glomerulonephritis (renal biopsy normal by light microscopy)
- Membranous nephropathy
- Immunoglobulin A (IgA) nephropathy
- Focal segmental glomerulosclerosis
- Focal necrotizing glomerulonephritis (associated with syndrome of rapidly progressive glomerulonephritis)
- Mesangiocapillary glomerulonephritis.

Minimal change glomerulonephritis

These patients (usually children between 2 and 6 years) typically present with rapid-onset nephrotic syndrome. The condition is very rarely associated with impairment of excretory renal function and is occasionally secondary to drug use (particularly non-steroidal anti-inflammatory drugs (NSAIDs)) or malignancy (e.g. lymphoma).

Severe oedema may be present but without associated hypertension.

Management of care

Diuretics will clear the oedema. Most patients respond to high-dose corticosteroids, but relapse is common as the dose is reduced, and up to 50% of patients remain corticosteroid-dependent. In these patients, alkylating agents such as cyclophosphamide are sometimes successful. Ciclosporin is also effective (Macanovic & Mathieson 1999).

Prognosis

Subsequent relapses in the condition can be treated with similar protocols. Patients do not usually develop chronic renal failure.

Membranous glomerulonephritis

These patients typically present with proteinuria which may be asymptomatic or severe enough to cause nephrotic syndrome. Microscopic haematuria, hypertension and/or impaired excretory renal function may also be associated. It is seen in adults rather than in children. Onset is insidious and the disease develops slowly, over the course of 20 years in some cases.

There is widespread thickening of the capillary wall in the glomerulus (but without proliferation of the cells) which seems to result from the deposition of immune complexes in the kidney. This can occur as a result of drug use (particularly NSAIDs, gold and penicillamine), secondary to tumours (e.g. carcinoma of bronchus or breast), infection (particularly hepatitis B) or hypothyroidism.

Management of care

The prognosis of the secondary forms of the disease depends on the prognosis of the underlying condition. Complete resolution may be expected on withdrawal of the offending drug, whereas membranous glomerulonephritis, which is secondary to a tumour has a poorer prognosis unless the tumour is eradicated.

At least 25% of patients undergo spontaneous remission of proteinuria without treatment. For those with a poorer prognosis, a combination of treatment with a steroid and an immunosuppressant (chlorambucil) given in alternating cycles may prove beneficial. There is a particular risk of thrombosis in membranous glomerulonephritis, so anticoagulants may also be prescribed (Macanovic & Mathieson 1999).

Prognosis

GFR may be normal for the first few years, but then may slowly deteriorate as the sclerosis of the glomerulus increases. If no primary cause of the disease is found and eradicated, dialysis or organ transplant may be inevitable in the long term.

IgA nephropathy

This is the most common type of glomerulonephritis worldwide. Patients present with haematuria, sometimes with associated proteinuria, hypertension and impaired renal excretory function. The immunoglobulin IgA is deposited in the glomerulus, and there is sometimes proliferation of the glomerular cells. The cause of the deposits is not known, but it seems the problem is in the IgA system rather than in the kidney. An associated glomerular change is seen in Henoch–Schönlein purpura, a condition more common in children which is associated with a purpuric rash, joint and gastrointestinal involvement.

Management of care
There is no proven treatment for this form of glomerulonephritis, although in patients with heavy proteinuria, steroids may be used successfully to reduce the protein loss. Antihypertensives (for example, angiotensin-converting enzyme (ACE) inhibitors) may also be used.

Focal segmental glomerulosclerosis
This condition is named after the areas of scarring which occur in the glomeruli. The sclerotic changes affect some glomeruli but not others (focal) and may affect only parts of each glomerulus (segmental). The patient will typically present with nephrotic syndrome (hypertension, haematuria, impaired excretory renal function).

Management of care and prognosis for the patient
Treatment with prolonged courses of corticosteroids may induce remission of nephrotic syndrome, but the disease often progresses and end-stage renal failure develops in about 50% of patients within 10 years.

Focal necrotizing glomerulonephritis
Also known as rapidly progressive glomerulonephritis, this condition is associated with rapid but progressive deterioration in renal function and the presence of oliguria or anuria. Haematuria and proteinuria also occur. If pulmonary haemorrhage is present, this is known as Goodpasture's syndrome. Without effective treatment, end-stage renal failure will develop in weeks and months, rather than years.

Acute inflammation in the glomerulus is the underlying cause, sometimes with the formation of crescents when the glomerulus is squashed by cells which fill the Bowman's space. In some cases, antibodies to the glomerular basement membrane are present but, in most cases, no immunoglobulin is identified in the glomerulus.

Management of care and prognosis
If specific antibodies are identified (by a serological test), plasma exchange followed by corticosteroid and immunosuppressant therapy will remove the offending antibodies and prevent further proliferation. The prognosis in these cases is directly related to the amount of damage already done to the glomeruli.

Mesangiocapillary or membrane-proliferative glomerulonephritis
Three subtypes of this condition are recognised, identifiable only by electron microscopy. In all cases the presentation of the patient is similar, with

proteinuria, haematuria, hypertension and impaired renal function. There are no known causes. All types tend to have a progressive course, and up to 50% of patients develop chronic renal failure within 10 years.

Treatment focuses on blood pressure control and use of corticosteroids.

Postinfection glomerulonephritis

Poststreptococcal glomerulonephritis (for example, following a throat infection) was a common cause of renal failure in the preantibiotic era and is still common in some parts of the world. Immune complexes which arise following infection with group A haemolytic streptococci deposit in the glomerular capillary wall, resulting in proteinuria, haematuria and hypertension.

Glomerulonephritis may complicate infection with a range of organisms. Infection with *Staphylococcus*, influenza B, hepatitis B and C and human immunodeficiency virus (HIV) may all result in renal damage.

Pyelonephritis

This is a bacterial infection of kidney tissue, with the infection beginning in the lower urinary tract and ascending to the kidney(s). Acute pyelonephritis is commonly associated with pregnancy, obstruction, instrumentation or trauma to the urinary tract and in patients with a chronic illness.

Chronic pyelonephritis is the result of repeated infections of the urinary tract. There is widespread destruction of nephrons and replacement with scar tissue, which eventually causes end-stage renal failure. For the majority of patients, the disease starts in early childhood and is due to ureteric reflux and infection, but symptoms of the disease may not present clinically until adulthood. In adults, chronic pyelonephritis is a complication of obstruction in the renal tract, because stone formation and structural abnormalities both cause stasis of urine.

Clinical features and management of care

The patient will present with pyrexia and rigors and loin pain over the affected kidney(s). Symptoms of a lower urinary tract infection may also be present.

Antibiotics can be given to treat the acute phase of the infection, but there is little evidence to prove that prophylactic antibiotics slow down the onset of chronic renal failure. A high fluid intake (up to 3 L day^{-1}) is important.

Disease progression and prognosis

If the chronic infections are only affecting one kidney, the disease is usually prolonged but benign. Bilateral chronic infection will ensure that chronic renal failure is of rapid onset.

Reflux nephropathy is a congenital anatomical abnormality where there is incompetence of the sphincter at the junction of the ureter with the bladder, allowing the reflux of urine back up the ureter and into the renal pelvis. Infection may develop and the formation of scar tissue will eventually cause chronic renal failure. If identified early, surgical correction will be needed. Recurrent urinary tract infection during childhood should always be fully investigated and treated.

Polycystic kidney disease

Polycystic kidney disease is one of a number of cystic diseases of the kidney. Polycystic disease refers to two hereditary cystic diseases—autosomal recessive polycystic kidney disease and autosomal dominant polycystic kidney disease. Both conditions may occur in children, although the recessive disease is more commonly seen in this age group. The following descriptions will refer to autosomal dominant polycystic kidney disease, one of the most common genetic disorders which is responsible for approximately 10% of patients with end-stage renal failure.

Genetics

The autosomal dominant form of the disease is one of the most common genetic disorders, affecting an estimated 80/100 000 of the population (Davison et al 1999). The condition occurs equally in men and women and is transmitted by both sexes. If one parent is affected, 50% of the offspring will develop the disease, although symptoms may not develop until patients reach their 20s. The mean age of starting dialysis treatment is 57 years. However, by the age of 80, virtually all individuals who carry the gene will manifest some form of the disease.

Three genes appear to be responsible for the condition: currently, location of two of the genes is known (Murcia et al 1998). Work is also in progress to identify genes responsible for the recessive form of the disease (in which two copies of the affected genes must be inherited, one from each parent).

Pathology

Both kidneys are considerably enlarged and consist of a compact mass of cysts which are scattered equally throughout the cortex and medulla (Fig. 2.24). The cysts increase in size and eventually rupture, allowing

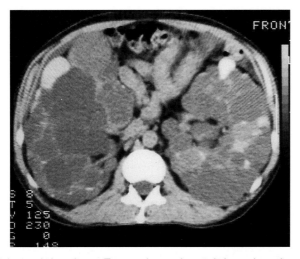

Figure 2.24 Polycystic kidney disease. Two very large polycystic kidneys, shown by computed tomography. (From Davison AM, Cumming AD, Swainson CP et al. Diseases of the kidney and urinary system. In: Haslett CC, Chilvers ER, Hunter JAA et al (eds) Davidson's principles and practice of medicine. 18th edn. Edinburgh: Churchill Livingstone, 1999:417–470, with permission.)

infection and scar tissue formation, and reducing the number of functioning nephrons. The enlarged cysts compress the normal renal tissue and hypertensive changes and glomerulosclerosis occur. Cysts are filled with watery fluid which may be clear, blood-stained from a recent haemorrhage, brown from an old haemorrhage or filled with pus (Figs 2.25–2.27).

Liver cysts may be found in patients with polycystic kidneys and there is also a significant association with aneurysms of the cerebral arteries.

Clinical features and management of care

1. Pain: the patient may complain of abdominal distension or discomfort following minor physical trauma and this may cause frank or microscopic haematuria. Pain in the flank is associated with the large cysts rupturing and any blood clots that are passed will cause the patient to experience colic. Mild analgesia may be sufficient to relieve discomfort, but pain caused by cysts rupturing or from clot retention may require opiates.

2. Haematuria and proteinuria: microscopic or frank haematuria is seen in more than 50% of patients. Chronic blood loss does not usually result in anaemia since the erythropoietin production by the kidneys is increased. Patients may be advised to alter their lifestyle if they are prone to physical abdominal trauma which may cause cysts to rupture. Mild proteinuria is always present in the mid to late stages of the disease and may be the first

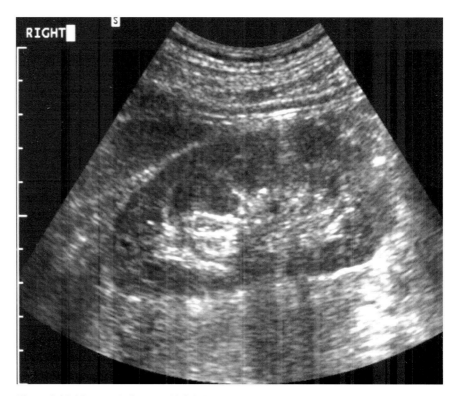

Figure 2.25 Ultrasound of a normal left kidney.

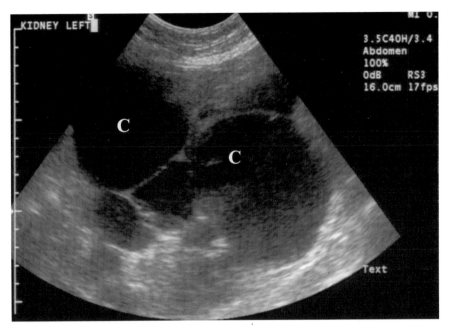

Figure 2.26 Ultrasound of a polycystic kidney showing how the normal tissue is replaced by multiple fluid-filled cysts (C).

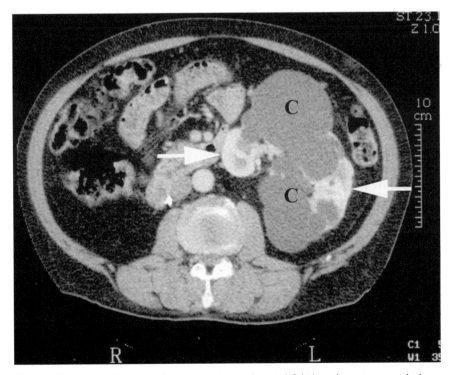

Figure 2.27 Computed tomography scan showing a polycystic left kidney; the cysts are marked by C. The white arrows point to normal renal tissue. The right kidney has been removed.

abnormality that draws attention to the condition during a routine medical examination.

3. Urinary tract infections: repeated urinary tract infections are common complications, and may affect the cysts. Unnecessary urological investigation should be avoided and female patients should receive health education regarding perineal hygiene. All patients should be advised on the importance of a high fluid intake to prevent urinary stasis and how to recognise the signs of a urinary tract infection.

4. Hypertension: secondary hypertension is common in patients with polycystic disease and may deteriorate as end-stage renal failure approaches. It is treated aggressively, not only because it may accelerate deterioration of renal function, but because it may increase the risk of intracerebral haemorrhage in these patients (Ecder et al, 2000).

Multisystem diseases affecting the kidney

The kidney may be affected in many ways by disease processes which are not directly associated with renal function. This vulnerability is, in part, due to the high blood supply of the kidneys; together the kidneys receive 25% of the cardiac output. The glomerular capillaries, because of their filtering properties, come into close contact with all blood constituents.

The effects of diabetes mellitus and of systemic infections in the kidney have already been mentioned. The following are some more examples of multisystem diseases which may affect the kidney.

Systemic lupus erythematosus

This is an autoimmune inflammatory disease which affects joints, blood vessels, skin and the nervous system, as well as the kidneys. Glomerular inflammation may result in proteinuria, haematuria and hypertension; renal involvement often occurs within 3 years of diagnosis of the disease. Non-renal manifestations of the disease are usually present, such as arthralgia, rash and haematological disorders.

Renal amyloidosis

Amyloidosis is the term given to a group of chronic infiltrative disorders characterised by the presence of deposits of an abnormal protein called amyloid. Two groups of protein deposit exist, AL amyloid or AA amyloid, but renal involvement occurs with both. AA amyloid deposits are a complication of many chronic inflammatory diseases, occurring in up to 10% of patients with rheumatoid arthritis; AL amyloid deposits may occur secondary to myeloma or as the primary condition, AL amyloidosis. This is a systemic disease which affects the heart, peripheral nervous system, liver and kidney.

A common site of deposition of the insoluble amyloid fibrils is in the walls of the renal arterioles and glomerular capillaries. The result is usually nephrotic syndrome followed by progressive renal failure.

Scleroderma or systemic sclerosis

This is a multisystem condition which causes gradual hardening and tightening of the skin and increased binding to subcutaneous tissue. Renal involvement is one of the less common but most serious complications of the disease and, in the past, was a major cause of mortality. Patients often present with the features of malignant hypertension and rapidly deteriorating renal function. Diastolic pressure may exceed 130 mmHg. Antihypertensives, particularly ACE inhibitors, improve the renal outlook of these patients, but there is no treatment for the underlying condition.

Polyarteritis nodosa

More common in men than women, this condition usually presents in later life. It is characterised by widespread inflammation of small and medium arteries and aneurysm formation. Thrombosis in these arteries can lead to complications which particularly affect the gut, peripheral nervous system and kidneys. The renal presentation is that of progressive renal impairment caused by renal infarction and hypertension. Treatment is with corticosteroids, and renal prognosis depends on early diagnosis and treatment since organ damage is irreversible.

REFERENCES

Ambrus JL, Nagaraja R, Sridhar R. Immunological aspects of renal disease. JAMA 1997, 278:1938–1945.

American Diabetes Association (1999) Clinical practice recommendations. Available: www.diabetes.org. 31 Oct 2001.

Ansell D, Feest T (eds). UK Renal Registry report. Bristol: UK Renal Registry, 2000.

Couser WG. Seminar. Glomerulonephritis. Lancet 1999; 353:1509–1515.

Davison AM, Cumming AD, Swainson CP et al. Diseases of the kidney and urinary system. In: Haslett CC, Chilvers ER, Hunter JAA et al (eds) Davidson's principles and practice of medicine. 18th edn. Edinburgh: Churchill Livingstone, 1999:417–470

Eadington D, Plant, W, Winney R. Chronic renal failure. The Practitioner 1993; 237:64–69.

Ecder T, Edelstein CL, Fick Brosnahan GM et al. Progress in blood pressure control in autosomal dominant polycystic kidney disease. Am J Kidney Dis 2000; 36:266–271.

Fogo A. Nephrotic syndrome: molecular and genetic basis. Nephron 2000; 85:8–13.

Gabriel R Renal involvement in systemic disease. Update 1993a; 46:647–654.

Gabriel R The causes of chronic renal failure. Update 1993b; 47:203–210.

Goldberg L The kidney in systemic disease. Medicine 1999; 27:108–112

Lacombe C, Bruneval P, Da Silva Jh et al. Production of erythropoietin in the kidney. Semin Hematol 28 (suppl 3):14–17

Lawrence DR,. Bennett PN. Clinical pharmacology. 6th edn. Edinburgh: Churchill Livingstone, 1987.

Macanovic M, Mathieson PW. Glomerulonephritis. Medicine 1999; 27:59–62.

McLaughlin K, Jardine AG, Moss JG. ABC of arterial and venous disease. Renal artery stenosis. Br Med J 2000; 320:1124–1127.

Murcia NS, Woychik RP, Avner ED. The molecular biology of polycystic kidney disease. Pediatr Nephrol 1998; 12:721–726.

Ritz E, Rychlik I, Locatelli F et al. End-stage renal failure in type 2 diabetes: a medical catastrophe of worldwide dimensions. Am J Kidney Dis 1999; 34:795–808.

Scoble JE. Renovascular disease. Medicine 1999; 27:100–102.

Steffes MW. Diabetic nephropathy: incidence, prevalence, and treatment. Editorial. Diabetes Care 1997; 20:1059–1061.

Whitworth JA, Lawrence JR (eds) Textbook of renal disease. 2nd edn. Edinburgh: Churchill Livingstone, 1994.

Psychological perspectives

3

Juliet Auer

■ **CONTENTS**

■ **LEARNING OUTCOMES FOR THIS CHAPTER**

- To appreciate the far-reaching effects of renal failure on every aspect of life
- To explore the psychological pressures experienced by patients and carers
- To demonstrate differences between stresses of treatment in different age groups
- To emphasise the importance of information-giving to promote active involvement of patient and carer
- To evaluate the multidisciplinary approach to patient care
- To promote understanding of the reasons for non-adherence to dialysis therapy
- To explore issues surrounding withdrawal from treatment and the sympathetic management of the dying patient.

INTRODUCTION

Ever since dialysis and renal transplantation were introduced in the USA in the late 1950s and early 1960s, and in the UK in the mid-1960s, psychologists and psychiatrists have been involved in studying the impact of living on a life-supporting machine or with a donor kidney, and with the problems encountered by patients, their families and also the staff who support them over years of survival against the odds (Abram 1969, 1970, Abram et al 1971, Kaplan de Nour & Czackes 1968, Shambaugh & Kanter 1969).

Much research has been done into psychological aspects of dialysis and the quality of life of these patients and numerous studies have been published by those most active in this field over the past 20 years, particularly Atara Kaplan de Nour, Roberta Simmons, Norman Levy, Howard Burton, Nancy Kutner and Roger Evans. As dialysis came to be offered to a wider age range in the 1980s, the adjustment of elderly patients has been studied by Westlie et al (1984), Kline et al (1986), and Neu & Kjellstrand (1986) in North America, and by Auer (1986) and Quarello et al (1992) in Europe, concluding that there is no reason why there should be any age limit to treatment, and that many patients in their eighth and even ninth decade should achieve good quality of life. In the 1980s and 1990s, as concern grew over the seemingly limitless demands of the healthcare budget, a number of studies focused on cost–benefit aspects of quality of life on dialysis, and the need to ration resources (Gudex 1986, Loomes & McKenzie 1989, Stanton 1999, Williams 1985). In the view of the health economist, dialysis is an expensive way of prolonging a life that may lack quality by objective measures, such as vocational rehabilitation and functional capacity. These conclusions, however, raise questions about the validity of objective measures in an area that may be better approached from a subjective stance; that is, do patients see their life on dialysis as worthwhile?

In the present chapter, a brief overview of some of the important findings is given, but chiefly attention is drawn to some of the everyday experiences of patients, gathered largely from working in a busy dialysis and transplant unit over a 20-year period. This will allow the reader to recognise some of the patients' reactions and the reasons for them, and provide a practical insight useful to those working with patients and families.

Every aspect of life is affected by renal failure and its treatment, and the effects spread to all those closely involved with the patient. Greater understanding of the day-to-day stresses and concerns of patients allows staff in renal units to respond with appropriate support. This needs to begin as early as possible, to prevent problems, whether practical (as in employment or finances), or emotional (as in relationship problems and unnecessary fears about prognosis or treatment: Bradley & McGee 1994).

THE PREDIALYSIS STAGE

Unfortunately, only about half of the patients who enter renal replacement programmes are followed in a predialysis clinic during the decline of their renal function towards end-stage. The remaining patients present acutely in end-stage renal failure (ESRF), or in acute-on-chronic renal failure, previously undiagnosed, which progresses rapidly to end-stage. Older patients (>70 years) with acute renal failure are less likely to regain function than those less than 70 years of age. Those patients who have time to adjust over a period of months, or even years, to the fact that dialysis and/or transplantation will become necessary, seem to adjust more smoothly to treatment.

Increasingly, renal units are using this time to good effect, by preparing patients for the transition from chronic renal failure to ESRF and the need for dialysis, not only medically but also psychologically and socially. Such predialysis education may even delay the need for dialysis (Binik et al 1993), perhaps as a result of promoting better understanding of antihypertensive medication.

The subjects that need to be addressed vary according to age and circumstances, but may include:

• the importance and purpose of medication and diet

- choosing the treatment best suited to the patient's social situation and lifestyle
- problems with employment and finances due to the illness
- problems with housing, taking treatment needs into consideration
- role changes within relationships and effects on family members or carers
- difficulties in sexual and affectionate relationships (Stout et al 1985)
- effect of ESRF on leisure activities and holidays.

In the case of younger patients, the effects can be far-reaching and devastating to contemplate, involving disruption of the overall life plan, including career prospects, marriage and having children. Older patients usually face less fundamental losses.

Predialysis and pretransplant groups

With few exceptions, the more information and preparation that can be provided, the better patients are able to adjust, especially if the knowledge acquired enables them to choose the treatment modality best suited to their circumstances (Bradley & McGee 1994). This preparation also benefits the spouse or carer, who is often more worried than the patient, having not always had the opportunity of talking to the doctor on clinic visits. Spouses are affected by the effects of the illness on the patient. These effects may include:

- lethargy and tiredness
- inability to concentrate
- irritability
- apathy/depression or anxiety
- reduced ability to show affection or sexual interest
- withdrawal and lack of communication
- constant complaints about symptoms such as itching, loss of appetite or breathlessness.

Spouses have frequently expressed frustration that symptoms are minimised or not reported to the medical team on clinic visits. Patients who are trying to come to terms with their own feelings often find it hard to spare extra energy to cope with the feelings of those close to them. They also feel guilty that the illness is affecting others, making it hard to relate to those they are 'letting down'. As a result, many spouses, who are facing the same worries about the future as the patient, feel unsupported and unappreciated.

Some units run predialysis and pretransplantation groups to assist both patients and their families during this period. In the author's renal unit, predialysis counselling was undertaken on an individual basis by the dietitian, social worker and nurses until the mid-1980s. This always included a visit to the patient's home by the social worker to assess which type of treatment was most likely to suit the individual's requirements. A social report was then prepared for medical and nursing staff, assessing the housing, way of life, employment, social supports, financial position and any particular strengths and weaknesses inherent in the patient's situation. Such factors are far better explored away from the hospital in the patient's own environment. Ideally, this would still be the practice in most cases, but the increase in workload in renal units, certainly in the UK, has made it impractical to visit all patients at home before the need for dialysis treatment.

The solution chosen in an increasing number of units is to invite patients and families to attend sessions where as much information and teaching as possible can be given, to the greatest number, in the most time- and cost-effective way. In some hospitals these groups are run by nursing staff, in others by the social worker. The most effective groups seem to be run on a multidisciplinary basis, with input from medical, nursing, dietetic and social work staff, and include teaching from established dialysis and transplant patients themselves (Bradley & McGee 1994).

There are a number of different agendas and types of communication that can be used in an information group:

- straightforward teaching— information about the causes and effects of renal failure, and the methods of treatment—medication, diet and dialysis/transplantation
- group support
- reassurance—the dispelling of myths about renal failure and treatment, ensuring that the patient's concerns are realistic, focusing on the real problems rather than rumours or hearsay (e.g. a number of patients have asked whether it is true that one can only survive a short period on dialysis and can expect to die unless transplanted quickly)
- encouraging active participation in treatment, by establishing a climate of cooperative interaction between patients and staff, rather than passive acceptance
- Introducing topics and encouraging questions, especially on subjects that many patients feel inappropriate to raise with busy medical staff at clinic appointments. This gives validity to a number of concerns that patients and relatives may consider outside the scope of the unit, for example:
  — depression
  — anxiety
  — relationship difficulties
  — body image
  — sexuality.

Once these are placed on the agenda, patients feel able to approach staff for individual discussion if necessary.

In order to fulfil a number of these criteria at once, patients are taught partly by staff and partly by other patients, thus giving the role of 'patient' both status and an active and positive connotation. It also means that the information given has greater credibility, since it comes from someone who has first-hand experience. The informal support provided by the experienced patient to those not yet receiving dialysis is reassuring and valuable (Klang et al 1999). Questions to 'patient teachers' are often more freely expressed and wider-ranging than those put to staff. The overall impression created is one of teamwork, with the patient as part of the team rather than the passive object of attention.

A continuous ambulatory peritoneal dialysis (CAPD) exchange may be demonstrated by a patient, using a minimum of special equipment (i.e. no special work surface, bag warmer or hospital drip stand), allowing a brief overview of what is involved from a technical point of view. This demonstration gives a clear message that the treatment is portable, flexible and does not require either a clinical setting or the 'safety' of home. It is also shown to be something that can be done without embarrassment in front of others. All these messages are relayed without even needing to be mentioned. Most of the demonstrators used are middle-aged (50s plus), and are in employment, at least part-time—again giving a positive image of the treatment. Demonstrators are often asked whether they 'skip a treatment from time to time' or break the rules—and they usually give a truthful answer in the affirmative, in spite of the presence of staff—again helping to set the atmosphere for honest and realistic interaction with members of the team.

The teaching session includes a visit to the haemodialysis unit, where predialysis patients and relatives are encouraged to talk to patients on dialysis. Many have not previously entered the unit, and most are relieved and pleasantly surprised to find that the treatment is neither painful nor terrifying. The message conveyed by seeing patients eating, reading, dozing, knitting or watching television during treatment is a powerful one, emphasising the normality that is possible under these circumstances rather than the clinical procedure itself. It is also reassuring for those in the predialysis stage to be told that only a small amount of blood is outside the body at any one time. They see a number of different types of dialysis access and haemodialysis machines, and can be introduced to patients preparing for home treatment. There is often animated discussion with those on treatment, and many practical questions are asked, diverting thoughts from the general dread of needing a life-support treatment towards the reality of coping effectively with the situation.

By presenting the options for treatment, patients feel involved in the choice of dialysis modality. In some cases there are strong medical arguments for the choice of one or other type of dialysis but patients should, nevertheless, feel that they have been presented with as much choice and information as possible. It is also empowering to patients to be given some control over a situation that has, in many ways, removed their options and self-determination—there can be few more limiting experiences than dependence on a life-support system. The patients who appear most successful, in the sense of making the most of a life that is being sustained against the odds, are those who maintain a sense of control over their treatment rather than being at the mercy of their situation. There is increase in confidence in patients encouraged to perform self-monitoring of weight and blood pressure rather than relying on staff. The more empowered patients feel, the less dependent and helpless they will feel. The goal is to give the patient as much self-respect and self-determination as possible, in a life that seems ruled by the illness and by healthcare professionals (Kutner 1994). A sense of control over the situation should include the knowledge and ability to 'bend the rules' within safe limits from time to time, for example missing an occasional CAPD exchange in order to attend a special event or knowing how to overstep the dietary restrictions for a special occasion without risking hyperkalaemia or serious fluid overload. These well-considered events should not be considered as non-compliant behaviour; rather, as the exceptions that prove the rule. It can be hard for staff to encourage flexibility, fearing abuse of any latitude allowed; yet, as in parenting, it is important to encourage an attitude of sensible and responsible independence. Slavish adherence to limiting regimes is probably responsible for more problems and unhappiness than occasional well-judged 'lapses'.

How much information should be presented?

The information presented at this type of meeting needs to cater for a mythical 'average' patient, neither giving unrealistically high expectations by presenting an exceptionally fit, active and well-adjusted patient as an example, nor offering the point of view of a very depressed and disabled patient.

It is useful for those in the predialysis phase to hear from somebody who has experienced problems with one type of dialysis and has subsequently done well on another. It is also beneficial to introduce a transplant patient who has experienced the failure of a first graft and has later had a successful one.

Honesty is an important part of the contract between the patient and the team, and for this reason the possible complications of treatments, such as CAPD peritonitis, hernias, leaks, need for resiting catheters, failure of a fistula to develop, or the side-effects of immunosuppression posttransplant, need to be openly discussed where appropriate. Staff are not helping or respecting patients if they are overprotective or overoptimistic about what they have to offer. Staff may use denial when interacting with patients—indeed, patients are likely to feel a 'failure' if staff present an idealised picture and they do not 'achieve' in line with expectations (Kaplan de Nour 1983). It is, however, possible to be honest without being unduly negative, and to present a balanced picture of possible benefits and drawbacks.

The philosophy behind information groups is therefore to present a realistic but not over-detailed picture, which sets the scene for a cooperative and interactive relationship with the team. It is always stated that individual problems and questions can be discussed on a one-to-one basis with an appropriate member of staff following the session or in clinic. The timing of sessions is quite important, since an adjustment period of at least 6 months is desirable. This allows time for considerations such as:

- negotiating with employers to arrange changes in hours or duties that will fit the future demands of treatment
- making adaptations to housing or moving house—this is especially important for older patients, who may wish to apply for sheltered accommodation or for a transfer to a bungalow or ground-floor flat

(letters from the hospital can often expedite such arrangements in the UK)
- early application for relevant Social Security benefits (e.g. disability living allowance) to minimise financial problems.

Although there is no hard and fast rule, it is usually appropriate to invite those with a creatinine of 300–400 mmol l l⁻¹, and whose renal function is declining, to attend information groups.

THE PSYCHOLOGICAL IMPACT OF RENAL REPLACEMENT THERAPY

Access surgery

The reality of approaching dependence on dialysis is brought home to the patient by the creation of venous and/or peritoneal access. The anxious response to this admission for surgery can therefore seem out of proportion to the procedures themselves, which are comparatively trivial. The creation of access is an unmistakable signal that dialysis treatment is imminent. It is also therefore the appropriate time for final psychological preparation. During admission for access the patient can be given literature and information, talk to the dietitian about current and future nutrition and to the social worker or nurse counsellor about feelings, psychosocial, housing, employment, family or financial concerns. It is also a good time to discuss future leisure activities and holidays, because the patient is usually most aware of contracting horizons and limitations at this point, and needs to be reminded that the object of dialysis is to enable life to be lived and to provide a life that is worth living, not simply to keep the patient alive to be dialysed.

To provide good psychological support and preparation involves spending time with patients and however good one's communication skills and intentions, there is seldom the chance to do all that one would like. In this situation there is sometimes the temptation to abandon even the attempt to talk to patients about their concerns, on the grounds that if it cannot be done 'properly' it is not worth doing at all. This is very far from the case. Excellent and sensitive counselling can often be given with two minutes of listening and responding to a particular worry, provided one remains aware of needs and fears, and able to pick up the cues provided.

The creation of haemodialysis access is often a disfiguring experience for patients. Staff become so used to seeing central venous catheters, fistulae and grafts that they can forget that these cause turned heads and curious glances outside the hospital. Women in particular are sensitive to the appearance of access sites, not because of greater vanity, but because their normal clothing is less likely to cover the arms, shoulders and neck than a man's shirt and jacket. Most patients will have seen the well-developed fistulae of long-standing haemodialysis patients at clinic visits, and these can be off-putting. Staff, particularly nursing staff, need to recognise the patient's feelings, advise on clothing, and help to make the lines and dressings as unobtrusive as possible.

Some haemodialysis access surgery is performed under local anaesthetic, and can take a long time. In spite of adequate premedication it can be an anxious and uncomfortable time for the patient, who may benefit from the presence of a familiar nurse to talk to during the procedure.

The Tenckhoff catheter in preparation for peritoneal dialysis (PD) is less noticeable to the outside world but arouses many private concerns, mostly involving body image and the reaction of the spouse or partner. Many patients fear that they will no longer be attractive to their partner, partly because of the catheter itself and partly because of abdominal distension which changes the figure. Some patients, aware of the problems of colostomies and ileostomies, fear that the catheter will have a detectable smell. Before patients leave hospital it is useful for the nurse to make sure that the partner has seen the exit site and understands about the dressing and taping of the catheter securely to the side, whether or not the partner will be involved in assisting with treatment. It should be possible to explain to the couple at this stage that CAPD need not interfere with sexual relations. Some nurses feel comfortable with addressing this subject, while others do not, particularly if the couple are old enough to be the nurse's parents. If possible, discussions touching on sexuality should be left to someone who is at ease with the topic, since reluctance or embarrassment is hard to disguise and easily transmitted to the patient.

Haemodialysis in hospital

Patients go through a recognisable series of stages following the diagnosis of renal failure, similar to the responses to bereavement described by Kubler Ross (1970). These responses represent a process of adjustment to loss, starting with shock and numbness, followed by denial, bargaining, grief and anger, before reaching a degree of acceptance. Abram (1970) identified a second process of adjustment to the start of dialysis treatment. The stages may overlap, or fluctuate, as with the stages of bereavement, but can usually be identified by both staff and the patients themselves. At its most simple, the process has three phases:

First phase—euphoria

Initially there is usually a sense of relief, for several reasons. First, after months or years of waiting in a kind of limbo, the hurdle of dialysis has been reached and cleared. Second, the patient may feel the benefit of treatment immediately, especially if uraemia was symptomatic, causing nausea and itching, or if breathlessness from pulmonary oedema was a problem. Third, the experience of haemodialysis is usually less traumatic than the patient had expected.

Second phase—depressive reaction

The second stage follows fairly quickly. The novelty of treatment wears off, the limitations, frustrations and the time involved begin to take their toll and the realisation that this situation will continue indefinitely starts to sap patients' reserves of endurance. In addition, although no longer frankly uraemic, patients are aware that dialysis cannot make them feel fully well. Tiredness, lack of energy and enthusiasm for life, irritability, poor sleep and low-grade depression make life on dialysis hard to tolerate, especially for those who expected to feel miraculously better. The partner and family are also likely to feel the strain and relationships may suffer. The effort of trying to continue with work while under these pressures may seem to be too much, and the patient doubts whether employment will be possible, and fears the financial and family consequences if work has to be abandoned. Those who had been full of determination not to let dialysis affect or interfere with their lives have to concede defeat—it is not possible to remain unaffected. This stage may last weeks or months, and needs to be handled with tolerance and understanding by all staff.

Third phase—realistic adjustment

If adjustment goes to plan, the patient gradually accepts the inevitable limitations, while making the most of the remaining possibilities. Hobbies, habits and roles at home may have to change. Alternative sources of satisfaction and enjoyment need to be discovered and exploited, but all this takes time and may need to be actively encouraged by staff. In the interim, support and consistency from the team provide the framework within which the patient learns to come to terms with a changed lifestyle.

It is not surprising that during this period of adjustment the patient may be low in mood, irritable, quick to take offence and sometimes unwilling to follow medical advice. It is easy for staff to find this unattractive and 'ungrateful', especially when dialysis is a scarce and expensive resource, and staff are themselves highly pressurised and doing their best. Most patients do not find the dialysis itself a difficult ordeal, unless there are persistent problems with access or cramps, or frequent battles over excessive interdialytic weight gain. The factors most likely to produce irritation are delays, especially caused by the transport system or machines not being ready, changes of schedule due to pressures on dialysis places, and the unpredictability of minor setbacks such as access problems. The time involved in the whole process becomes a central focus for many patients, who resent the proportion of their life now dedicated to dialysis, in spite of the fact that it is dialysis that is making life possible at all. Some frustration is directed at staff, but patients are usually anxious not to alienate those who are caring for them, and to be 'good'. As a result, the spouse and family may take the brunt of the negative feelings and often lament that on hospital visits, the patient claims that all is well yet complains of numerous physical problems at home (Auer 1990b).

This pattern of reaction in the early months of haemodialysis applies to all age groups, but the negative effects are undoubtedly felt more by younger patients, who find the constraints more burdensome. It is normal for people in their 20s and 30s to be fully occupied with jobs, courtship and marriage, families and the fulfilment of ambitions. For the young person with renal failure, life had lain ahead of them, and that life plan has been brutally altered without the provision of an acceptable alternative. The only chance of re-establishing the course of events lies in the uncertain hope of receiving a good transplant. Sadly, this is not a planned event with a time scale within which to work (unless a living related donor is contemplated). Life for most of the young patients is therefore perceived as being 'on hold', and the longer the wait for a transplant, the more frustrated and downhearted they can become.

The young person

Many young patients find it hard to make relationships with the opposite sex, feeling that they have little to offer a prospective partner, and those who have a boy- or girlfriend often find their fears justified, when relationships break up under the strain of the situation. Research such as the Oxford–Manchester study (Auer 1990a) suggests that younger patients and particularly young men, find dependence on dialysis particularly frustrating, perhaps because society expects men to be more active, aggressive and ambitious in forging a role in life. It is certainly evident to those working in renal units that young male patients express more dissatisfaction, and are more likely to show this in non-compliant, self-destructive and despairing behaviour.

The middle-aged person

Middle-aged patients have usually established a role for themselves, and have achieved a number of their goals, such as marriage, family, a career and a home. From this base they are often, but not always, better able to adjust to limitations. For them, however, there is the fear of losing what has been achieved, and being unable to carry out responsibilities to those who depend on them. Role changes within the family threaten the identity, pride and self-image of the patient, who does not wish to become a burden or liability. It is, however, comparatively rare for well-established relationships to break up in these circumstances. There is a taboo against leaving a sick partner that holds many couples together even in the most difficult situations. Marriages are, however, put under pressure, especially when sexual contact becomes diminished or non-existent.

The older person

Reasonably fit elderly people are in some ways the most satisfied group (Auer 1986, Westlie et al 1984). The attitude of many elderly patients is that they have already 'had a good life' and have reached an age when death would not be unlikely in any case. They have not been cheated of a normal lifespan by their illness. To be given the chance of a further few years due to dialysis is a bonus to those who still have an appetite for life. Those in their 70s and 80s probably do not want to pursue very strenuous activities, preferring a little gardening, cooking and the company of friends and family. Those who live alone and feel isolated regard the trips to the hospital for treatment as a welcome social activity. A number who have never had help with daily living—home adaptations and home help or meals from Social Services—receive this for the first time following contact with the hospital. Staff should however remain sensitive to the problems of elderly patients, particularly depression, and be aware that the patient may wish to discuss the option of withdrawal from treatment. If patients know that this is an option and understand that the Unit would support them and their families following such a decision, this knowledge is often enough to give them the will to carry on. Knowing that one is in control of the situation, rather than trapped in a system, is reassuring. (See section on withdrawal from dialysis, on p.93.)

Home haemodialysis

A number of patients, especially those for whom an early transplant is unlikely and who wish to continue full-time work, opt to perform haemodialysis at home. Although the numbers entering home haemodialysis programmes are declining overall, this is still a good option for those who have strong motivation and good reasons for wanting the flexibility of this type of dialysis (Courts 2000). It is rarely the best treatment for very frail elderly patients, especially if assisted by an elderly spouse who may find the treatment stressful to learn and to supervise. From the psychological point of view, it is essential to offer good back-up to home patients, including respite treatment in hospital to give the spouse or assistant a break from time to time. It is also advisable, wherever possible, to ensure that at least two home assistants are available in case one is ill or wishes to be away at a certain time. As was stated earlier, patients may be far more negative and demanding towards family members than is evident in the unit, and one should not therefore underestimate the burden that the spouse may be carrying.

Early research comparing quality of life on different types of renal replacement therapy suggests that home haemodialysis offers the greatest scope for pursuing normal life, including employment, with quality-of-life scores comparable to those of transplanted patients. More recently, Lunts (1999) describes how home haemodialysis is a viable and often optimal therapy for many patients.

Peritoneal dialysis

Those on PD usually experience the same phases of psychological adjustment as haemodialysis patients, that is, an initial honeymoon period, followed by a depressive phase that may last for weeks or months. The chief difference between the two treatment patterns is that the patient on PD is performing dialysis at home, rather than being in regular contact with nurses in the Unit. The depression is therefore less likely to be noticed or openly discussed with staff. Patient, and spouse or carer, often suffer in silence during this period of adjustment. The problems are greatly reduced if the Unit has community nurses able to do regular home visits.

PD training

The greatest dilemma in teaching the techniques of CAPD and other PD therapies is to strike a balance between promoting a consistent, safe and meticulous technique, while encouraging enough flexibility and latitude to enable the patient to explore the potential for freedom that the treatment allows. Younger patients who opt for PD in order to carry on with full-time employment are likely to use the possibilities fully, after a short period of 'feeling their way'. Most take holidays away from home, go away for week-ends, and can tell stories of unlikely places in which they have successfully performed an exchange. It is harder to encourage elderly patients to do the same. Many feel that it is unsafe to attempt an exchange in unfamiliar sur-roundings and develop an almost superstitious fear of altering the circum-stances of the exchange in any way. Some say that performing the four daily exchanges has become a way of life in itself rather than a means to an end.

Patients who are doing well on PD and making the treatment work for them may show this by devising compact travelling exchange kits, with ingenious ways of warming and hanging the bags, and portable surfaces that can be kept clean, such as a large plastic table mat. Such patients will be proud to show staff how they have found ways of solving problems. They also display confidence in the way they dress, finding flattering but convenient clothing, and taking trouble with grooming. In contrast, the patient who is doing less well and may benefit from advice and counselling takes little pride in appearance, seldom or never travels with the treatment, and becomes house-bound and isolated. Extrovert characteristics seem to be a great benefit, since such patients are not too shy or inhibited to perform exchanges in places where they may be seen by others. A few patients are so shy that they would rather not be seen dialysing even by family members, particularly children and grandchildren. Because they regard the exchange as an excretory function (which is, in many respects, true) they feel that it should be performed in private. (Those on haemodial-ysis may not see the treatment as excretory, even though the same process of waste removal is taking place.) The PD nurse who is sensitive to signs of good or poor adjustment to treatment is able to reinforce and encourage sensible and flexible use of this type of dialysis.

The individual and intensive training needed to prepare a patient to perform PD safely at home allows the formation of a strong supportive bond with the nurse, probably a closer relationship than that formed in the haemodialysis unit. In a recent survey of 65 patients (33 on CAPD and 32 on haemodialysis) who started treatment in the last year in the author's unit, the question 'Do you feel that you receive enough information about your treatment?' received a 'Yes' from 94% of CAPD patients and 69% of haemodialysis patients. Similarly, the question 'Do you feel you receive enough support?' received a 'Yes' from 85% of CAPD patients and only 63% of haemodialysis patients. This probably reflects good initial contacts with CAPD staff, and a sense of continued support via phone calls to the unit whenever required. This 'accessibility' of the PD nurse is important, because patients discharged home on PD might otherwise feel more isolated and unsupported by the unit than those attending for regular haemodialysis. Visits from a community nephrology nurse are a regular procedure in some units, and are much appreciated by patients and spouses. At the very least, a visit to the patient's home is desirable before PD therapy starts. The equip-ment takes up a lot of space, and it may be impossible to store a month's supply of fluids at a time. Such initial assessment visits should ideally be made by the social worker, occupational therapist and a community renal nurse together, so that advice can be given on performing exchanges, possible adaptations to the home if needed and any community support that may be available.

GENERAL PROBLEMS AFFECTING PSYCHOLOGICAL WELL-BEING

Sexual problems and low fertility

Renal failure affects both sexual desire and the ability to engage in sexual intercourse. Estimates of the problem are likely to be inaccurate due to unwillingness to discuss this symptom—often the unwillingness is more on the part of staff than of patients—however, it is generally accepted that 70% of male patients suffer from a degree of impotence, and a similar proportion of female patients have problems with arousal and reaching orgasm. The reasons for this are likely to be multifactorial.

Physical causes may include the following factors:

- hormone imbalance
- anaemia leading to tiredness
- the effect of drugs, especially some antihypertensive medication
- vascular problems affecting blood flow to the genital area
- neuropathy, especially in those with diabetes, lowering sensitivity to sexual stimuli.

Psychological causes often compound and contribute to the problem:

- depression
- poor self-image/body image
- role changes, leading to dependence and lack of confidence in sexual identity
- sense of guilt towards the partner.

When sexual relations are rare or absent, affectionate touching and cuddling frequently stop as well, leading to further impoverishment of the physical relationship.

Physical problems leading to impotence in men can often be successfully treated. Efficient dialysis and treatment of anaemia with erythropoietin may be enough to restore sexual function. If there are still problems with getting or maintaining an erection, there are several possible approaches to treatment. These include vacuum devices, insertion of prostaglandin pellets into the penis, injections into the base of the penis, and the drug sildenafil (Viagra) which is now licensed for the treatment of male renal patients. It is important that men with sexual problems are referred for help, because the effect of impotence on confidence and identity, let alone relationships with the spouse or partner, seriously affects well-being and happiness (Case Study 3.1).

■ CASE STUDY 3.1

The 40-year-old wife of a long-standing haemodialysis patient contacted the renal sexual counsellor, due to her extreme frustration. She explained that they had not had intercourse for over 2 years. She felt angry and irritable, both with her husband and her children. She also felt guilty, because it was not her husband's fault that he had kidney failure and no longer showed any interest in sexual relations.

During discussion with the couple, the counsellor asked the patient if he ever had an erection. He replied that he occasionally had a partial erection, in the early hours of the morning. The patient's wife was astonished, and asked why he had not told her about this. The patient pointed out that she had been taking sleeping pills for a long time, and was hard to wake, let alone sexually arouse, at 5 or 6 o'clock in the morning! The patient's wife immediately stopped taking the sleeping pills and the couple were able to report successful love-making a week later.

It is often useful for patients and their spouses to talk to a counsellor, because they start to communicate about their problem, which may be easy to improve or solve with simple adjustment in behaviour.

Treatment of loss of desire in women has received far less attention. There are currently trials of sildenafil to study whether increased blood supply to the genital area improves sexual response and lubrication, but in 2001 the drug is not yet licensed for treatment of female sexual problems. If female patients feel able to engage in intercourse, it is possible to maintain the physical bond with their partner, even if they do not themselves experience sexual satisfaction (Case Study 3.2). Artificial lubrication may be necessary to prevent discomfort.

■ CASE STUDY 3.2

In conversation with the renal counsellor, a female haemodialysis patient, aged 45, mentioned that her husband was 'very good and caring' towards her, and never asked for sexual relations. The counsellor suggested that, if she felt able to do so, the patient should initiate love-making herself, even though she was no longer able to get aroused. This would be a way of reassuring her husband of her love, and thanking him for his care and consideration. The patient was sceptical about this, but a few months later called into the office. She said that she had taken the advice and just wanted to say 'thank you', because the effect upon the relationship had been very beneficial. 'He was so thrilled', she said, 'it has really brought our marriage to life again'.

It is also possible that it prevented this husband from getting so frustrated that he looked elsewhere for the physical warmth he needed.

In women, the major issue affecting self-image is loss of fertility (irregular or absent ovulation and menstruation, and the knowledge that, while on dialysis, conception is unlikely and a successful pregnancy even more so).

Psychological problems leading to difficulties in sexual relationships are often much improved following discussion with a counsellor. This should preferably involve both partners, to achieve communication between the couple. It is often very reassuring for the fit partner to receive confirmation that it is the illness, rather than a decrease in affection, that is the cause of reduced or absent sexual interest. If affectionate touching has ceased it can be encouraged, strengthening the physical bond, and in some cases, occasional successful love-making results, with or without penetration.

Most of the problems described here are improved or eliminated following a successful transplant, although vascular problems and neuropathy associated with diabetes may continue to compromise sexual activity.

Body image

Both dialysis treatment and transplantation affect body image, making patients feel different, unattractive and ill at ease within their own bodies.

Access surgery often results in multiple scarring, involving the arms, chest and abdomen. A fistula which is regarded as 'very good' by nursing staff can be seen as a horrible disfigurement by the patient, who may try to conceal it from friends and the curious stares of strangers. Staff become so used to central lines that they forget the response to these outside the hospital. Patients with fistulae and grafts have even been thought to be drug addicts by the public, due to the effects of multiple cannulation.

The Tenckhoff catheter is less evident to outsiders, but patients may be convinced that they look strange and that everybody is aware of this. Many feel embarrassed in front of their partners and feel that nobody could find them attractive anymore. Some even imagine that the catheter smells offensive and that others are repelled. Most of these problems are subjective and reflect the patients' own attitude to and disgust with their own body.

Following transplantation, the immunosuppressive drugs, especially steroids, change the face, so that patients may feel they no longer recognise their image in the mirror as being the person they knew (Case Study 3.3). In addition, the texture of the skin and hair changes and hair grows in unwanted places, such as the eyebrows and cheeks. It is important to reassure patients that, as a general rule, these effects become less obvious as the drugs are reduced. However, in those cases where appearance remains changed, ongoing support and advice may be necessary.

■ CASE STUDY 3.3

Following a transplant, a middle-aged man chose to grow a beard. When complimented on this, he replied that he had been forced into the decision, because he was unable to bear seeing his reflection in the mirror when shaving.

'It is no longer me that I see. I cannot recognise the face in the mirror and this frightens me', he said. After a year, when the effects of the immunosuppressive drugs had decreased, he was able to shave off his beard.

It is common to assume that women are more affected than men by their body image, but this is by no means always the case.

Confidence and a sense of our own identity depend on a clear image of how we appear, both to ourselves and to others. If the integrity of this self-image is violated in some way, by drugs, surgery or even the distortions we mistakenly apply to ourselves, it can lead to severe psychological damage.

Awareness of early death

Those who have a life-threatening illness such as renal failure live on 'the edge', maintained on a life-support system. Such patients are bound to be more than usually aware of the fragility of life and the possibility of early death. Although there are some who spend many decades on dialysis or with a transplant, and approach a normal span of life, statistically these are the exception. For the young patient, the diagnosis is more devastating than for someone in their 70s or 80s, who could expect to die within a decade in any case. Most patients cope by putting the thought out of their minds as far as possible, but there are gloomy reminders on visits to hospital, when friends or acquaintances are found to have suffered complications or died. Most wonder whether they will be next. Dialysis patients form a close community who know, better than most, 'not to ask for whom the bell tolls, for it tolls for thee'.

This predicament can lead to mental conflict—whether to make hay while the sun shines, by living life to the full and risking the consequences, or to live a restricted life observing all the rules—maybe a longer life, but without the fun or range of experiences that others can enjoy. The most successful patients seem to be those who find a coping mechanism by balancing between the two extremes. Sadly, patients cannot control everything that happens, even if they try to follow all advice. The condition is 'perverse' and frustrating (Hooper, 1994). More than most of us, those with renal failure have to learn to live with uncertainty about the future.

The young patient with no ties or emotional attachments is often considered to be at a disadvantage, but, paradoxically, the happiness of marriage and children carries its own price in suffering—there is so much more to lose (Case Study 3.4).

■ CASE STUDY 3.4

A man of 38, who had been on haemodialysis since the age of 14, was referred during an admission for a hip replacement. He had been very active and had always managed to stay in employment as well as doing voluntary work. Bone disease had made him increasingly disabled and he had recently started to use a wheelchair. A few years ago he had married and he and his wife had had a child by donor insemination. He was thrilled at the birth of the child—a little boy, now aged three—and was a devoted father. Now, with time on his hands due to his hospital admission, he had become acutely aware of the possibility—in fact, the likelihood—of early death, which would prevent him seeing this child grow to adulthood. He wanted to care for his wife and son over the span of a normal marriage, but the illness had denied him this natural expectation. 'It was bad enough', he said, 'when I only had myself to worry about. When I got married, I had my wife's needs and feelings to take into account. She would suffer by my death. Now that I have a child, it is the greatest joy of my life, but he is so little and vulnerable. How can he understand about my illness? The thought that I will not be there to protect him and see him grow up is absolutely unbearable'.

There is no answer or true comfort to offer in this situation. The counsellor suggested that he should write letters to his son, to be kept for the future, saying the things he would like the child to know. These could be tailored to different ages,—perhaps a letter for a 5-year-old, a 10-year-old, and so on. In this way he could be sure that the boy was aware of his father's love and concern, even if he was no longer living.

Failure to take medical/nursing advice—non-adherence

Few patients take all the advice that is given by medical and nursing staff or follow instructions all the time. This probably represents a healthy and adaptive sign rather than otherwise, unless, of course, patients put themselves at serious risk. Those with renal failure have little chance of disguising the fact that they are failing to follow advice, because blood results, blood pressure and weight gain reveal underdialysis and diet and fluid abuses, as well as failure to take medication.

Within reason, such 'non-adherence' may be a good sign. Obsessional concern with the illness and treatment is not a desirable outcome. However, persistent non-adherence to a dangerous level, often for no discernible reason, is cause for serious investigation. The commonest causes appear to be:

• a lack of understanding, either of the instructions themselves, or of the implications of not following them. Much of the advice to renal patients takes into account that the condition is long-term. There is often no immediate perceived consequence of failure to take advice, e.g. drugs to protect the bones, or antihypertensive medication. This can lead to the patient assuming that the drugs are having no effect. The long-term effects on the heart, produced by habitual fluid overload, are also hard to appreciate. The patient may feel that fluid abuse merely leads to a short lecture and a little longer on dialysis, and regard this as a worthwhile price to pay for a good night out. On an occasional basis, this may be a sensible attitude, but it easily becomes a habit

- depression—apathy about treatment and life in general. Since life is barely tolerable it really does not matter greatly if one takes risks with it
- a negative, and in some ways emotionally regressed sense of defiance, often directed against what is seen as 'nagging' by staff. Many adult patients will not have been 'told what to do' in a motherly or teacher-like fashion since they were children
- denial—underlying denial there is often desperation. The patient is aware of the reality of the situation but cannot bear to face it squarely. Acting as if the painful situation does not exist enables the patient to maintain a fantasy that is bearable. Denial is not always dysfunctional. It can be a useful coping mechanism. In dying patients, for example, those who maintain hope and act as if life is going to carry on may make things easier for themselves (and those around them), although there may be problems in realistic communication of feelings and planning for the future. Denial in the dialysis situation may however make it impossible for patient and relatives to discuss the illness on a realistic basis and can become a threat if it leads to behaviour that is a risk to life (Case Study 3.5).

■ **CASE STUDY 3.5**

A young man of 28 was referred due to serious abuse of his fluid limits. He frequently attended for dialysis with 5–6 L of fluid weight gain, which was beginning to cause cardiac enlargement.

During discussion of the long-term effects of this, he said: 'It is as much as I can do to think about surviving from day to day. I cannot even *begin* to think about several years in the future. Whatever I do, I probably won't live that long in any case, so I might as well enjoy things today'. After further discussion of his attitudes to treatment and underlying feelings, he added: 'I *hate* the way the nurses nag me. I wonder how they would cope? They make me really angry. So now, when I come in with several kilos extra fluid, I think … 'that's one in the eye for staff!'

If adherence becomes a battle between the patient and the staff, it is a battle that is already lost. Patients can only be told the consequences of their actions. After that, it is up to them to decide what to do.

One can only sympathise with both nurses and patients in the whole subject of non-adherence. Dialysis nurses are in a highly stressful job with a high technical component and limited time to interact with individual patients, yet have prolonged contact, over months or years. They are unable to 'cure' their patients, and therefore have very specific target outcomes, gaining their satisfaction and measuring their own success by the efficiency and efficacy of the dialysis process. Nurses who have one or a number of patients who seem to be wilfully denying them that satisfaction are at high risk of engaging in a personal battle, which can culminate in frustration, anger and burn-out. One patient is often singled out as the nurse's personal crusade, waged, of course for the good of that patient, and therefore utterly justified. Sadly, we do not like our 'failures', but cannot let go of them either! The struggle is therefore likely to descend to the level of the school playground. 'Go on, kill yourself,—see if I care!' becomes the nurse's unspoken response to the patient's 'One in the eye for the staff!'

The depressive reaction is most commonly seen in older patients and defiance and denial are usually seen in younger patients. All these reactions seem to be indirect appeals for help and need to be treated as such. Anger from staff, threats of dire consequences or lectures on the behaviour expected of a dialysis patient are unlikely to be helpful. Naturally, patients need to be given a clear explanation of the reasons for the rules that are set, and the possible results and risks that they run in choosing to break those rules, but they also need to have their underlying motives and feelings explored and respected. Some of the causes for distress may be alleviated by counselling, changes in medication, adjustment of dialysis regime or other measures. It is always helpful to focus on what can be had or done, not what cannot.

WITHDRAWAL FROM DIALYSIS

This decision may be taken by a patient at any age, but is most frequent in elderly patients, who are sometimes very poorly adjusted to life on treatment. This may be due to depression following bereavement or experiencing additional medical problems such as stroke, malignancies, amputations and ischaemic heart disease, which further restrict their quality of life. Such patients may wish to withdraw from dialysis, a subject that needs sympathetic exploration. If found to be a considered and serious wish rather than an expression of frustration or an oblique request for a particular problem to be recognised, such requests to withdraw from treatment should be supported and respected. Dialysis may prove to be an intolerable burden to those who have other reasons to feel that life no longer offers any opportunities and satisfactions. Some bitterly resent the limitations of the ageing process, cannot adjust to being a 'spectator' and wish only to turn back the clock. In a minority of cases, it is overwhelmingly the fear of dying rather than a wish to live that makes the patient continue with dialysis, making it hard to achieve any real life satisfaction.

It is common for renal unit staff to feel that the treatment of very frail older people, especially those with multiple medical problems, by means of a scarce and expensive resource such as hospital haemodialysis, is unjustified. If little or no subjective quality of life results, it would be hard to disagree. It is very important that we explore the attitudes of elderly patients, and do not carry on with treatment which is giving no quality of life, remembering, however, that quality of life is a subjective matter, and only the person concerned can tell whether life is worth living. One can be surprised both by the apparently full life which is unacceptable to one patient, and by the apparently burdensome life which is regarded as worthwhile by another. Respecting these views can be difficult, especially in the case of the patient who seems to have a good life, yet wishes to discontinue treatment. Kaplan De Nour (1994) concludes that the answer to the question 'Is it all worth the effort—is machine-dependent life worth living?' lies in the psychological condition of the patient rather than any objective quality of life.

SPECIAL PROBLEMS OF PEOPLE FROM ETHNIC MINORITIES

Members of Asian and Afro-Caribbean ethnic groups have a higher incidence of renal failure than the Caucasian UK population (Bradley 2000). This seems to be connected to the greater prevalence of diabetes in the Asian community, especially in those past the age of 40, and a higher incidence of hypertension in the Afro-Caribbean population.

In order to allow patients from cultural backgrounds other than the UK to obtain equal benefits from the healthcare system, it is important to be aware of factors that could affect the situation. These include:

- language and understanding
- dietary differences
- attitudes to illness
- family relationships.

It is difficult enough for members of the multidisciplinary team to communicate fully and effectively with those of the same cultural background and language, let alone those who have language problems and different cultural concepts. It is necessary to remain sensitive to the effects of ethnicity, both on understanding and attitudes to illness and treatment (Allison et al 1983).

Language
The most obvious of these is language. Elderly Indian, Pakistani and Chinese patients, for example, often rely on younger family members for the translation of interviews with medical and nursing staff, and to relay information on symptoms and feelings. Medical advice and information are also given via a third party and may suffer in translation. It is advisable to have a qualified interpreter for any sensitive and important communication, since family members may be too involved to give an impartial and accurate interpretation, relaying nuances of meaning.

All patient information material needs to be available in translation, but it is necessary to check reading ability rather than assuming that by giving a leaflet one has imparted the information.

Diet

Diet, which plays a major role in the management of renal disease, can be a source of considerable problems. Most renal diets are based on native UK eating habits, and are hard to adjust to the religious and cultural requirements of other countries. Many Asian patients prefer to have food brought in by the family during hospital admissions. Those on PD who are vegetarian, have a greater need to maintain adequate protein intake, and sometimes find it hard to do so when pulses are their major source of dietary protein. Specialist dietetic advice is necessary to achieve good serum albumin levels in such diets (Ch. 9).

Attitudes to illness

It is usual for Asian families to take a major part in the everyday care of a sick family member (whether at home or in hospital), and for a number of relatives, both young and old, to spend a lot of time at the bedside. Staff used to the less involved attitude of many native UK families may find this unusual or inconvenient, especially if there is a lack of space and facilities on the ward.

Attitudes to illness, and even the conceptual understanding of disease and treatment, may differ from culture to culture, needing the sensitive understanding of the nurse. Cause and effect may be differently perceived. Religious acceptance of illness as a predestined fate to be accepted without attempts to change matters is a further concept that may cause misunderstandings. Culturally acceptable responses to illness may also differ from country to country. An Asian patient will often cover the whole body, including the head, with a blanket, making some staff and other patients uneasy and puzzled. Accepted responses to pain may also differ from one ethnic group to another, leading to an over-or underestimation of the subjective suffering involved.

Some ethnic groups may have religious or cultural beliefs about cadaver or living related grafts. Even if these problems do not apply, the likelihood of a well-matched graft is reduced for patients from an ethnic minority, whose tissue type may be uncommon in the UK. There are major initiatives by the Department of Health to promote both cadaver and living related donation of kidneys in the ethnic minority population, in the hope of increasing transplantation rates in these groups—the fastest-growing section of the transplant waiting list in the UK.

It is important that all members of the team remain sensitive, both to the needs of the patients and families and to their own attitudes.

Family relationships

The family structure and hierarchy should also be taken into account, since some cultures regard any major decision as traditionally the preserve of the senior male member of the family present, leading to an unwillingness on the part of a female patient to determine her own preference or accept responsibility without consultation with a husband, father, uncle or son.

It can be difficult to understand Asian family structure and relationships since, in many families, anyone with a family connection tends to be designated 'a cousin', even, in some cases, where there is no relationship. (In native

UK culture the same pattern leads us to call close family friends 'uncles' and 'aunties', without explaining that the title is 'honorary'.) Many patients have relatives, including spouses, in their country of origin and like to visit them every few years. It can therefore be very traumatic to have an illness that precludes travel due to lack of medical facilities at home. If elderly parents die, and the patient is unable to return for the funeral, there can be great distress, not only because of the natural pain of bereavement, but because of the religious implications of duty and respect which carry greater significance than in western culture.

TRANSPLANTATION

From what has already been said about the stresses of life on dialysis, it is obvious that, for many patients, dialysis is a period of 'marking time' while awaiting transplantation. Almost every study of quality of life so far has shown that successful transplantation offers the best chance of leading a near-normal life, and is associated with the highest perceived life satisfaction. Objectively, the quality (although, contrary to the belief of some patients, not the quantity) of life is greatly increased. Successful transplantation is associated with a number of benefits, including:

- higher chance of employment
- greater energy
- improved mental alertness and concentration
- freedom from a restrictive diet
- the return, in most cases, of sexual capacity
- the possibility of child-bearing.

It would, however, be misleading to regard even successful transplantation as a panacea. Following transplantation, the patient with ESRF needs to feel that life is wonderful. A successful transplant is, after all, the nearest to normality that the patient will ever achieve, and has often been the long-awaited 'answer' to the patient's problems, so from a psychological point of view the patient has a need to feel that life has been transformed. The reality is sometimes rather different. Those who want to return to employment find that, although declared fit by the doctor, the view of prospective employers is less enthusiastic. Many find it hard to get a job in competition with others. Financially, the position is therefore worse than on dialysis, because, in the UK, Benefits Agency disability benefits are often withdrawn, and the patient can only claim basic unemployment benefit. Relationships sometimes become strained, because less tolerance is now shown by spouses and families. The individual requiring dialysis has every right to claim that life is a burden, but gradually and subtly, sympathy is withdrawn from the transplant patient, who should after all be 'grateful for the gift of life' which, whether this is actually stated or not, is seen to have been won at the cost of the death of a cadaveric donor, or through the sacrifice of a living relative. This can be a hard gift to accept, carrying with it a burden of responsibility to make the suffering of others worthwhile.

Patients who lose their grafts quite often feel that they have let down not only the team caring for them, but also the donor and donor family.

Immediately posttransplant, provided all goes well, there is usually a euphoric phase, possibly accentuated by steroid immunosuppression, and the sudden 'clearing of the mind' reported by many patients, which has never been fully explained. This is mixed with anxiety that rejection will occur and the graft will be lost. One of the hardest aspects of this stage is the sudden removal of conscious control. Dialysis patients have been conditioned to be very much in control of their health through adherence to diet and fluid restrictions, a regular treatment regime, scrupulous care of access and weight and blood pressure measurement. After a transplant, the situation changes dramatically. Apart from regularly taking immunosuppressive medication and attending for follow-up, patients' contribution to the survival of the graft is minimal. They are, as it were, at the mercy of factors beyond conscious control—their own immune response and the effects of the foreign body which now needs to become accepted as part of the self. It is no wonder that many patients become acutely superstitious (the natural human response to forces that cannot be influenced by reason or action). Anxiety can reach almost obsessional levels, and may become displaced from the transplant itself to attach to other health concerns.

The side-effects of immunosuppression for some may cause little distress, but for others have a considerable psychological effect and, in a very few, produce a psychotic response. The commonest effects are upon body image. Cushingoid changes in the appearance are distressing to both sexes. Facial hair and changes in hair texture are more distressing to women. Many men choose to grow a beard following transplant, chiefly to disguise the 'moon face'. Weight gain as a result of appetite increase on steroids compounds the body-image problem. Ciclosporin has many advantages as an immunosuppressive agent, but patients can be very distressed by the tremor sometimes associated with this drug.

A good counselling programme should be provided, including access to advice on facial hair removal, treatment for changes in skin texture and advice on skin care to help avoid malignant changes stimulated by exposure to sun. The creation of a positive body image after transplantation is every bit as important as on dialysis.

Counselling may also be needed to help with emotional oversensitivity at this time. Both male and female patients who regarded themselves as previously emotionally controlled are sometimes surprised to find themselves liable to tearful episodes and mood swings, partly due to the drugs and partly due to the very considerable inner turmoil created by the experience of transplantation. The need for sympathetic reassurance and support from the transplant team in the early stages cannot be overestimated.

It is comparatively common for young women who are keen to have children to become pregnant soon after having a transplant. Often they are unmarried and unsupported. It seems that the desire to have a baby overrides all other considerations for these women and that rational arguments and advice are unlikely to have any part to play against such an imperative. Fear of losing the graft, damaging their own health, risking stillbirth or a seriously premature child, let alone the problems of trying to care for a baby without the security of a permanent relationship, seem completely unimportant. Grafts can be lost due to the strain of pregnancy, especially when undertaken less than a year after transplantation. While it is essential to counsel young women on the risks, advise on birth control and advocate a reasonable delay before becoming pregnant, it seems unlikely that this will prevent some of them from seizing what they see as their only chance of having a child, regardless of the consequences. It is a further way of ratifying their 'normality' following the very artificial and restricted life on dialysis. In the few cases where termination is performed, the feelings of ambivalence are likely to be severe, and may even be directed against the graft itself, whose survival has been protected at the expense of the child.

Graft loss

The patient whose graft is rapidly rejected experiences an acute disappointment, but is in many ways better able to recover and come to terms than the patient who has several months of unsatisfactory graft function before finally returning to dialysis. In such cases there may have been heavy courses of methylprednisolone or monoclonal antibodies, numerous biopsies and possibly further surgery to no avail, resulting in a state of physical debility and mental anguish far worse than before the operation. Such patients often say at the time that they regret ever having tried transplantation, yet the great majority return to the transplant list within a few months.

PATIENTS WITH MULTIPLE PATHOLOGY

There are increasing numbers of patients now receiving dialysis for whom renal failure is the most treatable aspect of a serious systemic illness, such as diabetes, scleroderma, primary amyloid or myeloma. A further large patient group consists of those with generalised vascular disease. The complications of these underlying conditions are responsible for many long hospital admissions and a great deal of the morbidity and mortality of patients on dialysis programmes.

The patient with diabetes can be particularly hard to counsel and distressing to nurse. As the disease reaches its late phases, one has no sooner supported a patient through the loss of one limb, when the next becomes problematic. Eyesight may already have been poor, only to be followed by total blindness. Autonomic neuropathy may then lead to diarrhoea and incontinence, and inability to maintain blood pressure when changing position.

As with all those on renal replacement therapy, there are two important aspects for nursing and other staff to consider: the psychological impact of the illness and the practical arrangements that may be necessary to enable the patient to spend time at home. Patients who are aware that their underlying condition is fatal, and that dialysis is a means of prolonging life in the short term, need every help to spend as little time in hospital as possible.

This entails involving community nursing, occupational therapists, physio-therapists and care managers from Social Services to provide a package of care. This may involve visits from home-care staff several times a day, the provision of meals, day centre attendance, respite care in nursing homes and the provision of equipment such as stair lifts, rails and ramps for wheelchair access.

There is occasionally some conflict with community nurses and carers, who express the opinion that the patient is not well enough to be out of hospital, and that it is 'too risky' for the patient to be at home. In their opinion the patient might fall, sustain fractures, succumb to a massive haemorrhage or a cardiovascular crisis or have some other medical emergency. This is, of course, true, but the philosophy of renal units can be at odds with the 'normal' world. Our patients would all have perished without renal replacement. They are alive against the odds, and for them, a degree of risk is an acceptable price to pay for seizing the chance to experience life outside the hospital. A more lengthy admission is unlikely to reduce the chance of sudden and maybe fatal complications. If patients are happy to take that risk, they need our support.

The strain on spouses and family members is considerable. Many will have jobs and family responsibilities, and may feel guilty if they do not put the patient's needs above their own. Support needs to be given to relatives in this situation, to reduce guilt wherever possible. This entails allowing opportunities for the expression of feelings and encouraging relatives to set aside time for themselves. Some will, for example, visit daily from long distances during the patient's admissions to hospital—a time when there is the chance for carers to recharge their own batteries, take much-needed relaxation or catch up with other tasks. This is also a time when unfinished business may need to be resolved. This may be in the form of reconciling old family differences and feuds to secure the future for those who will be left when the patient has died. Another aspect of this may be the desire of common-law partners to marry.

Staff need to be aware of the patient's state of mind, and ready to hear the message that the patient has had enough. It is not unreasonable to choose death from uraemia in preference to a short period of further suffering before succumbing to a more distressing end to life. Some, it is true, are never able to let go, but others may wish to do so while they are still capable of determining their own destiny through rational decision. It may, however, be hard to express this to staff who are unwilling to hear.

Acute renal failure and acute presentation in ERSF

Providing support

Patients with acute renal failure often come to the renal ward via intensive therapy units, following overwhelming illnesses. Illness severe enough to cause acute renal failure requiring dialysis or haemofiltration is always a crisis for patient and relatives, attended by high levels of anxiety. This is justified, since the mortality in such patients is very high. Once the precipitating illness is controlled and the patient's condition is stable, concern is transferred to the renal failure, and whether the kidneys will recover. During this period, patient and relatives often need emotional support from staff, and reassurance that renal function is expected to return in spite of the need for dialysis over several weeks. From the psychological point of view, it is important to help the spouse to visit as often as possible, both for the sake of the patient and the partner. It is always recognised that children need a parent to be with them, and that recovery is helped by the security this offers. It is seldom realised how lonely and frightened adults, especially if elderly, can become when seriously ill and separated from their partner and environment.

The patient is often admitted to a unit many miles from home, making visiting expensive. Help with transport costs should be sought from the Department of Social Security or charitable funding if hardship is suspected. It is not uncommon for the family of a critically ill patient, admitted for 3–4 weeks, to incur £300–400 in visiting costs. Staff need to explore the possibilities for inexpensive accommodation in or near the hospital for relatives of such patients. When the patient is finally ready to leave hospital, it is important for a care manager to assess the home circumstances, since the illness may have had permanent debilitating effects. Preparation for this may help to mitigate the emotional blow of returning home, and finding that, while home is the same as ever, the person who left it a few weeks ago has changed. Following leg amputations, patients may show a reluctance to go on a visit home to assess future ability to cope. The 'safe and familiar place' has lost its ability to reassure, because it now contains challenges and hazards. Sensitivity, honesty and understanding are needed to build the confidence of patients who feel, rightly, that they will 'never be the same again'.

Despite attempts to improve early referral rates, through liaison with GP practices, many patients are still seen in a renal unit for the first time when at the point of needing renal replacement therapy. For these patients, the adjustment process is condensed into a very short period. Both responses to the diagnosis and adjustment to treatment itself are experienced concurrently, leading to greater problems with acceptance. In a retrospective study of those starting dialysis during the previous year in a large UK renal unit, higher current levels of depression and anxiety were reported by patients who had started treatment acutely, without time for psychological preparation (Auer 1995).

SUMMARY

The care of those with renal failure is a highly specialised area of nursing, with unique satisfactions and unique stresses. There is no other field of hospital nursing that involves such intensive involvement with patients over such long periods. High technology may appear to predominate but in spite of, or because of, the dependence of the patient on complicated artificial life-support systems, it is the quality of the human relationships created between the patient and the professional team that determines the success of the whole undertaking. Clinical skills are not enough to give the patient on dialysis the chance to live to the best potential. The commitment of both patient and team is, quite simply, lifelong. As a result, it is an unusually close relationship with all the benefits and disadvantages that this implies. Those who work in renal units have in common a sense of belonging to an extended family group. This is not to say that they are free of conflict, stresses and frustration—rather, the reverse. Staff as well as patients need support, and many units recognise this and have good support systems, some formal, some informal.

It is not possible for the renal nurse to avoid a degree of personal involvement. Total detachment from a patient with whom the fight for survival is shared over months, years or even decades is scarcely a realistic proposition. Hospital staff cannot help but admire the tenacity and courage of patients and their spouses, feel frustrated by them and for them, and experience anger, exhausted patience, great sadness at battles lost and great happiness at battles won.

REFERENCES

Abram HS. The psychiatrist, the treatment of chronic renal failure and the prolongation of life. Am J Psychiatry 1969; 126:57.

Abram HS. Survival by machine: the psychological stress of chronic haemodialysis. Psychiatr Med 1970; 1:37.

Abram HS, Moore GL, Westevelt FB. Suicidal behaviour in chronic dialysis patients. Am J Psychiatry 1971; 127:1199–1204.

Allison M, Gregg D, Randell E et al Social work with patients suffering from kidney disease and with their families. Birmingham: British Association of Social Workers, 1983.

Auer J. Psychological aspects of elderly renal patients. In: Stevens E, Monkhouse P eds., Aspects of renal care, vol. 1. Eastbourne: Baillière Tindall, 1986:200–208.

Auer J. The Oxford–Manchester study of dialysis patients: age, risk factors and treatment method in relation to quality of life. Scand J Urol Nephrol 1990a; 131(suppl.):31–37.

Auer J. Psychological problems in chronic illness. In: Badawi M, Biamonti B, eds., Social work practice in health care. Cambridge: Woodhead Faulkner, 1990b.

Auer J, Charters V, Brownson A et al. Support and counselling pre-dialysis and on dialysis—need and outcome. Paper presented at EDTNA/ERCA conference, Athens. 1995.

Binik YM, Devins GM, Barre PE et al. Live and learn: patient education delays the need to initiate renal replacement therapy in end stage renal disease. J Nerv Ment Dis 1993; 181:371–376.

Bradley J. Ethnic susceptibility to renal disease. Br J Renal Med 2000; 5:4.

Bradley C, McGee H. Improving quality of life in renal failure: ways forward. In: McGee H, C. Bradley eds., Quality of life following renal failure. Chur: Harwood Academic Publishers, 1994:275–299.

Courts NF. Psychosocial adjustment of patients on home hemodialysis and their dialysis partners. Clin Nurs Res 2000; 9:177–190.

Gudex C. QALYs and their use by the health services. Discussion paper 20. York: University of York Centre for Health Economics, 1986.

Hooper G. Psychological care of patients in the renal unit. In: McGee H, Bradley C, eds. Quality of life following renal failure. Chur: Harwood Academic Publishers, 1994:181–196.

Kaplan De Nour A. Staff–patient interactions. In: NB Levy, ed. Psychonephrology. vol. 2. New York: Plenum, 1983.

Kaplan De Nour, A. Psychological social and vocational impact of renal failure. In: McGee H, Bradley C, eds. Quality of life following renal failure. Chur: Harwood Academic Publications, 1994:33–42.

Kaplan De Nour A, Czackes, JW. Emotional problems and reactions of the medical team in a chronic hemodialysis unit. Lancet 1968; ii:987.

Klang B, Bjorvell H, Clyne N. Predialysis Education helps patients choose dialysis modality and increases disease-specific knowledge. J Adv Nursing 1999; 29:869–876.

Kline SA, Burton HJ, And Akhtar M. The elderly patient on dialysis— psychosocial considerations. In: Oreopoulos DG, ed. Geriatric nephrology. Boston: Nijhoff, 1986.

Kubler Ross E. On Death and Dying. London: Tavistock. 1970.

Kutner NG. Is there bias in treatment for renal failure? In: McGee H, Bradley C, eds. Quality of life following renal failure. Chur: Harwood Academic Publications, 1994:161.

Loomes G, McKenzie L. The use of QALYs in health care decision making. Soc Sci Med 1989; 28:299–308.

Lunts P. Rediscovering home haemodialysis. Returning choice to patients. EDTNA/ERCA J 1999; XXV:40–41.

Neu S, Kjellstrand CM. Stopping long-term dialysis. N Engl J Med 1986; 314:14–20.

Quarello F, Piccoli GB, Bonello F et al. Dialysis in the elderly: ten year experience in a large population. Geriatr Nephrol Urol 1992; 2:190–191.

Shambaugh P, Kanter S. Spouses under stress: group meetings with spouses of patients on haemodialysis. Am J Psychiatry 1969; 125:7.

Stanton J. The cost of living: Kidney dialysis, rationing and health economics in Britain, 1965–1996. Soc Sci Med 1999; 49(9):1169–1182.

Stout JP, Auer J, And Kincey J. Sexual and marital relationships and dialysis patients. Perit Dial Bull 1985; 7:97–99.

Westlie L, Umen A, Nestrud S, et al. Mortality, morbidity and life satisfaction in the very old dialysis patient. Trans Am Soc Art Intern Organs 1984; 30:21–31.

Williams A. Economics of coronary artery bypass grafting. Br Med J 1985; 291:326–329.

FURTHER READING

McGee HM, Bradley C. Quality of life following renal failure. Chur: Harwood Academic Publishers, 1994.

Stein A, Wild J (eds). Kidney failure at your fingertips. London: Class Publishing, 2001.

Acute renal failure

Tim Armstrong   Gemma Bircher

4

■ CONTENTS

■ LEARNING OUTCOMES FOR THIS CHAPTER

- To understand the different types and causes of acute renal failure (ARF)
- To help and support the patient and family during an episode of ARF
- To describe the signs and symptoms of ARF
- To analyse the nutritional requirements of those with ARF
- To evaluate the various treatment options for ARF.

INTRODUCTION

Since the kidney has multiple functions, the patient with ARF will often present the nurse with a complex scenario (Sinert et al 2001). Despite the availability of various dialysis treatments and different drug therapies, these patients face a mortality rate of up to 50% and, for those who are critically ill, up to 85% (Chen et al 2001).

ARF has often been defined as a sudden deterioration in renal function that results in the inability to excrete the products of metabolism. In turn, this produces a rise in blood urea and other nitrogen waste products (Dauguirdas 2000). Depending on its severity and duration, ARF is often transient in nature and, with careful nursing care, the patient can regain normal renal function. However, without appropriate specialised treatment, the patient may be denied the opportunity to make a full recovery and a precipitation of further impairment may lead to chronic or end-stage renal failure (ESRF).

The aim of this chapter is to emphasise the vital role the nurse plays in the delivery of care for the patient in ARF. The importance of the nurse–patient role is vital to the well-being of the patient, whereby the nurse can monitor the patient for complications, participate in emergency renal replacement therapy, assess the patient's progress and response to treatment, and provide physical and emotional support. In this central role the nurse can maintain close links with the patient's family, which can be instrumental to a family-centred approach to the patient's treatment. The alliance between the patient, the family and the nurse is paramount in keeping the family informed of the patient's condition, assisting them to understand treatments and providing psychological support. Figure 4.1 gives an overview of the signs and symptoms of ARF.

However, in recent years, the intensive care nurse has taken over from the renal nurse in caring for those requiring continuous renal replacement therapy (CRRT). Specific nursing activities for CRRT are therefore beyond the scope of this book, but further reading can be found at the end of this chapter.

Mortality

It is important for nurses and carers to be able to understand that ARF is a serious condition that should never be underestimated. Constant improve-

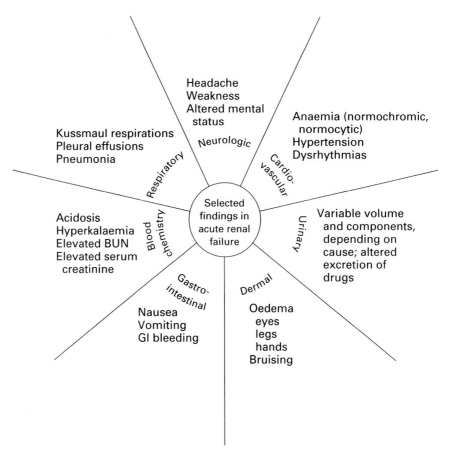

Figure 4.1 Signs and symptoms of acute renal failure. BUN, blood urea nitrogen; GI, gastrointestinal. (From Brundage D. Renal disorders. Mosby, 1992 with permission from Mosby.)

ments in dialysis technology, combined with a growing chronic renal failure population and limited funds, have put clinicians under pressure to try and predict the outcomes of treatment. Whilst improvements in technology have enabled there to be greater comfort and survival, there are greater monetary costs (Peeters & Rublee 2000). A number of attempts have been made to predict the outcome of ARF but due to its complex and erratic nature, this has been difficult to predict (Levy et al 1996).

However, it can be seen that there are a number of patient groups in whom ARF has a particularly high mortality rate. For example, the mortality rate of those patients whose ARF is caused by burns can be as high as 96% (Cantarovich & Verho 1996). The need for rapid identification of the cause of ARF and those patients at highest risk is essential so that the current course of treatment can be adopted (DuBose et al 1997). Therefore it is vital for the nurse to play a major role in assisting physicians in the treatment options available for this fragile group of patients.

Classification

ARF may be divided into three major categories, in which each category has a physiological location of the insult (Table 4.1):

- prerenal—relates to the ineffective perfusion of the kidneys, which are structurally normal
- renal (intrinsic)—damage to the renal parenchyma, sometimes secondary to prerenal problems
- postrenal—disordered urinary drainage of both kidneys or of a single functioning kidney.

In addition, an acute impairment may present in the patient with existing chronic renal failure, which may lead to further structural damage; this presentation is often referred to as acute-on-chronic renal failure.

Prerenal acute renal failure

Prerenal causes of ARF are directly related to hypoperfusion states or a decline in the blood supply to the kidneys. The structure of the kidneys is normal. However, when the renal blood supply is restricted, glomerular filtration is reduced, causing decreased perfusion of the kidneys. The net effect is a decreased blood flow to the glomeruli, which therefore leads to ineffective filtration because of inadequate blood flow. Without an effective renal plasma flow rate the glomeruli are unable to filter waste from the blood but the structure of the renal tubules remains intact (Fig. 4.2).

In this prerenal state, urine osmolarity is high and sodium low, which is consistent with renal hypoperfusion and well-preserved renal function. If at this state, renal blood flow can be restored, then normal renal function will return. However, if the prerenal state is prolonged, then this may lead to ischaemic damage due to poor perfusion, which in turn may lead to acute tubular necrosis (Sinert et al 2001).

The importance of early recognition, diagnosis and treatment is vital in prerenal failure, in order to prevent the condition progressing to renal failure with a degree of parenchymal damage.

Table 4.1 Acute renal failure: major causes and aetiology

Stage	Major causes	Aetiology
Prerenal	Cardiovascular	Congestive cardiac failure
		Myocardial infarction
		Cardiogenic shock
		Cardiac tamponade
		Pulmonary embolism
	Vasodilation	Sepsis
		Anaphylaxis
	Hypovolaemia	Haemorrhage, including blood loss due to surgery
		Burns
		Gastrointestinal loss
		Renal loss
Renal (intrinsic)	Glomerulonephritis	Poststreptococcal infection
		Systemic lupus erythematosus
		Haemolytic–uraemic syndrome
		Wegener's granulomatosis
		Goodpasture's syndrome
	Vascular	Vasculitis
		Hypertension
		Eclampsia of pregnancy
		Renal artery stenosis
		Renal vein thrombosis
	Intratubular	
	Pigment	Myoglobin (see rhabdomyolysis)
	Proteins	Myeloma
	Crystals	Nephrotoxins (see nephrotoxicity)
Postrenal	Obstruction of lower urinary tract	Prostatic hypertrophy
	Obstruction of upper urinary tract	Ureteric obstruction (clots, extrinsic compression, calculi)

Renal (intrinsic) failure

This cause is sometimes referred to as intrinsic or intrarenal failure and is associated with structural damage to the glomeruli and renal tubules. The difference between pre- and postrenal failure and intrinsic failure is that in intrinsic failure the correction of the aetiology will not guarantee the complete recovery of renal function because of damage to the nephron itself. Here the episode of ARF may run a lengthy duration and can often lead to ESRF.

The clinical course of intrinsic renal failure is often complex and, depending upon underlying disorders, the recovery may be prolonged for up to 6 weeks. As illustrated in Table 4.1, there are a wide variety of causes for intrinsic renal failure that may involve multisystem disease or originate from a primary renal disorder, but often involve complicating severe illness that causes vasomotor nephropathy.

Some specific causes are now discussed.

Decreased blood supply caused by:

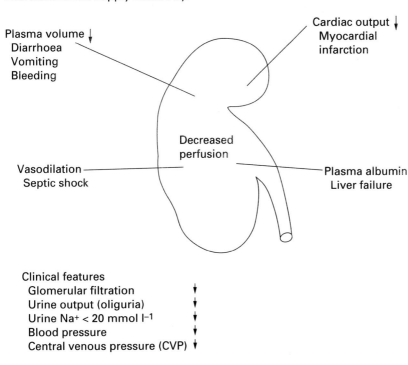

Plasma volume ↓
Diarrhoea
Vomiting
Bleeding

Cardiac output ↓
Myocardial
infarction

Decreased
perfusion

Vasodilation
Septic shock

Plasma albumin
Liver failure

Clinical features
Glomerular filtration
Urine output (oliguria)
Urine Na+ < 20 mmol l⁻¹
Blood pressure
Central venous pressure (CVP) ↓

Drowsiness, confusion, weakness,
dry mucous membranes,
loss of skin turgor, thirst.

Figure 4.2 Prerenal failure.

Acute interstitial nephritis

This condition often follows exposure to drugs in the form of antibiotics, analgesics and non-steroidal antiinflammatory agents. Infections can cause a very similar clinical and pathological picture and these include *Salmonella*, *Streptococcus*, *Meningococcus*, leptospirosis and many viral disorders.

Other categories of interstitial nephritis are caused by systemic disease such as systemic lupus erythematosus and sarcoidosis or present as the primary disease.

Clinical features

Fever, rash, arthralgia, back pain, and eosinophilia are clinical features of acute interstitial nephritis.

ARF may not develop for some weeks but in some cases renal dysfunction may occur within a few hours after exposure to a causative drug.

Rhabdomyolysis

A major cause of ARF is toxic in nature. Rhabdomyolysis is a result of the release of muscle contents, including myoglobin, into the plasma.

Rhabdomyolysis is often caused by trauma, for example a crush injury or pressure-induced muscle necrosis. This causes damage to muscle that allows the pigment myoglobin to be released into the plasma. Myoglobin is a red respiratory agent and in high plasma levels becomes nephrotoxic.

Clinical features
The urine is often brown or coffee-coloured due to the presence of myoglobin. Patients often present with acute illness with fever, weakness, pain and nausea and vomiting.

Renal failure and liver disease
ARF is often associated with acute liver injury that may result from:

• paracetamol overdose
• circulatory shock
• severe leptospirosis sepsis.

It may also be seen in surgery on the biliary tract.

For the patient with advanced liver disease the onset of renal failure is often referred to as hepatorenal syndrome. Septicaemia, fluid and electrolyte imbalance or hypovolaemia from gastrointestinal haemorrhage are common causes of the syndrome. These patients often require intensive care and the appropriate choice of therapy is of utmost importance (Rialp et al 1996).

Cortical necrosis
Cortical necrosis may follow any course of intensive or prolonged ischaemia. The condition is also associated with sepsis, shock, transfusion reactions and burns.

Renal biopsy reveals pathology of patchy necrosis of the glomeruli, tubules and small vessels of the renal cortex. The renal medulla remains intact but the renal cortex becomes infarcted and calcifies, and this may be seen on plain abdominal X-ray.

The return of renal function is often slow but if cortical necrosis is extensive, recovery is unlikely and the patient may become dialysis-dependent.

Acute tubular necrosis
Acute renal failure due to ischaemic changes or toxic renal injury presents a clinical syndrome which is often referred to as acute tubular necrosis. It is a very common cause of ARF and has a high mortality rate of around 50%. It causes damage to the tubular portion of the nephron. Unfortunately, despite 35 years of haemodialysis, little progress has been made in altering the outcome for acute tubular necrosis (Lieberthal & Nigam 2000).

Although the aetiology of acute tubular necrosis can vary, the common factor is that there is a reduction of oxygen and nutrients to the active tubular cells, which results in a lack of cell function and patchy necrosis. The tubular cells will regenerate at the basement membrane level. The aim is to keep the patient alive and well during this regeneration phase. An almost full recovery can be made provided the appropriate and timely treatment is undertaken (Pusnani & Hazra 1997). Most intrinsic renal failure is caused by ischaemia through exposure to toxic agents, such as drugs or bacterial endotoxins.

Nephrotoxicity

In any patient with acute renal failure, particularly acute tubular necrosis, a potential causative effect could be a therapeutic agent. Therapeutic agents can affect the kidney in any of the three categories listed, as illustrated in Table 4.2 (Coffman 1998).

Ischaemic acute tubular necrosis is often associated with inadequate perfusion to the kidney, in that the efferent and afferent arterioles are unable to maintain their autoregulatory function, and this leads to a fall in the glomerular filtration rate. This interruption in blood flow to the kidney may be due to surgical intervention, e.g. aortic repair, and is quite likely to cause ischaemia (Weldon & Monk 2000).

Postrenal failure

Postrenal conditions obstruct the flow of urine. Obstruction will not cause renal failure except for in those with a solitary kidney; therefore the obstruction has to be bilateral in order to cause failure. The rapidity of recovery will depend on the duration and completeness of the obstruction.

The urinary tract may be obstructed by three mechanisms:

- obstruction from within (e.g. ureteric stones)
- disease of the wall
- obstruction from outside.

As with all renal failure, it is important to find the cause and start treatment as soon as possible since in theory, all postrenal failure is reversible (Barrat 2000).

Table 4.2	
Clinical syndrome	**Causative agents**
Prerenal	Ciclosporin, radiocontrast, amphotericin B, ACE inhibitors, NSAIDs
Intrinsic: acute tubular necrosis	Aminoglycosides, amphotericin B, cephalosporins
Acute interstitial nephritis	Penicillins, cephalosporins, sulphonamides, rifampicin, NSAIDs, interferon, interleukin-2
Postrenal	Aciclovir, analgesic abuse Other heavy metals, including gold, lithium, mercury, silver

ACE, angiotensin-converting enzyme; NSAIDs, non steroidal antiinflammatory drugs.

MANAGEMENT OF ACUTE RENAL FAILURE

Since the normal kidney is essential to homeostasis of the body, particularly with regard to volume, electrolyte balance, acid–base balance and excretion of nitrogenous waste products, loss of these functions can lead to hyperkalaemia, volume overload, acidosis and uraemia.

The first step in good management is to detect any degree of renal failure. It is important to screen fully those patients at risk from renal failure prior to any invasive event (Alkhunaizi 1996).

Hyperkalaemia

Hyperkalaemia is often a fatal complication in ARF. The failing kidney is unable to excrete potassium effectively when the patient is oliguric (<400 mL urine day^{-1}) or, worse, anuric (no urine). It is further complicated by the very complex treatment of an individual who is often infected, hypoxic and requiring blood transfusions and potassium-containing drugs.

Haemodialysis is the most efficient treatment for hyperkalaemia but this may take time if vascular access is required. Other alternatives are available:

- oral or rectal potassium exchange agents in the form of calcium resonium
- the administration of intravenous insulin and dextrose will help move potassium ions back into the intracellular compartment and away from the extracellular compartment. It is important to monitor the patient's blood sugar, since hypo-hyperglycaemia can occur.

Volume overload

Successful volume homeostasis permits maintenance of a constant internal circulatory and extracellular volume despite consumption of varying quantities of water and salt intake and variable invisible losses of water.

The presence of oedema may be seen in the feet, legs and sacral area. This is often pitting in nature. The skin is particularly at risk at this stage and extra care must be taken. Shortness of breath and especially orthopnoea are indicative of pulmonary oedema.

Each patient in ARF should have an individual prescription for fluid and sodium intake. As a generalisation, the fluid intake volume should equal the daily urine output plus 300–500 mL. Patients with a large insensible loss, such as happens with burns, obviously need a larger fluid intake and special care should be taken. It is important that the patient and family are involved in accurate fluid balance.

Metabolic acidosis

The presence of ARF must not lead the nurse to think that it is the only cause of acidosis until other causes have been eliminated, e.g. ketoacidosis, lactic acidosis.

Acidosis in renal failure occurs when the renal tubules fail to regenerate bicarbonate and secrete hydrogen ions into the urine. In turn this causes an acid–base imbalance.

It is possible, since most acid comes from the breakdown of dietary protein, to reduce the level of acidosis by limiting the level of intake of protein. Another alternative is to infuse sodium bicarbonate but one has to be aware of fluid overload and hypernatraemia. The most efficient way of treating acute acidosis is bicarbonate haemodialysis.

Uraemia

The accumulation of nitrogenous waste products will produce acute uraemia and symptoms of uraemia often include nausea, vomiting, hiccups; bleeding risks; infection risks; neurological problems; irritability, confusion and twitching. As previously mentioned, it is necessary to begin appropriate dialysis.

Dialysis in acute renal failure

The purpose of dialysis is to prevent morbidity and to support the kidney during its recovery phase. The amount and frequency of dialysis are dictated by the severity of the patient's condition (Dauguirdas 2000).

Indications for dialysis:

- Uraemic symptoms, e.g. pericarditis
- Volume overload
- Hyperkalaemia
- Metabolic acidosis
- 'Space-making', e.g. nutrition, transfusions.

When prescribing acute dialysis, certain factors need to be considered and these include time on dialysis (possibly only 2 h for the first treatment), frequency (daily dialysis may be required), potassium concentration of dialysate (3 mmol l^{-1} may be necessary), a biocompatible dialyser and good fluid balance control. For those patients who are too haemodynamically unstable for conventional haemodialysis, CRRT is advisable and this is discussed later in the chapter.

THE CLINICAL COURSE OF ACUTE RENAL FAILURE

The clinical course of ARF can be divided into four stages or phases:

- initiating stage
- oliguric stage
- diuretic stage
- recovery stage.

Types of urine output can be found in Table 4.3.

Initiating stage

This occurs when the kidneys are injured and when diagnosis is made and treatment established. It can last anything from hours to days (Venkataraman & Kellum 2000).

Table 4.3 Types of urine output

Anuria	No urine output
Oliguria	< 400 mL day^{-1}
Non-oliguria	> 400 mL day^{-1}
Polyuria	Normal or high urine output

Oliguric stage (Fig. 4.3)

This can last from 5 days to over 15 days. When ARF persists for weeks, endocrine problems, such as reduced erythropoietin production, are noticed. Functional renal changes occur, such as decreased tubular transport, reduced urine formation and lowered glomerular filtration. Renal healing will begin to occur, with the basement membrane being replaced with fibrous scar tissue and the nephron clogged with inflammatory products. The patient is particularly susceptible to bleeding and infection.

Diuretic stage

With continued healing the kidney begins to regain most of its lost function, but this depends on the severity of the initial injury. The signs and

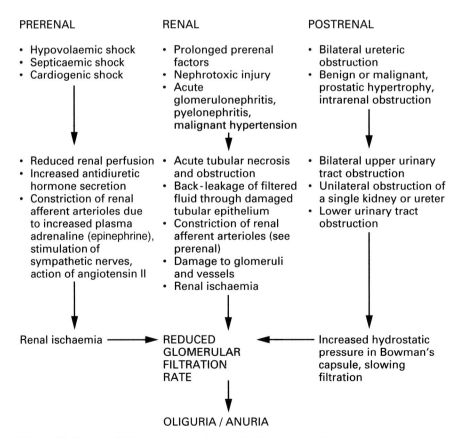

Figure 4.3 Acute renal failure: mechanisms involved in the genesis of oliguria.

symptoms of the original condition begin to disappear. Urine output can begin to increase back to normal levels of up to 3 L day^{-1}.

Recovery stage

The recovery stage can last from several months to over a year. The basement membrane is restored to its previous structure; scar tissue will remain but is not clinically significant. The kidneys respond in a regulatory excretory function to the body's needs.

As previously, the mortality rate for ARF is very high and appropriate treatment and management are essential (Fiaccadori et al 2000).

NUTRITIONAL MANAGEMENT OF ACUTE RENAL FAILURE

Approximately 40% of patients with ARF have been reported to be malnourished (Fiaccadori et al 1999) and protein-calorie malnutrition has been implicated as one of the factors contributing to the high mortality rate seen in ARF (Brivet et al 1996, Mault et al 1983). However, feeding these patients can be a challenge because optimal nutritional therapy is hard to define and metabolic derangement is often present.

ARF is often associated with accelerated protein breakdown, which unfortunately may be difficult to suppress, even with adequate nutritional intake. The cause of this excessive protein catabolism is multifactorial—uraemic toxins, underlying disease, hormonal changes, metabolic acidosis, insulin resistance and nutrient losses during renal replacement therapy will all play a part (Druml 1998). Changes in water, electrolyte and acid–base metabolism are invariably complicated by alterations in protein, carbohydrate and lipid metabolism.

Hyperglycaemia is common due to a combination of insulin resistance and accelerated hepatic gluconeogenesis, resulting from the conversion of amino acids released during protein catabolism into glucose (Campbell 1999). In addition, lipid metabolism is altered, with an impaired ability to use free fatty acids and triglycerides due to decreased activity of lipoprotein and hepatic triglyceride lipases (Druml et al 1992).

The aims of nutritional support are to:

* preserve lean body mass/prevent or minimise malnutrition
* stimulate immunocompetence
* repair tissue damage
* preserve organ function
* maintain biochemistry/fluid balance
* enhance recovery.

Requirements

As patients with ARF are a heterogeneous population, nutrient requirements need to be calculated on an individual basis. It has been shown that renal failure does not have an influence on energy expenditure per se (Bouffart et al 1987, Schneeweiss et al 1990) and therefore requirements need to be determined by the underlying disease. The most common method involves calculation of the patient's basic metabolic rate (BMR) from standard equations which are based on age, gender and weight (Schofield 1985). Modifications to cover stress, activity, the energy requirements of feeding and temperature can be added to the BMR (Elia 1990). To avoid overfeeding, the provision of carbohydrate energy during the dialysis therapy also needs to be taken into account. Dextrose absorption during renal replacement therapy varies with the type of dialysis therapy, from zero or very little in conventional intermittent haemodialysis, to the equivalent of approximately 500–900 kcal absorbed during continuous arteriovenous haemodialysis, with 1.5 and 2.5% dialysate solutions respectively (Sigler & Teehan 1987). The rate of glucose oxidation is approximately 4 mg kg^{-1} min^{-1} (Wolfe et al 1979) and in critical illness this should not be exceeded. Glucose overload is more likely when fat-free total parenteral nutrition (TPN) solutions are administered or if the dextrose calories from the dialysate solutions are not accounted for. If TPN has been instigated then the changes in lipid metabolism associated with renal failure should not prevent the use of lipid emulsions.

The optimal requirement for protein is more influenced by the illness causing the ARF, the associated complications, extent of protein catabolism and the type and frequency of dialysis. Patients may range from being in a non-catabolic state to being critically ill and hypercatabolic and protein requirements will range from 1.2 to 1.5 g kg^{-1} day^{-1} (Campbell 1999). Account should also be taken of the losses of amino acids during renal replacement therapy.

The electrolyte content of the nutritional prescription should be adjusted based on each individual patient and whether the patient is on renal replacement therapy. Sodium should not be greatly restricted unless oedema is present. If the patient is being dialysed then sodium will be removed from the patient, enabling a balance to be achieved.

Serum levels of potassium, magnesium and phosphorus are generally elevated in patients with ARF but can decrease as a result of intracellular shifts associated with carbohydrate delivery and losses incurred during treatment with continuous renal replacement therapy. Frequent monitoring to assess the need for supplementation is essential.

The requirements for micronutrients are not well documented in ARF. Many of the recommendations are extrapolated from work conducted with patients with chronic renal failure. There is a potential, in patients with chronic renal failure, for toxicity of some fat-soluble vitamins and minerals which are renally excreted. However, one study involving 8 patients with ARF demonstrated, with the exception of vitamin K, deficiencies of fat-soluble vitamins (Druml 1998). Most centres will supplement fat-soluble vitamins with caution. Due to dialysis losses there is a potential for deficiency of water-soluble vitamins (B vitamins and folic acid) with the exception of vitamin C. Large doses of vitamin C have resulted in oxalate deposition and supplementation of no greater than 200 mg day^{-1} is recommended (Druml 2001). The requirements for trace elements in ARF are not well defined.

Patients with ARF are frequently anuric and hence monitoring of fluid balance and restriction of intake is often necessary. The development of continuous renal replacement therapy has allowed fluid to be more easily managed without the need for the reduced fluid allowances that previously meant having to limit nutritional support.

Route of feeding

The enteral route for feeding is generally considered to be cheaper, safer and more physiological than feeding intravenously and is therefore the feeding method of choice. However in the critically ill patient it may not be possible to feed enterally and either TPN or a combination of both methods may be considered.

The development of concentrated low-electrolyte feeds has proven invaluable in allowing delivery of optimal protein and calories with the minimum of fluid and electrolytes. However, these special feeds are not normally needed if the patient is receiving continuous renal replacement therapy.

Novel substrates

The use of novel substrates in acute illness to modulate the stress response is an area of research which is expanding. Glutamine, recognised as a conditionally essential amino acid, has many functions. One of its major roles is as an oxidative substrate for rapidly replicating cells such as the gastrointestinal mucosal cells and immune cells—lymphocytes and macrophages. Glutamine may play a vital role in the maintenance of intestinal integrity and function and has been shown to reduce infectious complications (Houdijk et al 1998). Arginine, nucleotides and omega fatty acids, thought to aid the immune system, are now available in specialised enteral feeds but the evidence for their benefit has been mixed (Beale et al 1999, Mendez et al 1997). What is apparent is that the outcome of using novel substrates in patients with ARF needs further research.

CONTINUOUS RENAL REPLACEMENT THERAPY

The use of CRRT has developed enormously during recent years. The first therapy of this type was continuous arteriovenous haemofiltration, described by Kramer et al in 1982. This became a popular method of managing the fluid and electrolyte balance of patients in intensive care with ARF. Patients who required more efficient fluid and electrolyte clearance remained dependent on intermittent haemodialysis treatments performed by renal nurses.

The 1990s witnessed both an evolution of the treatments and a concomitant devolution of the responsibility of prescribing and monitoring renal replacement therapy. The nurses in the intensive care unit have developed their skills, taking on additional responsibilities which were once the domain of the renal nurse. It is recognised that intermittent haemodialysis may be contraindicated in patients with ARF who are critically ill.

Complications such as cardiovascular instability, sepsis and multiorgan failure make conventional treatments difficult.

There are a large variety of treatment options available and choice will depend on physician preference, nurse expertise and availability of the appropriate equipment.

Today the options fall broadly into three categories: continuous haemofiltration, continuous haemodiafiltration and continuous haemodialysis.

When performed continuously over 24 h, they allow optimal values to be obtained for urea and fluid exchange control, and electrolyte and acid–base balance.

Continuous haemofiltration

Continuous arteriovenous haemofiltration

Continuous arteriovenous haemofiltration has been performed in intensive care since the early 1980s (Kramer et al 1982). This procedure provides a simple method of removing fluid from the patient and, at the same time, convective removal of solutes. It is rarely used today as more advanced techniques have been developed, but its main benefit is that it was relatively simple to use.

Continuous venovenous haemofiltration

Continuous haemofiltration with the aid of a blood pump provides solute removal by convection. It offers high-volume ultrafiltration using replacement fluid, which can be administered in a variety of concentrations according to the patient's biochemistry. The pump guarantees adequate blood flow to maintain required ultrafiltration rates. This method can be performed using several litres of replacement fluid each hour. The addition of a blood pump to the circuit removes the necessity for arterial access and provides a more reliable and controllable method of delivering treatment (Fig. 4.4).

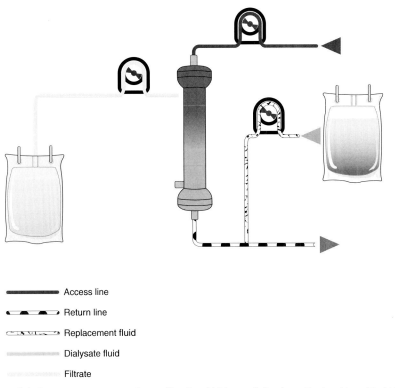

▮▮▮▮▮ Access line

◀▬▬▶ Return line

⟶ Replacement fluid

▭▭▭ Dialysate fluid

⎯⎯⎯ Filtrate

Figure 4.4 Continuous venovenous haemofiltration. (With permission from Gambro Hospal Ltd, UK.)

Continuous haemodiafiltration

Continuous arteriovenous haemodiafiltration

If the blood flows with continuous arteriovenous haemofiltration are satisfactory but clearance of urea is inadequate, the addition of dialysate will provide a concentration gradient and increase the clearance of small molecules by diffusion. A pump will be needed to deliver the dialysate at the required flow rates: as a result, the relative simplicity of continuous arteriovenous haemofiltration becomes a more complicated procedure. Good arterial access is a major challenge for this type of therapy. As a consequence, venovenous techniques have largely replaced arteriovenous systems.

Continuous venovenous haemodiafiltration

To increase the efficiency of small-molecule clearance, a dialysis solution is continuously pumped through the filter in a countercurrent direction to the blood. Small-molecule (urea) clearance by diffusion is more efficient. It is possible to use a standard blood monitor for the extracorporeal circuit and then use infusion pumps to administer dialysate and replacement fluid (Fig. 4.5).

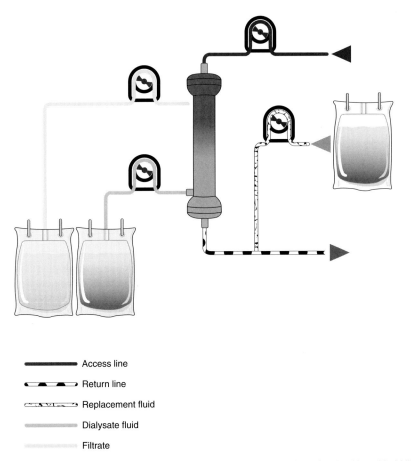

Access line

Return line

Replacement fluid

Dialysate fluid

Filtrate

Figure 4.5 Continuous venovenous haemodiafiltration. (With permission from Gambro Hospal Ltd, UK.)

Continuous venovenous haemodialysis

This method incorporates the same principles as intermittent haemodialysis but operates at a greatly reduced rate. From the nursing perspective, the use of fully automated systems provides a reliable and easy method of monitoring the fluid balance of patients who are critically ill. This allows

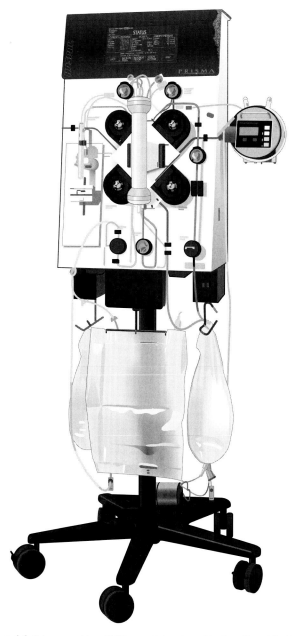

Figure 4.6 Prisma machine. (With permission from Gambro Hospal Ltd, UK.)

nurses more time to dedicate to direct patient care. An example of an integrated system for continuous fluid management and automated renal replacement therapy is the Prisma machine (Fig. 4.6).

The machine comprises a basic blood module with blood pump, venous and arterial pressure monitoring and an air detector. The fluid monitor has two integral pumps—one to remove fluid from the filter and the second to pump replacement fluid to the patient. The replacement fluid and the ultra filtrate are suspended on a weigh scale, which calculates and controls a linear patient weight.

With such accurate fluid control, the nurse does not need constantly to measure and record fluid loss and replacement as with previous methods. The ultrafiltration rate and physiological solutions are prescribed by the physician based on available clinical data (fluid state, biochemistry).

Nursing interventions for CRRT can be found in the further reading section at the end of this chapter.

Plasma exchange

Therapeutic plasma exchange is an intensive treatment used to treat a variety of immunological and non-immunological disorders, including Goodpasture's syndrome, Wegener's granulomatosis and antiglomerular basement membrane disease. The circuit is similar to that described for haemofiltration, except that the filter is replaced with a plasma filter which separates the plasma containing antibodies and immune complexes whilst retaining the red blood cells. A colloid substitute such as human albumin solution is infused into the patient to replace the plasma removed. Regimes for plasma exchange vary greatly depending on physician preference and clinical need.

SUMMARY

The impact of ARF on patients and families is often unexpected and, despite new technology, it remains a serious disease with a high mortality rate. The key aim of care is to balance humanistic caring skills with the technological and clinical expertise required to optimise the patient's survival and quality of life. All patients require nutritional support to maintain protein stores. In ARF it is not renal insufficiency per se that determines the need for nutritional support but the type and severity of the underlying disease and the degree of associated hypercatabolism. Understanding the nutritional requirements, careful interpretation of nutritional assessment and familiarity with the various forms of renal replacement therapy will greatly improve the success of nutritional therapy, although the optimal nutritional regimen has not yet been defined. The renal nurse now has much less of a role in the care of the acutely ill person with ARF, as many patients are managed in the intensive care unit. However it is imperative that renal nurses keep up-to-date with new technologies as they may often act in a supportive role for those intensive care nurses who are new to filtration therapies.

REFERENCES

Alkhunaizi AM. Management of acute renal failure: new perspectives. Am J Kidney Dis 1996; 28:315–328.

Barrat J. Outcome of acute renal failure following surgical repair of ruptured abdominal aortic aneurysms. Eur J Vasc Endovasc Surg 2000; 20:163–168.

Beale RJ, Bryg DJ, Bihari DJ. Immunonutrition in the critically ill: a systematic review of clinical outcome. Crit Care Med 1999; 27:2799–2805.

Bouffart Y, Viuale JP, Annat GM et al. Energy expenditure in the acute renal failure patient mechanically ventilated. Intens Care Med 1987; 13:401–404.

Brivet FG, Kleinknecht DJ, Loirat P et al. Acute renal failure in intensive care units—causes, outcome, and prognostic factors of hospital mortality: a prospective, multicentre study. Crit Care Med 1996; 24:192–198.

Campbell IT. Limitations of nutrient intake. The effect of stressors: trauma, sepsis and muliple organ failure. Eur J Clin Nutr 1999; 53 (suppl. 1):S143–S147.

Cantarovich F, Verho MT. A simple prognostic index for patients with acute renal failure requiring dialysis. Renal Failure 1996; 18:585–592.

Chen YC, Hsu HH, Kao KC et al. Outcomes and APACHE II predictions for critically ill patients with acute renal failure. Renal Failure 2001; 23:61–70.

Coffman TM. Primer on kidney disease. 2nd edn. USA: National Kidney Foundation, 1998.

Dauguirdas JT. The handbook of dialysis. 3rd edn. Philadelphia: Lippincott Williams & Wilkins, 2000.

Davies SP, Reaveley DA, Brown EA et al. Amino acid losses in patients with acute renal failure. Crit Care Med 1991; 19:1510–1515.

Druml W. Protein metabolism in acute renal failure. Mineral Electrolyte Metab 1998; 24:47–54.

Druml MD. Nutritional management of acute renal failure. Am J Kidney Dis 2001; 37: (suppl. 2):S89–S94.

Druml W, Fischer M, Sertl S et al. Fat elimination in acute renal failure: long–chain vs short-chain triglycerides. Am J Clin Nutr 1992; 55:468–472.

Du Bose TD, Warnock DG, Mehta RL et al. Acute renal failure in the 21st century: recommendations for management and outcomes assessment. Am J Kidney Dis 1997; 29:793–799.

Elia M. Artificial nutritional support. Med Int 1990; 82:3392–3396.

Fiaccadori E, Lombardi M, Leonardi S et al. Prevalence and clinical outcome associated with preexisting malnutrition in acute renal failure: a prospective cohort study. J Am Soc Nephrol 1999; 10:581–593.

Fiaccadori E, Maggiore U, Lombardi M et al. Predicting patient outcome from acute renal failure comparing three general severity of illness scoring systems. Kidney Int 2000; 58:283–292.

Houdijk APJ, Rijnsberger ER, Janse J et al. Randomised trial of glutamine-enriched enteral nutrition on infectious mortality in patients with multiple trauma. Lancet. 1998; 352:772–776.

Kramer P, Bohler J, Kehr A et al. Intensive care potential of CAVH. Trans Am Soc Artif Organs 1982; 28:28.

Levy EM, Viscoli CM, Horwitz EI. The affect of acute renal failure on mortality. A cohort analysis. JAMA 1996; 275:1489–1494.

Lieberthal W, Nigam SK. Acute renal failure II. Experimental models of acute renal failure: experimental but indispensable. Am J Physiol Renal Physiol 2000; 278:F1–F12.

Mault JR, Dechert RE, Clark, SF et al. Starvation: a major contribution to mortality in acute renal failure. Trans Am Soc Artif Intern Organs 1983; 29:390–395.

Mendez C, Jurkovich GJ, Garcial I et al. Effects of an immune-enhancing diet in critically injured patients. J Trauma 1997; 42:933–940.

Peeters P, Rublee D. Analysis and interpretation of cost data in dialysis: review of western European literature. Health Policy 2000; 54:209–227.

Pusnani ML, Hazra DK. Early haemodialysis in acute tubular necrosis. J Assoc Physicians India 1997; 45:850–852.

Rialp G, Roglan A, Betbese AJ et al. Prognostic indexes and mortality in critically ill patients with acute renal failure treated with different dialytic techniques. Renal Failure 1996; 18:667–675.

Schneeweiss B, Graninger W, Stockenhuber F et al. Energy metabolism in acute and chronic renal failure. Am J Clin Nutr 1990; 52:596–601.

Schofield WN. Predicting basal metabolic rate. New standards and review of previous work. Hum Nutr Clin Nutr 1985; 44:1–19.

Sigler, MH, Teehan BP. Solute transport in continuous hemodialysis. A new treatment for acute renal failure. Kidney Int 1987; 32:562–571.

Sinert R, Salomone JA, Talavera F et al. Renal failure, acute. *EMed* J 2001; 2:5.

Venkataraman R, Kellum JA. Novel approaches to the treatment of acute renal failure. Expert Opin Invest Drugs 2000; 9:2579–2592.

Weldon BC, Monk TG. The patient at risk for acute renal failure. Recognition, prevention and preoperative optimisation. Anaesthesiol Clin North America 2000; 1:705–717.

Wolfe RR, Allsop JR, Burke JF. Glucose metabolism in man: responses to intravenous glucose infusions. Metabolism 1979; 28:210–220.

FURTHER READING

Adam SK, Osbourne S. Critical care nursing: science and practice. Oxford: Oxford University Press, 1997.

Baker LRI, Hurst MJ, Rudge CJ et al. Practical procedures in nephrology. London: Arnold, 2000.

Challinor P, Sedgewick J. (eds) Principles and practice of renal nursing. Cheltenham: Stanley Thornes, 1998.

Grassmann A, Uhlenbusch-Körwer I, Bonnie-Schorn E et al. Good dialysis practice: composition and management of hemodialysis fluids. Lengerich: Pabst Science, 2000.

Jacobs C, Kjellstrand CM, Koch KM et al. Replacement of renal function by dialysis. 4th edn. Dordrecht: Kluwer Academic, 1996.

Levy J, Morgan J, Brown E. Oxford handbook of dialysis. Oxford: Oxford University Press, 2001.

Neilson EG. Immunologic renal diseases. Philadelphia, PA: Lippincott,/Williams & Wilkins, 2001.

Vander AF. Renal physiology. 5th edn. New York: McGraw-Hill, 1995.

Whitworth JA, Lawrence JR. Textbook of renal disease. 2nd edn. Edinburgh: Churchill Livingstone, 1994.

USEFUL WEBSITES

www.kidney.org/professionals/doqi/
DOQI guidelines

www.edtna-erca.org
European Dialysis and Transplant Nurses Association/European Renal Care Association

www.hdcn.com
Hypertension, Dialysis and Clinical Nephrology

www.kidney.org/
National Kidney Foundation

www.renal.org/
Renal Association

www.renalreg.org/
Renal Registry

www.renalweb.com/
Renal Web

www.usrds.org/
US Renal Data System

Predialysis care

Judith Hurst

5

■ LEARNING OUTCOMES FOR THIS CHAPTER

- To evaluate the role of the nurse in the prevention of renal failure
- To assess and care for those with reduced renal function
- To have insight into the preparation of those with reduced renal function for renal replacement therapy (RRT).
- To reflect and evaluate best practice guidelines on predialysis to ensure evidence-based care for those with reduced renal function.

INTRODUCTION

This chapter will investigate care required for those with reduced renal function before renal replacement therapy (RRT) commences. Renal nurses are often involved with the technical, monitoring and evaluative aspects of RRT for those with end-stage renal failure (ESRF). However, many patients may experience reduced renal function for many years before reaching the stage of needing RRT. This chapter will discuss the potential for renal nurses to expand their scope of practice so that the predialysis group of patients can expect to thrive on RRT for many years. The prevention of renal failure, the planning for RRT and considerations when introducing the patient to the renal unit for the first time will be explained and explored.

PREVENTING RENAL FAILURE

In the past 30 years the development of multidisciplinary nephrology care has advanced greatly in the management and treatment of ESRF. But what of the progress of the renal team in preventing individuals ever reaching ESRF in the first place? It can be argued that for any number of reasons, this is one area of care provision that has not demanded extensive resources for research and development. The measures that are presently employed to slow the progression of ESRF for those with renal insufficiency will be discussed. These measures must be considered within the context of what is realistically possible in a future of limited resources, expensive treatments and reduced numbers of skilled renal multiprofessional care personnel.

In the past 10 years the rate of acceptance on to RRT programmes has doubled, and is likely to continue to rise steadily in the future (Kissmeyer et al, 1999). Early detection and treatment of known factors that lead to renal failure, either in the form of deteriorating renal failure per se, or chronic renal failure as a complication of another disease process, are well documented to halt or slow the progression to ESRF (Hoy et al 1999). Of all those commencing some form of dialysis, approximately 30–50% present for the first time to the renal team, and require dialysis within days or weeks (Jungers et al 1993). For many of these patients predialysis treatment may have delayed or prevented further deterioration of renal function. This is particularly significant for those groups of patients who have a high incidence of renal failure in their ethnic group, or their existing disease presentation (Hoy et al 1999, Kissmeyer et al 1999). In order for this preventive care to come to fruition for the individual, there must be early detection of the reducing renal function and appropriate referral to the nephrology team.

Evidence-based clinical guidelines for the management and treatment of those with diabetes mellitus and hypertension are clear in their suggestions for care and treatment to reduce the numbers of those persons eventually requiring RRT due to nephrological complications (British Hypertension Society (BHS) (1999) cited in Ramsay et al (1999a); Diabetes Care and Complications Trial (DCCT) (1993)). These suggestions will be discussed in more detail below as significant numbers of people already experiencing these conditions make up the present RRT population. However, in order to identify and address renal insufficiency within the population as a whole, there appears to be a lack of clinical guidelines to assist medical general practitioners (GPs) and healthcare personnel in other clinical areas of the hospital and the community.

Some studies have been completed in other countries to assess the potential cost–benefit analysis of mass screening for renal failure indicators at the primary care level. In 1983 a total of 107 192 individuals over 18 years of age were identified and asked to participate in a mass screening programme in Japan. Serum creatinine levels were monitored for 10 years and records kept of those who developed ESRF in that time. Logistical regression analysis on the risk of ESRF was performed to determine the significance of serum creatinine levels in comparison to other variables. The results of this study found that serum creatinine demonstrated prognostic significance, whereas other factors such as hypertension were not necessarily a significant predictor of ESRF. Clinical predictors and baseline serum creatinine levels were also able partly to explain gender differences in the incidence of ESRF in Japan (Iseki et al 1997). This study suggests that simple tests can be useful in identifying the incidence and progression of ESRF in a general population, and those predictors may already be familiar to the renal professional.

Whilst the work in Japan was studying the general population, the work of Hoy et al (1999) in Australia concentrated on the Aboriginal population who are known to have high levels of cardiovascular death (CVD) and ESRF. A criticism of the Japanese study may be that it would be very expensive and time-consuming to test whole populations for renal failure indicators when other screening programmes may have a greater impact on overall public health. However, Aborigines have a CVD rate which is five times that of non-Aborigines, and an incidence of ESRF which is greater than 20-fold and rising. Hoy's team were able to screen 90% of the adults in this community in the Northern Territory, treat the identified hypertension, advise on cessation of smoking, treat identified diabetes mellitus and lipid levels and advise on alcohol intake. The 1- and 2-year evaluation points have thus far demonstrated an estimated 50% fall in the incidence of ESRF alone (Hoy et al 1999).

This study is therefore in contrast to the Japanese study where limited screening resources are targeted to vulnerable ethnic groups. In the UK, African-Caribbean groups show high incidences of hypertension and ESRF, and the various Asian communities show high levels of ESRF and type 2 diabetes mellitus by pathology, but may require insulin therapy for glucose control (Roderick et al 1994). The potential predeterminants to progression of ESRF are multifactoral but well known. The costs of the screening and treatment here clearly outweigh the costs of treating the complications and comorbidities in an incremental crisis approach. It can therefore be argued that one part of preventing ESRF is to direct resources to groups within the population with a high incidence of ESRF. With the development of renal nursing practice, there is a role in the UK for the experienced renal trained nurse to be involved in collaborative projects with practice nurses and community nurses to target vulnerable populations. Nephrologists could also be involved in preventive nephrology within the community as well as at the hospital.

The Renal Association (1997) recommends that joint clinics between nephrologists and other specialists may seek to manage an individual's care collaboratively. Whilst this has been demonstrated to be of immense value, the benefits are often restricted to hospital inpatients or to those individuals who have already been referred to a nephrologist. If the estimate made by Jungers et al (1993) is correct, that up to 50% of our patients commencing dialysis present just before they require RRT, then there appear to be huge numbers of individuals with reduced renal function who are not being referred to the nephrology team for preventive treatment to halt, or slow down, the progression of their recent renal dysfunction. The investigations and treatment that individuals experience when they are referred will be discussed later in this chapter. These figures would suggest that around 50% of these individuals are not having their access for RRT planned and matured in advance, and appear not to have full access to education and psychological and social preparation before they become unwell and require RRT.

Kissmeyer et al (1999) considered whether it is really feasible to screen for renal patients in the UK at the primary-care level. The team assessed nearly 17 000 individuals from 12 practices in Inner and Greater London, identifying around 15.5% as having hypertension, diabetes, or both. When auditing the records of these individuals, some do not seem to have had all the recommended monitoring schedules implemented. However, the team found a prevalence of >110 000 patients per million with renal insufficiency in this group. Whilst this may seem unusually high, it may be indicative of just how much undiagnosed renal insufficiency is present in this very racially diverse location. Only 28% of the subjects had been referred to a nephrologist. Kissmeyer et al (1999) identified the high prevalence of chronic renal sufficiency that exists in those with hypertension and/or diabetes alone, and that it is feasible to detect renal insufficiency at a primary-care level. Indeed, this could be extended to identifying known factors that may lead to ESRF, but an effective system must be coordinated across a region, and ethnic identities and underlying potential disease processes identified.

Already GPs are required to complete a urinalysis at initial registration to their surgery to screen for diabetes mellitus. A screening programme across the population would have to have some incentive for GPs to ensure completion, and would require present renal services to provide resources and a management framework to deal with all the extra potential referrals they seem likely to receive. However, in the present context of ever-increasing difficulties in meeting the present need for RRT, a major effort to identify and treat predialysis precursors must reduce the burden on present services. Indeed, for the individual who has been treated for a period of time, fewer complications of the underlying disease processes will mean a better quality of life on dialysis.

STANDARD STATEMENTS AND GUIDELINES UNDERPINNING GENERAL NEPHROLOGY CARE

Early diagnosis and prompt treatment of renal disease processes may prevent progression to ESRF and the need for RRT. Comorbidities are reduced and the prognosis and quality of life on RRT are improved (Vora et al 2000). However, as discussed above, this is only possible with prompt referral to a nephrologist or joint management of the individual by the GP and the nephrologist. At present there are no clear guidelines for when an individual should be referred to a nephrologist, but the Scottish Intercollegiate Guidelines Network (SIGN 1997a, b) recommend treatment strategies for patients with identified haematuria and/or proteinuria.

The Renal Association (1997) recommends referral to a nephrologist when:

- major renal syndromes are identified (e.g. chronic or acute renal failure, acute glomerulonephritis, recurrent renal stones)
- proteinuria and/or haematuria is identified on urinalysis
- there is raised plasma creatinine (>150 μmol^{-1} L) without apparent cause that may or may not be symptomatic
- persistent microhaematuria is identified even if renal function is normal, particularly if the patient is under 40–45 years of age, or there is associated proteinuria and/or hypertension. Older patients with haematuria should always be referred for urological opinion

- frank haematuria is present in patients under 45 years of age
- persistent proteinuria is identified with normal renal function
- there is refractory hypertension and abnormal urinalysis and/or elevated plasma creatinine concentration
- the patient has known polycystic kidney disease. Even if there is normal renal function, the patient and close relatives will need counselling and advice on the treatment and management of this genetic disease
- patients have unusual urinary tract infections or an unusual presentation, e.g. with hypertension, in adult males, or during pregnancy
- patients have diabetes mellitus and with proteinuria
- pregnant women have known renal disease.

For the renal nurse, these recommendations may seem very medically oriented and beyond their scope of practice influence. However, it is important to understand what these parameters are, particularly the significance of urinalysis and observations such as blood pressure in the context of renal insufficiency. Being able to share this knowledge with trained nurses performing these tasks in other areas of practice can only enhance knowledge, and may prompt further investigation when abnormal results are found.

DIABETES MELLITUS

Good blood glucose control in individuals with diabetes mellitus has been shown to prevent or slow down the progression of renal failure as a complication of this disease process (DCCT 1993). More recent research has also indicated that tight blood pressure control is also beneficial (United Kingdom Prospective Diabetes Study Group 1998). The American Diabetes Association (1999) has published a position statement on diabetic nephropathy. This position statement provides evidence-based guidelines on the detection, prevention and treatment of early nephropathy.

There is continued debate as to whether those with reduced renal function should follow a reduced-protein diet to slow the progress of renal failure. There are those who feel that reducing protein intake may have the desired renal effect (Klahr et al 1994, Levy et al 1996), but cause patients to become malnourished. This appears to put them in a disadvantageous position when faced with the rigors of RRT. Others argue that continuing with normal or higher levels of protein in the diet would be a precursor to cardiovascular disease and hyperlipidaemia which are the major causes of death in the ESRF population. See Chapter 9 for further discussion on this issue.

Lifestyle advice that is culturally sensitive, including and encouraging cardiovascular exercise, has been identified as a necessary strategy for ultimate success in blood pressure control (Box 5.1). Use of medication and the pursuit of tight glycaemic control for those with diabetes (Hood & Gennari, 1996) are important, but all these factors must come together. Benefit from

■ BOX 5.1

Greenhalgh et al (1998) interviewed older people with diabetes about their understanding of their diabetes and their adherence to the treatment prescribed. One elderly Muslim could not understand why his doctor kept asking him to 'do more exercise'. 'But I do ... I pray five times a day.' What the diabetes care team had failed to understand was that in this man's culture and language, 'exercise' meant spiritual exercise, and to create a sweat with cardiovascular exercise was considered unseemly. Sweat was for manual labourers. Also this paper highlighted that women who are restricted in their dress code and their ability to go out and about unaccompanied need very careful consideration to interpret the general lifestyle recommendations that are published.

exercise that encourages cardiovascular fitness is particularly recommended for those with diabetes mellitus.

Monitoring and control of cholesterol and lipid levels

This may require medication as well as dietary intervention. These levels may not directly affect the progression of renal function, but may exacerbate the CVD as a comorbidity. The current recommendations are that statin therapy is indicated up to age 70 years when serum cholesterol is greater than or equal to 5.0 mmol L^{-1}, and for secondary prevention (when there is already evidence of CVD), when cholesterol levels are >5.0 mmol L^{-1}, and the 10-year coronary heart disease risk is greater than or equal to 30 (Scottish Intercollegiate Guidelines Network 1999, Joint British Recommendations 1998, Standing Medical Advisory Committee 1997).

Control of blood pressure

The control of systemic hypertension and the primary disease are the only interventions proven to prevent the progression of renal failure (Klahr et al 1994, Ramsay et al 1999b; Box 5.2). Again, lifestyle advice must be part of the care, as it is well known that to continue smoking whilst receiving hypertensive treatment obliterates any cardiovascular morbidity effects that the treatment is trying to achieve.

■ BOX 5.2

Whilst a treatment target blood pressure is 140/85 mmHg for all ages, it is thought that many of those with diabetes may need these figures to be lower to achieve the same clinical benefits (i.e. 120/70 mmHg, Ramsay et al 1999). There is evidence that the use of angiotensin-converting enzyme (ACE) inhibitors may prevent diabetic nephropathy or slow its progression (Ramsay et al 1999b, United Kingdom Prospective Diabetes Study Group 1998).

Complications affecting the eyes and feet

Whilst this may not be directly related to renal function, complications may indicate reduced micro- and macrovascular competency which also affects the kidneys (United Kingdom Prospective Diabetes Study Group 1998).

Monitoring and treatment of microalbuminuria

As renal insufficiency progresses, protein in the form of microalbuminuria (30–300 mg 24 h^{-1}) may be identified in the individual's urine. This can be identified by specialised dipstick testing (which may be unreliable) or early-morning urine (EMU) testing. This is an indication of deteriorating renal function. Debate continues as to the cost and long-term benefit outcome when testing for microalbuminuria. Some diabetologists advocate only testing for microalbuminuria in those with diabetes under 40 years of age. The renal opinion is markedly different to this. The majority of those that present in ESRF are aged in their mid-60s, so to monitor microalbuminuria in only younger patients misses those who go on to develop ESRF (Strojek et al 2001).

OUTREACH AND JOINT CLINICS

The kidney is involved in hypertensive disease and diabetes mellitus and collaboration amongst those who assist these individuals in care delivery may be able to halt the progression to ESRF. The kidney may also be involved in other systemic immunological disorders such as vasculitis and systemic lupus erythematosus, often later on in the disease progression. Monitoring the use of nephrotoxic agents such as non-steroidal anti-inflammatory drugs and the use of contrast media in individuals who have reduced renal function or who are at high risk of ESRF is very pertinent. Again, collaboration between nephrologists and those delivering care for these individuals can assist in the review of care delivery, often in joint clinics (Renal Association 1997).

Hence, joint clinics may happen regularly, as in the case of diabetes and hypertensive care, but may be less regular, depending on patient populations in rheumatology, and antenatal clinics, for example. There is a definite role for the experienced renal nurse to be involved in these formal structures, and also to assist other nursing colleagues to identify renal complications and precursors.

ACCESS TO RENAL SERVICES

It is necessary to be mindful of the access the general population has to renal services. A number of recent studies have evaluated acceptance rates to renal services assessing geographical, gender and ethnic variations. In the UK, Roderick et al (1999) found that age was a major determinate of acceptance, with a seven-fold higher rate in males over 64 years compared to younger men, and acceptance rates in females were much lower again. Amongst Asian and African-Caribbean groups, acceptance rates were high, but generally there was an inverse relation of acceptance with distance to the main renal unit. Roderick et al conclude that local need and supply factors influence service use, and pressure to expand renal services needs to be aimed at areas with large ethnic minority populations and those living long distances from existing renal units.

Ozminkowski et al (1998) reviewed access to cadeveric transplantation services, asking if the prevalence of transplantation as a form of RRT would still demonstrate the same picture in the USA if information about health status, attitudes about treatment and socioeconomic measures were levelled across the patient group. They concluded that simulations of their data demonstrate that, if this levelling were to happen, waiting list spots or transplants per 1000 patients would shift from advantaged to disadvantaged persons where socioeconomic decisions no longer influenced the decision-making process. Whilst we can talk of clinical statements to guide referrals, we must also be aware of our own professional discriminations that may prevent access to the services an individual may require. Indeed, Jassal et al (1998) demonstrated that the elderly renal patients they studied were better served by transferring acute care facilities and expertise to the outpatient or community environment, rather than expecting patients to travel to the main nephrology centre many miles away. As a result of this reallocation health needs and treatment issues were addressed sooner, and by the renal experts, resulting in less crisis management and better overall control of potential complications.

PREVENTION OF THE PROGRESSION TO ESRF

Criteria for referring patients for nephrological assessment and opinion have been highlighted. However, the nephrology team needs to consider how to assess and treat an individual to prevent further loss of renal function.

Individuals who have progressive renal failure will undergo regular follow-up to prevent further loss of renal insufficiency where possible and prevent complications. Indeed, this time is also ideal to start to prepare the person physically and mentally should RRT be necessary at some point in the future. Early referral and assessment will include diagnostic imaging, renal histopathology, dietetic and urology expertise. Some individuals referred will have conditions that are reversible or easily controllable. Others with more marked loss of function (plasma creatinine >300 μmol L^{-1}) may have lower potential for reversal and be cared for in a low-clearance clinic. It is in this environment that the following strategies will be employed.

Control of systemic hypertension

In chronic renal failure, hypertension may also be the result of increased cardiac output because of sodium retention and fluid overload, or as a complication of severe anaemia. Vasopressor functions of the kidney and the production of renin can also have a major role in the development of hypertension.

Optimal dietetic management of protein and calorie intake

Some of the controversy surrounding restricting protein intake is discussed above and also in Chapter 9. Supporting patients and their families is an important role of the nurse, especially in terms of coping psychologically and financially. Of course, if protein is restricted then the production of urea as the byproduct of protein metabolism is also reduced. It must be understood that when urea and plasma proteins are used as markers of nutritional status, these may be obscured by dietary restriction advice or lack of appetite due to anorexia and nausea. Whilst we may weigh patients and record lean body mass and plasma protein levels, they may still prove to be a subjective assessment of the patient's nutritional status in chronic renal failure. Heimburger et al (2000) suggest that hand-grip muscle strength should be added to the present recordings as a less subjective measurement of nutritional status than, say, albumin or fat mass.

Control of serum bicarbonate within normal levels

As an individual becomes more uraemic the pH balance in the internal environment starts to become more acidic. The body's natural response to this is to produce bicarbonate, metabolised from the liver and activated by the kidney, which acts as a buffer to return the pH to more neutral levels. However, if the kidney is defective, this process is thwarted and supplementary bicarbonate may be administered. The nurse must be aware that administering bicarbonate may result in plasma volume expansion and hypertension which should be reported. The safest way to control bicarbonate balance is with dialysis. Hence, if this condition is not adequately controlled then commencement of dialysis may be indicated. (See below for further discussion of acid–base balance.)

Control of cardiovascular disorders

Left ventricular heart failure is seen in all those with renal failure and may be the result of chronic anaemia, hypertension and volume overload seen in renal failure. However, studies into cardiovascular function by Raine et al (1993) and, more recently Amann et al (1999) indicate that left ventricular hypertrophy in renal failure is independent of the long-term complications associated with ESRF. There appears to be another aspect of the renal disease process that causes these cardiac effects.

Whilst there is thought to be little influence of lipid levels on the progression of renal failure, recommendations centre around cholesterol concentrations, as cited for the non-renal population. From a holistic point of view, cardiac health and prevention of CVD as a complication and comorbidity for renal patients is paramount.

Management of bone disease

Renal failure causes an abnormality of vitamin D metabolism, causing deficient calcium levels, skeletal damage and bone pain. Refer to Chapter 2 for further information on the underlying physiological processes.

The aim of care is to keep calcium and phosphate levels within normal ranges, preventing hyperparathyroidism. After correcting the acidosis, plasma phosphate and calcium levels can be controlled with oral phosphate binders, calcium supplements and dietary restrictions.

Supplementation of vitamin D for those in the predialysis phase is a controversial subject in the current literature. Some recommend that vitamin supplements should be started at early stages of renal insufficiency (Baker et al 1989), whilst others use supplementation much later in the renal disease process. Serum parathyroid levels are indicative of renal bone disease, and interpretation of those results is splitting opinion at present. For the nurse, taking regular samples and understanding the significance of the results are essential, and the information should be shared with other members of the multidisciplinary team. If supplementation is to be started early, then parathyroid levels need to be kept as near to the normal physiological levels as possible.

Control of anaemia

Anaemia in chronic renal failure is usually normocytic and normochromic and due to primary causes such as reduced production of erythropoietin production, uraemic toxins inhibiting erythropoiesis and haemolysis due to uraemic changes to the red cell membrane. The individual will become more anaemic as renal failure progresses, as three types of cells in the blood are affected:

- erythrocytes—causing anaemia
- leukocytes—causing immunosuppression
- platelets—causing bleeding tendencies.

It is now recommended that early treatment with erythropoietin will help to combat the side effects of anaemia (Ritz & Eisenhardt, 2000). Hence if the anaemia is corrected the lethargic and cardiac complications are managed. However, until recently erythropoietin has not been used extensively for patients before the end-stage phase of renal failure, largely due to the high costs of supplying this hormone. Of course the costs of supply must be compared to the costs of caring for a person with chronic anaemia side-effects. The increased mortality and morbidity rates of those with a haemoglobin level of $<10 \, \text{g} \, \text{dL}^{-1}$ are well documented (National Kidney Foundation Disease Outcome Quality Initiative (DOQI) 1997). By the time the patient has reached ESRF with uncorrected haemoglobin, the nurse is caring for someone who is very weak and has a short concentration span. This is often a confusing and frustrating time for the patient and the accompanying lethargy of anaemia hampers giving information and understanding at the start of RRT. The nurse must be very clear as to the symptoms of anaemia in the individual, and personalise care accordingly. Should erythropoietin be prescribed, than the nurse has a monitoring role in assessing its benefit, and in educating the patient and carers in its administration and supply. Whilst target haemoglobin levels have been suggested for those who are receiving RRT, this has thus far not been possible for the predialysis group. However, the effects of a drop in the haemoglobin levels and the effects on mortality and morbidity rates are evidenced in the DOQI guidelines (1997) and by Fink et al (2001). Treatment of anaemia must also include correcting contributing factors to anaemia, e.g. gastrointestinal bleeding, iron deficiency and Vitamin B_{12} deficiency and maintaining adequate calorie intake and nutritional status. Persistent anaemia may be indicative that the individual needs to start RRT. Chronic uraemia can predispose to pericarditis where the patient will present with a pericardial rub. If this is not treated by reducing the urea with dialysis, a life-threatening cardiac tamponade may develop.

Control of gastrointestinal disorders

These disorders are common in chronic renal failure, especially as the individual approaches end-stage. The person may experience anorexia, nausea and vomiting, hiccups, a metallic taste in the mouth and, for those with diabetes, exacerbation of gut complications presenting as episodes of diarrhoea. Bleeding from the gut may be seen in the advanced stages of chronic renal failure causing haematemesis or melaena. Urea is excreted in the gut, and broken down, releasing ammonia which acts as an irritant. Some medications may give unpleasant side-effects, e.g. heartburn with phosphate binders and oral iron supplementation. However, the DOQI guidelines (1997) recommend intravenous iron therapy as the most efficient way to build up iron stores in conjunction with erythropoietin. Oral iron supplementation has been found to be ineffective and troublesome to patients (Van Wyck 2000). Constipation is common. Fluid intake is reduced, as is the residue in the diet as part of reducing potassium intake. Generally, the person with renal disease is less physically active due to the effects of a chronic illness causing lethargy and tiredness.

Patient education is required on those medications taken to relieve the symptoms which are safe in chronic renal failure, as many preparations which can be bought without a prescription may cause complications in renal patients. If nausea, vomiting and weight loss are persistent because of uraemia, dialysis may be the only effective treatment available.

Treatment of dermatological disorders

Generalised uraemic pruritus is a distressing symptom in patients with chronic renal failure, with often little relief from drugs. Deposits of calcium and phosphorus in the skin and sweat glands excreting urea are thought to be the causative factors of pruritus, but dry skin and drug allergies must not be overlooked as causes. Platelet defects and capillary permeability, both complications of renal failure, can cause bleeding and bruising of the skin, especially if there is continued scratching. Many patients with advanced renal failure have a yellow tinge to their skin which is a combined result of hypermelanosis and the deposition of pigments in the skin (urochrome and carotene) that are usually excreted by the kidneys. Although medications may be of some help, commencement of dialysis may be the only long-term relief.

Control of volume disorders

During the progression of renal failure some nephrons remain intact whilst others continue to be destroyed. The remaining undamaged nephrons hypertrophy and produce an increased volume of filtrate with increased tubular reabsorption, even though there is a reduction in the glomerular filtration rate. This process allows the kidney to continue to function until three-quarters of the nephrons are destroyed. In patients with chronic renal insufficiency with blood urea levels above 40 mmol L^{-1}, the solute load becomes greater than can be reabsorbed, producing an osmotic diuresis accompanied by polyuria of up to 3 L in a 24-h period. The urine is dilute as the kidney's concentration ability is lost and the patient will have nocturia. As more nephrons are destroyed, oliguria with the retention of waste products is evident. The individual develops a wide range of biochemical, haematological and endocrine disorders and the clinical features of fluid overload.

Changes in fluid allowance may be required in association with diuretics. Loop diuretics such as furosemide (frusemide) will increase sodium excretion from the kidney and so prevent sodium retention. During episodes of polyuria, volume replacement should be administered to prevent further reduction in renal perfusion and worsening of kidney function. When volume overload is unresponsive to treatment the commencement of dialysis is indicated.

Control of potassium disorders

Excess potassium is normally removed by renal excretion, but as chronic renal failure progresses, excretion of urinary potassium decreases because of a reduced glomerular filtration rate caused by tubular defects in diseases such as diabetes mellitus, ultimately resulting in hyperkalaemia. Hyperkalaemia (indicated as a potassium of above 6.0 mmol L^{-1}) can occur in chronic renal failure following episodes of acute illness, infection or non-adherence to dietary restrictions. Chronic metabolic acidosis also causes potassium to shift out of the cells and into the extracelluar fluid, giving rise to hyperkaleamia.

If metabolic acidosis is present this should be corrected first, and this will then help to reduce the serum potassium to within safe limits. If chronic hyperkalaemia is present, dietary advice may be indicated, so high-potassium foods are avoided. Potassium-sparing diuretics should be discontinued as these drugs block the distal potassium transfer so that potassium is retained. If hyperkalaemia persists, this should be monitored very closely and managed in one of two ways—either conservatively or with dialysis. Conservative management of hyperkalaemia may involve the use of exchange resins (e.g. calcium resonium). Oral resins are not absorbed but exchange potassium for calcium or sodium from the gastrointestinal tract. The choice of calcium or sodium depends on the level of hypercalcaemia or fluid overload in the individual. Serum calcium should be monitored in patients with chronic renal failure, and exchange resin therapy discontinued when the serum potassium falls to 5 mmol L^{-1}.

Acute hyperkalaemia may be managed using a glucose and insulin infusion where insulin shifts potassium back into the cells and glucose prevents hypoglycaemia. The effect of reducing the potassium can last up to 2 h, so it is a short-term measure, but may be life-saving. Intravenous calcium gluconate may be used to reduce the cardiotoxic effects of potassium, protecting cardiac muscle and preventing arrhythmias. Intravenous infusion of sodium bicarbonate will temporarily reduce serum potassium, especially in patients with acidosis, but it should only be given when no fluid overload is present. Essentially dialysis is the safest and most efficient way of removing potassium out of the body, so the above measures may be used if a dialysis facility is not possible, or is not possible immediately. Dialysis can be repeated often if the potassium levels require it (e.g. in rhabdomyolysis) and side-effects associated with the conservative treatment can be avoided.

Control of acid–base balance

In normal health, acid–base balance is maintained by the excretion into the renal tubules of excess acid (hydrogen or H^+ ions) where the following processes then take place:

- Filtered bicarbonate is reabsorbed.
- There is increased production of ammonia that combines with H^+ ions and is then excreted in the form of ammonium salts.
- A titratable acid is formed.
- Tubular fluid pH is reduced.

In chronic renal failure a mild metabolic acidosis may be present as normal renal tissue is not sufficient to perform the above functions efficiently. Metabolic acidosis may also be worse in patients who have renal tubular acidosis.

The individual will present with:

- a blood pH of less than 7.35
- hyperkalaemia, as metabolic acidosis shifts potassium from the cells into the extracellular fluid
- signs of renal bone disease, as metabolic acidosis reduces the bone carbonate buffers, allowing calcium to be lost from the bones: calcium is more soluble in an acid environment
- gasping for breath caused by acidosis as the patient attempts to breathe off the excess acid through expired carbon dioxide.

Intravenous sodium bicarbonate may correct acidosis but the sodium may cause hypernatraemia, leading to fluid retention and hypertension. Essentially, metabolic acidosis can indicate terminal chronic renal failure and the most efficient and safest way to treat it is with dialysis.

Disorders of the central nervous system

In chronic renal failure, nervous system dysfunction can cause numerous mental disabilities such as poor memory function, loss of concentration and slower mental ability. Physical disabilities result in peripheral neuropathies affecting the legs and feet and may result in 'restless legs' and paraesthesia. More serious neurological problems may rarely be seen, where there is fluid overload and hypertension in advanced renal failure, in the form of convulsions and cerebral oedema. A 'uraemic flap' may be seen in very toxic patients, where the hands involuntarily flap from the wrists. Other electrolyte disorders, e.g. hyper-/hypocalcaemia, also cause shaking or an involuntary reflex when nerve points are stimulated. All these symptoms and complications can be avoided with the introduction of early dialysis.

Sexual function

In women, the loss of sexual function may take the form of infertility due to amenorrhoea and other menstrual abnormalities. Loss of libido may be present: if pregnancy does occur there is a high risk of miscarriage due to the effects of uraemia (Levy et al 1998). There is also risk to the mother's health as it is possible that renal failure will accelerate because of the extra workload on damaged kidneys.

In men, the incidence of infertility and impotence increases with age and the advancement of chronic renal failure. There are multiple causes of impotence which include poor nutrition, anxiety, side-effects of antihypertensive drugs and reduced plasma testosterone. The individual and partner should be given ample opportunity to express fears and talk about symptoms that are causes for concern.

With the wider use of erythropoietin to correct anaemia, fewer women with decreased renal function are experiencing loss of fertility and amenorrhoea. Successful pregnancy for couples where at least one partner has a degree of renal failure is becoming more common and requires careful planning and monitoring for a successful outcome (Giatras et al 1998). In some cases storage of sperm or eggs may be possible until such time as the renal failure is stabilised and a successful pregnancy is possible. Collaboration with obstetric medical and nursing colleagues cares for both the mother and the unborn child in these unusual medical circumstances (Jungers & Chauveau 1997).

PATIENT EDUCATION IN THE PREDIALYSIS PHASE

The need for good education and preparation of the individual and the family at all stages of chronic renal failure, and potentially heading towards ESRF, cannot be underestimated (King 1998). The psychological aspects of dealing with this chronic illness have been dealt with in Chapter 3, but it is worth reiterating the importance of education and information as part of the treatment protocol. It is essential that the patient and renal staff work in collaboration, not only to ensure the best care possible for the person, but also for the renal team to understand the care outcomes the patient has in mind. In Canada, a nationally agreed Core Curriculum for patient education in the predialysis period has been developed (Porter 1998). For some, it is very important to be able to continue in their present employment, and so education about RRT modalities must include consideration of how that dialysis is to be performed. For example, peritoneal dialysis that patients can perform for themselves, night-time machine-controlled dialysis or some form of home dialysis programme would be key to maintaining employment status. In this instance the employers need information and support to ensure that prejudices and fallacies about renal failure are dispelled and that the individual is not discriminated against in the work environment.

For some, the thought of attempting to understand any aspect of the RRT process is daunting and overwhelming. This may be due to the immediacy of the circumstances in which they commenced RRT, or indeed their locus of control and unique personal characteristics that mean the understanding healthcare professionals should take the lead in directing care. This in no way means that the individual absolves responsibility or plays no part in any of the decision-making processes about care and treatment. But it does mean that a greater understanding of the individual's psychological and personality profiles will enable a good working relationship to develop, and mutually agreed expectations to be identified (Brun 1997).

There may also be those for whom initiation of dialysis may not be feasible. The option of not commencing dialysis at all is discussed in Chapter 3.

The ultimate skill any renal healthcare professional can hope to achieve in the care of those approaching RRT is to be able to gain an understanding of each individual. That person is unique as regards personal hopes and aspirations for the future, the ability to understand the care and treatment strategies that lie ahead, and how the individual wishes to be involved in that care delivery. All too often, renal professionals of all kinds can be very focused on the pathological and technical aspects which dominate their understanding of their role as a renal practitioner. For the individual approaching RRT, the priorities may be quite different, and studies have revealed that information-giving should start very early on, when the individual with renal insufficiency comes into contact with renal healthcare professionals. Patients have reported that they do not mind who gives them the information that they deem they need, but it is vital that they have a trusting and ongoing relationship with that person, and that the information should not be censored, even though it may be hard to accept at times (O'Donnel & Tucker 1999). The emphasis seems to be on the quality of the relationship, rather than what information is given when and how.

WHEN SHOULD DIALYSIS COMMENCE?

The optimal time at which the individual concerned can benefit most from commencing RRT is controversial. Indeed, for some individuals fast-track transplantation may be possible. What is not disputed is the fact that the later in the progression of renal failure and its effects the patient has access to RRT, the poorer the outcome in terms of mortality and morbidity rates and quality of life experienced during this period (Bonomini et al 1985). The issues as to when a person is referred to the renal care team are not just medical, but may have more to do with access to services and resources available nearby. So, what benefits are there from referring an individual to the nephrologist early? In some instances, the rate of decreasing renal function may be slowed or halted. However, Jungers et al (2000) found that the prevalence of cardiovascular disease was nearly twice as high in patients who were referred less than 6 months before starting RRT than in those who had benefited from effective nephrological care for more than 3 years in the predialysis period. Considering that CVD is the major cause of death in ESRF patients, this is a significant finding.

Sesso & Belasco (1996) also found health benefits for those who had an early referral. Indeed, mortality rates were higher (×2.77%) in patients who were referred to a nephrologist within the 6 months before commencing than those who had had an earlier referral. Most of these deaths were of cardiac origin which 'could have been prevented with dialysis care'. Levin (2000) and Roubicek et al (2000) also found more access problems and reduced therapeutic options open for individuals who had had a late referral, indicating that their quality of life on dialysis must be compromised; the patients experienced more short-term morbidity, and presented with severe hypertension.

But how early is early? There are at present no set recommendations as to when dialysis should commence. Suggestions have been made that small amounts of dialysis should be commenced at a time such as when weekly urea clearance falls to that regarded as optimal for a dialysis patient, corresponding to a Kt/V of 2.2 and a creatinine clearance of about 15 mL min^{-1} (DOQI 1997). This amount of dialysis should increase as residual renal function falls. However, this incremental/intermittent dialysis is not currently usual practice as the accompanying resources required would have major organisational and financial implications for present renal services. Others would argue that dialysis may be delayed at this stage if all three of the following criteria are present: stable or increasing oedema-free body weight, protein intake greater than 0.8 g kg^{-1} day^{-1} and an absence of clinical signs and symptoms attributable to uraemia. The Renal Association (1997) therefore suggests that 'all patients who appear to have progressive renal insufficiency and plasma creatinine above 150 µmol/l and/or rapidly rising renal creatinine concentrations should be referred to a nephrology service for assessment and follow-up'.

Tattersall et al (1995) have shown why such high rates of early morbidity and poor quality of life in terms of being able to return to employment after diagnosis of renal failure exist. In the UK he showed that patients starting dialysis had a weekly Kt/V of 1.05. Comparing this with the DOQI guidelines (1997) and the Canada–USA (CANUSA) study (1996), which recommend a prescribed Kt/V of 2.0, it can be seen that at the start of dialysis in the UK, patients are functioning on half the Kt/V of what is considered optimal dialysis. This picture is repeated in the USA and Canada, where patients studied were seen to have a Kt/V of about one-third optimal dialysis (CANUSA 1996). So a rather bizarre situation occurs where patients are started on dialysis treatment at an endogenous Kt/V level that is lower than is expected to be optimal for patients who are already on dialysis.

Other benefits of starting dialysis early may also be seen in patients who have been in contact with the renal care team for a lengthy period before commencing dialysis. Patient education and preparation for the treatment trajectory ahead was seen to serve the individual better in the long predialysis period than in the short predialysis and early dialysis periods. Hayslip & Suttle (1995) demonstrated the benefit of early education not only in assisting the person to adapt to a new way of life, but also in the outcomes of adherence to predialysis treatments. Whilst it has been discussed above how certain medical interventions may slow the progression of renal failure, it is important that the involvement and incorporation of the patient in the treatment process are understood to be just as an important component as all the scientific treatment that can be done (Brun 1997). Informed choice and timely access creation and maturation and assessment of the most appropriate treatment modalities are essential for a quality of life on RRT. The renal care team needs to rethink its ideas about the commencement of early dialysis, and consider more a 'healthy start' to RRT (Lameire 1997; Box 5.3).

■ BOX 5.3 What is a nephrology assessment?

Essentially the nephrology care team is concerned about the present cause of renal insufficiency and its cause. All members of the multiprofessional team are involved to give a holistic approach to care.

The aim is to delay the progression towards end-stage renal failure and dialysis. Investigations into renal function and present kidney efficiency include:

- treatment of the underlying cause of the renal insufficiency (e.g. exacerbation of an acute illness, complication of a chronic illness, use of nephrotoxic agents, congenital abnormalities, etc.)
- blood pressure control (see discussion above)
- avoidance of nephrotoxic agents such as contrast media and non-steroidal antiinflammatory drugs
- possible dietary restriction of protein (see discussion above)
- management of other manifestations affecting other body systems caused by chronic renal failure
- imaging and assessing renal function.
- assessment of vascular competency generally and for potential access for haemodialysis
- X-ray and scans to view the kidney size and shape, and possible bone scans to assess the state of the skeletal structure for the effects of renal bone disease
- a sample of kidney tissue may be taken by biopsy to identify the underlying cause of renal failure and the state of the disease process. However, interpretation and accuracy of the results depend on the skill of the expert and are usually only carried out when access to a renal histopathology service is available and results are expected to inform treatment.

SUMMARY

This chapter has discussed epidemiological, medical and therapeutic methods of screening for, and preventing, ESRF. Clearly there is a need for renal professionals to invest research time and clinical practice expertise in this area of renal care delivery. Identifying when to start dialysis to achieve the best outcome for the individual concerned has been a long-neglected issue in renal care. Strategies must address renal care both within the acute hospital setting and in the communities within which levels of renal insufficiency are a major cause for concern. To rely solely on Kt/V and nutritional markers as guidance for the initiation of RRT may underserve variations in individuals of different countries and different racial groups. A more holistic approach that considers the clinical status of the individual, the economical, psychological, medical/legal and ethical aspects of care is surely the basis for a healthy start on dialysis. Clearly a healthy start on to RRT can only be initiated if early contact is made with the renal care team. It is in this area that the specialist renal nurse can play an important role. Outreach, collaborative working, education, research and specialist clinical skills of the renal nurse can assist in the promotion of renal health. By promoting renal health the renal care team will not only prevent more individuals reaching ESRF with complex comorbidities, but essentially stop them ever needing the scarce resources of RRT. Collaboration and building relationships across traditional medical specialty boundaries amongst health professionals will assist in this goal. Investing effort in creating collaborating and trusting relationships with those requiring renal services is the way to achieve the best outcomes for the individual.

REFERENCES

Amann K, Munter K, Wagner J et al. Treatment of cardiovascular changes in renal failure—ACE inhibition, endothelin receptor blockade or a combination of both strategies? Nephrol Dialysis Transplant 1999; 14 (suppl.) 4:43–44.

American Diabetes Association. Position statement on diabetic nephropathy. Diabetes Care 1999; 22 (suppl.1).

Baker LR, Abrams SM, Roe CJ et al. Early therapy of renal bone disease with calcitriol: a prospective double-blind study. Kidney Int 1989; 27 (suppl.):140–142.

Bonomini V, Feletti C, Scolari MP et al. Benefits of early initiation of dialysis. Kidney Int 1985; 17, (suppl.) 12:S57–S59.

Brun R. Preparation for dialysis treatment using the psychologist. Eur Dialysis Transplant Nurses Assoc–Eur Renal Care Assoc (EDTNA–ERCA) J 1997; 13:31–35.

Canada–USA (CANUSA) Peritoneal Dialysis Study Group. Adequacy of dialysis and nutrition in continuous peritoneal dialysis: association with clinical outcomes. Canada–USA (CANUSA) peritoneal study group. J Am Soc Nephrol 1996; 7:198–207.

Diabetes Control and Complications Trial Research Group. The effect of intensive treatment of diabetes on the development and progression of long-term complications in insulin-dependant diabetes mellitus. N Engl J Med 1993; 329:977–986.

Dialysis Outcome Quality Initiative (DOQI). Development of methodology for clinical practice guidelines. Nephrol Dialysis Transplant 1997; 10:2060–2063.

Fink JC, Blahut SA, Reddy M et al. Use of erythropoietin before the initiation of dialysis and its impact on mortality. Am J Kidney Dis 2001; 37:348–355.

Giatras L, Levy DP, Malone FD et al. Pregnancy during dialysis: case report and specific management guidelines. Nephrol Dialysis Transplant 1998; 13:3266–3272.

Greenhalgh T, Helman C, Chowdhury AM. Health beliefs and folk models of diabetes in British Bangladeshis: a qualitative study. Br Med J 1998; 7136:316.

Hayslip DM, Suttle D. Pre-ESRD patient education: a review of the literature. Adv Renal Replace Ther 3:217–226.

Heimburger O, Qureshi AR, Blaner WS et al. Handgrip muscle strength, lean body mass and plasma proteins as markers of nutritional status in patients with chronic renal failure close to start of dialysis therapy. Am J Kidney Dis 2000; 36:1213–1225.

Hood VL, Gennari FJ. End-stage renal disease. Measures to prevent or slow its progression. Postgrad Med 1996; 11:163–166.

Hoy W, Kelly A, Jacups S et al. Stemming the tide: reducing cardiovascular disease and renal failure in Australian Aborigines. Aust NZ J Med 1999; 29:480–483.

Iseki K, Ikemiya Y, Fukiyama K. Risk factors of end-stage renal disease and serum creatinine in a community-based mass screening. Kidney Int 1997; 3:850–854.

Jassal SV, Brissenden JE, Roscoe JM. Specialised chronic care for dialysis patients—a five year study. Clin Nephrol 1998; 8:84–89.

Joint British recommendations on the prevention of coronary heart disease in clinical practice. Heart 1998; 80(suppl. 2): S1–29.

Jungers P, Chauveau D. Pregnancy in renal disease. Kidney Int 1997; 52:871–885.

Jungers P, Chokroun G, Robino C et al. Epidemiology of end-stage renal disease in the Ile-de-France area: a prospective study in 1998. Nephrol Dialysis Transplant 2000; 12:2000–2006.

Jungers P, Zingraff J, Albouse G et al. Late referral to maintenance dialysis: detrimental consequences. Nephrol Dialysis Transplant 1993; 8:1089–1093.

King K. Education factors affecting modality selection: a National Kidney Foundation study. Eur Dialysis Transplant Nurses Assoc–Eur Renal Care Assoc (EDTNA–ERCA) J 1998;14:27–29.

Kissmeyer L, Kong C, Cohen J et al. Community nephrology: audit of screening for renal insufficiency in a high risk population. Nephrol Dialysis Transplant 1999;14:2150–2155.

Klahr S, Andrew S, Levey A. The effects of dietary restrictions and blood pressure control on the progression of chronic renal disease. N Engl J Med 1994; 330:877–884.

Lameire NH. Patient referral and dialysis initiation practices: a European perspective. Part two. Available: www.hdcn.com/symp/early/lameier2.htm 23 January 2001.

Levin A. Consequences of late referral on patient outcomes. Nephrol Dialysis Transplant 2000; 15 (suppl. 3):8–13.

Levy AS, Adler S, Cagguila AW et al. Effects of dietary protein restriction on progression of advanced renal disease in modification of diet in renal disease study. Am J Kidney Dis 27:652–663.

Levy D, Giatras L, Jungers P. Pregnancy and end-stage renal disease—past experience and new insights. Nephrol Dialysis Transplant 1998; 13:3005–3007.

O'Donnel A, Tucker L. Predialysis education: a change in clinical practice. How effective is it? Eur Dialysis Transplant Nurses Assoc–Eur Renal Care Assoc (EDTNA–ERCA) J 1999; 15:29–31.

Ozminkowski RJ, White AJ, Hassol A et al. What if socioeconomics made no difference? Access to a cadaveric transplant as an example. Med Care 1998; 9:1398–1406.

Porter E, Predialysis initiatives in Canada, Nephrol News Issues 1998; 11:15–16.

Raine AEG, Seymour A-ML, Roberts AFC et al. Impaired cardiac function and energetics in experimental renal failure. J Clin Invest 1993; 92:2934–2940.

Ramsay LE, Williams B, Johnston DG et al. Guidelines for the management of hypertension: report of the third working party of the BHS. J Hum Hypertens 1999a; 13:569–592.

Ramsay LE, Williams B, Johnson DG et al. British Hypertension Society guidelines for hypertension management: summary. Br Med J 1999b; 4:630–635.

Renal Association. Treatment of adult patients with renal failure. Recommended standards and audit measures. London: Royal College of Physicians, 1997.

Ritz E, Eisenhardt A. Early epoietin treatment in patients with renal insufficiency. Nephrol Dialysis Transplant 2000; 15 (suppl. 3):40–44.

Roderick PJ, Jones I, Raleigh VS et al. Population need for renal replacement therapy in Thames regional dimension. Br Med J 1994; 29:1111–1114.

Roderick P, Clements S, Stone N et al. What determines geographical variation in rates of acceptance on to renal replacement therapy in England? J Health Service Res Policy 1999; 7:139–146.

Roubicek C, Brunet P, Huiart L et al. Timing of nephrology referral: influence on mortality and morbidity. Am J Kidney Dis 2000; 7:35–41.

Scottish Intercollegiate Guidelines Network SIGN. Investigation into proteinuria in adults. Edinburgh: Royal College of Physicans of Edinburgh, 1997a.

Scottish Intercollegiate Guidelines Network SIGN. Investigation of microscopic haematuria in adults. Edinburgh: Royal College of Physicans of Edinburgh, 1997b.

Scottish Intercollegiate Guidelines Network. Lipids and the primary prevention of coronary heart disease. Edinburgh: SIGN, 1999.

Sesso R, Belasco AG. Late diagnosis of chronic renal failure and mortality on maintenance dialysis. Nephrol Dialysis Transplant 1996; 12:2417–2420.

Standing Medical Advisory Committee. The use of statins. London: Department of Health, 1997.

Strojek K, Grzeszczak W, Gorska J et al. Lowering of microalbuminuria in diabetic patients by a sympathicoplegic agent: novel approach to prevent progression of diabetic nephropathy? J Am Soc Nephrol 2001; 12:602–605.

Tattersall J, Greenwood R, Farrington K, Urea kinetics and when to commence dialysis. Am J Nephrol 1995; 15:283–289.

United Kingdom Prospective Diabetes Study Group. Tight blood pressure control and risk of macrovasular and microvascular complications in type 2 diabetes: UKPDS 38. Br Med J 1998; 317:703–713.

Van Wyck DB. Management of early renal anaemia: diagnostic work-up, iron and epoetin therapy. Nephrol Dialysis Transplant 2000; 15(suppl. 3):36–39.

Vora JP, Ibrahim HA, Bakris GL. Responding to the challenge of diabetic nephropathy: the history of detection, prevention and management. J Hum Hypertens 2000; 10:667–685.

Investigations in renal failure

Althea Mahon   Jane Hattersley

■ LEARNING OUTCOMES FOR THIS CHAPTER

- To explain the procedures commonly undertaken in the diagnosis of acute and chronic renal failure
- To evaluate the nurses' role in postprocedure care
- To gain knowledge and understanding of the investigations required in the diagnosis of renal impairment
- To provide a rationale for the use of those investigations and procedures.

INTRODUCTION

Patients referred to a nephrologist are subjected to a bewildering array of diagnostic tests and procedures. Nurses working in this area should familiarise themselves with these investigations in order to be able to explain these procedures to the patient adequately, and consent will then be truly 'informed'. The tests covered in this chapter include those involving blood and urine, invasive diagnostic investigations, X-rays, scans, isotope studies and methods of evaluating glomerular filtration rate. Investigations which are carried out prior to erythropoietin (EPO) therapy are discussed, as well as those used in cases of diminished or non-response to EPO therapy.

Some patients who have progressive renal disease show no specific signs or symptoms and do not feel unwell until the disease is well advanced. Abnormal results of blood and urine tests carried out at routine medical examinations, whether they be pre-employment, pre-life insurance or preoperative, or during visits to a general practitioner for other reasons, may warrant referral. Patients in acute renal failure (see Ch. 4) for whatever cause, also come under the remit of a nephrologist, and urgent diagnosis and treatment in this potentially life-threatening situation are vital. Sometimes only a large number of investigations will help make the diagnosis.

Nurses are responsible for the correct procedure of many investigations, so an understanding of the nature of these tests is vital, as is the ability to recognise abnormal results.

An individual with end-stage renal failure is subjected to constant investigations to monitor the effectiveness of dialysis treatment, with the objective of giving the patient maximum benefit from treatment with the minimum of side-effects, in order to maintain a reasonable quality of life.

VENEPUNCTURE

Traditionally, venepuncture has not been regarded as a procedure routinely performed by nurses in the UK; the exception was those nurses who were carrying out what was known as an 'extended role'. Collecting blood samples was considered to be the job of the medical staff and phlebotomists. However, in 1994, the UK Department of Health recommended that, while redefining nurses' activities, venepuncture should now be considered a routine nursing procedure, to be shared with the medical staff in the absence of a phlebotomist (Greenhalgh Report 1994). In the renal field, as urgent blood test results can be vital to successful treatment, nurses who can demonstrate competency have extended their scope of practice to include venepuncture (United Kingdom Central Council for Nursing, Midwifery and Health Visiting (UKCC) 1992).

Before embarking on the collection of blood samples there are several factors that should be considered:

- the safety of healthcare personnel
- the safety and comfort of the patient
- the correct collection system.

Safety of health care personnel
In order to keep the danger of blood-borne infection to a minimum, universal precautions should be observed at all times; that is, all patients' body fluids should be assumed to be carriers of infective organisms (Department of Health 1998). Disposable gloves (also aprons and eye shields in some situations) should be worn as appropriate and attention paid to proper hand-washing before and after each procedure.

Safety closed blood collection systems are now available, for example, the Sarstedt Monovette and Becton Dickinson Vacutainer. Closed systems avoid the need to transfer blood from syringe to laboratory sample tube, as the blood collection device fulfils both functions. Decanting blood from syringe to blood tube should only be carried out when absolutely necessary. Local protocol may demand that samples from patients known to be infected with human immunodeficiency virus (HIV) or hepatitis B or C and other contagious organisms should be identified with internationally recognised yellow biohazard labels and be processed at the end of a laboratory run. On completion of the procedure, no attempt should be made to resheathe the needle; it should immediately be discarded into a suitable sharps box. Needlestick injury is still an unnecessary form of accident (British Medical Association 1990).

Choice of vein

When carrying out venepuncture on a patient with renal disease, great care must be taken of veins as they may be needed in the future for fistula formation for haemodialysis. For this reason the cephalic vein in the forearm must be avoided for both venepuncture and intravenous infusion. The veins of the antecubital fossa should be used for venepuncture whenever possible, with the veins of the upper aspect of the hand as second choice, although this can be a painful site for the patient (Fig. 6.1). It is best to avoid the antecubital veins in those with diabetes due to difficulties with access formation. Arteriovenous fistulae sites should not be cannulated except for dialysis purposes, to exclude the slight danger of infection or haematoma which may render the fistula unsuitable for dialysis in either the short or long term.

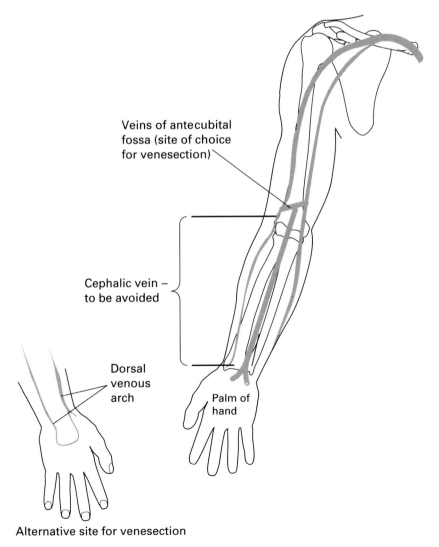

Veins of antecubital fossa (site of choice for venesection)

Cephalic vein – to be avoided

Dorsal venous arch

Palm of hand

Alternative site for venesection

Figure 6.1 Veins of the arm.

The correct collection procedure

Before attempting venepuncture, the correct method of collection according to local policy should be ascertained and all necessary equipment assembled. There are many designated tubes available; if blood is sent to the laboratory in the wrong tube it cannot be processed, time and money are wasted and unnecessary discomfort is caused to the patient in repeating the procedure. Check unfamiliar tests with the laboratory before commencing.

If difficulties arise in collecting a blood sample from a patient it is advisable that only two attempts should be made before calling for assistance from a more experienced member of staff.

Factors that can cause difficulties locating a vein include dehydration, hypotension, obesity and fragile veins.

Points for consideration

If difficulty is encountered in locating a suitable vein:

- Gently tap the chosen site.
- Ask the patient to open and close the fist several times.
- Inflate a sphygmomanometer cuff to a pressure between the patient's systolic and diastolic blood pressure proximal to the venepuncture site.
- Hang the arm down towards the floor for a few minutes.
- In cold weather, keep clothing intact until the last moment, or immerse the chosen arm in warm water to encourage peripheral circulation.

Haematoma formation can be prevented by applying adequate pressure to the puncture site until clotting occurs.

Blood samples from dialysis access needles or lines must be free of saline and anticoagulants (e.g. heparin), be free of clotted material, be blood directly from the patient and not the machine and must not be recirculated blood. Blood for any clotting tests should be taken predialysis from another site such as the back of the hand or antecubital fossa, as any heparin contamination will falsify the result.

Haemodialysis samples should all have 'pre-, mid- or postdialysis sample' clearly marked on the request form to avoid confusion.

The following items are important:

- Always check that the correct collection tube and request form are to hand.
- Know whether the sample has to be delivered immediately to the laboratory, or can be stored at room temperature, in a fridge or on ice.
- Check whether the patient should be fasting.
- Use minimum pressure with a tourniquet to avoid haemolysis, and also to minimise bruising of the patient.
- Ensure the sample is correctly labelled.
- Use biohazard labels for known contaminated samples (as per local protocol). However, all samples should be treated as potentially hazardous.

BIOCHEMICAL BLOOD TESTS

Normal values

These are listed in Table 6.1. These may vary locally and may be expressed in alternative units of measurement. Paediatric normal values should always be checked, as these vary with age.

Monitoring blood biochemistry of patients with renal disease is central to their diagnosis and ongoing care, as this reflects the kidneys' function in excreting the waste products of metabolism. Serum or heparinised plasma samples are suitable for most biochemistry investigations.

Blood to be separated for serum samples is collected in a plain clotting tube (no additives) or in a tube containing beads treated with a clotting activator.

Blood to be separated for plasma samples is collected in a tube containing lithium heparin or beads treated with lithium heparin. The beads form a layer between the blood clot and serum or plasma after centrifugation, which allows serum to be withdrawn by pipette (by mechanised or manual methods) for the appropriate analysis. Some tubes contain a gel for the same purpose to act as a barrier between cells and plasma or serum.

Renal profile

The following tests (urea, creatinine, sodium, potassium, calcium, phosphate, bicarbonate and albumin) are often requested together. The result is generated from one 5-mL blood sample in a plain or lithium heparin tube. Some centres may include other tests under this heading.

It is important to mention here that urea and creatinine levels may not show a significant increase until there is a 50% loss of kidney function. Therefore, they are not a sensitive test for early renal disease.

Urea

Urea is one of the principal end-products of protein metabolism. Urea is formed in the liver, carried by the blood and excreted by the kidneys in the

Table 6.1 Analysis of a normal blood sample

Urea (blood urea nitrogen)	Adult 2.5–6.4 mmol L^{-1} Child 1.1–6.4 mmol L^{-1}
Creatinine	Adult 70–120 μmol L^{-1} Child (increasing with age) 27–88 μmol L^{-1}
Sodium	135–147 mmol L^{-1}
Potassium	3.5–5 mmol L^{-1}
Calcium	2.2–2.6 mmol L^{-1}
Phosphate	0.8–1.5 mmol L^{-1}
Bicarbonate	22–30 mmol L^{-1}
Cholesterol	3.5–5.7 mmol L^{-1}
Total protein	60–80 g L^{-1}
Albumin	35–55 g L^{-1}
Glucose (fasting)	3.5–5.9 mmol L^{-1}

urine. Raised blood urea indicates failure of the kidneys and usually increases in tandem with creatinine levels in chronic and end-stage renal failure. However, serum urea levels may remain within normal limits whilst serum creatinine levels increase.

Urea can rise dramatically in previously healthy individuals who experience overwhelming infection or major crush injuries and are admitted to hospital in acute renal failure. A slight rise in urea may be seen if a very-high-protein diet is consumed, and in low-protein diets a lower level of blood urea may be observed. Certain drugs, such as corticosteroids and tetracycline, can cause a sudden rise in blood urea, especially if the patient already has chronic renal failure.

Non-renal causes of increased urea levels

- High-protein diet
- Chronic malnutrition—increased protein metabolism
- Gastrointestinal bleeds—increased protein absorption
- Dehydration—increased urea reabsorption.

A normal or low urea level is not necessarily indicative of adequate dialysis if a patient is malnourished with a low protein intake.

Creatinine

Creatinine is produced by the breakdown of creatine phosphate in muscle by catabolism and is excreted by the kidney. Raised creatinine can reliably be used as a specific indicator of kidney malfunction as it is fairly constant from day to day and rises steadily with progressive renal impairment. A higher level of serum creatinine may be expected with higher body weight, in males, and in those of Afro-Caribbean ethnicity.

Creatinine levels in patients with progressive renal failure may eventually rise to a level where it is considered expedient to commence dialysis. This may be in the region of 500–1000 µmol L^{-1} but varies with each patient, the symptoms experienced by the patient, and the policy of the renal unit. Patients with diabetes are usually commenced on dialysis earlier, sometimes with creatinine levels of 400–500 µmol L^{-1}. Creatinine levels can be plotted on a log graph at regular intervals over a period of time, and used as a predictor of the time when renal replacement therapy is likely to be necessary.

Sodium

Sodium is the principal electrolyte (Na^+) of the extracellular fluid of the blood, maintaining osmotic pressure, and is involved in acid–base balance and the transmission of nerve impulses. Sodium is taken into the body with the diet and is conserved or excreted by the kidneys. Hyponatraemia (<135 mmol L^{-1}) can be an indication of excess body fluid, and is also often present in burns, diarrhoea, vomiting, nephritis, neoplasms and diabetic acidosis.

Hypernatraemia (>148 mmol L^{-1}) can be an indication of dehydration and insufficient water intake, multiple myeloma, diabetes insipidus, metabolic acidosis or excessive intravenous isotonic fluids in renal failure. Patients may be proportionally hypernatraemic or hyponatraemic without an altered fluid state.

Potassium

Potassium is the principal electrolyte (K^+) of the intracellular fluid, with only low concentrations (2%) circulating in the extracellular fluid. Potassium is provided by the diet and excreted mainly by the kidneys, where regulation of the body potassium content occurs—a small amount is also lost in the faeces. Potassium is necessary to maintain nerve conduction and plays a major role in control of cardiac output. Potassium levels usually remain normal if a urine output in excess of 1500 mL day^{-1} can be maintained. Hypokalaemia (<3.5 mmol L^{-1}) may be found in cases of diarrhoea, vomiting, renal tubular acidosis, diuretic usage, intravenous fluid administration without added potassium, and when excess insulin causes an increase in the cellular uptake of potassium. Hypokalaemia can cause cardiac arrhythmias.

Hyperkalaemia (>5.5 mmol L^{-1}) may be seen in renal failure, burns, insulin deficiency, posttraumatic conditions (including surgery), disseminated intravascular coagulation or when potassium-sparing diuretics are used with Slow-K, and any condition where cell damage has occurred, causing leakage of intracellular potassium into the extracellular fluid. In patients with renal failure a potassium level >6.5 mmol L^{-1} may be a medical emergency requiring immediate instigation of dialysis or other treatments. If left unattended, the patient may suffer cardiac arrest caused by the arrhythmic effect of potassium build-up. Blood samples for accurate potassium analysis should be delivered swiftly to the laboratory or, if this is impossible, separated and stored, to prevent leaching of intracellular potassium into the serum, which results in a falsely raised level.

See Chapter 4 for hyperkalaemia treatments.

Calcium

Calcium (normal range total Ca^{+2} 2.2–2.6mmol L^{-1}) is provided by the diet, and is excreted by the kidneys. Most body calcium is found in the skeleton but a small proportion is circulated in the blood. About 50% of serum calcium is protein-bound and 50% is ionised. Ionised serum calcium is responsible for muscle contraction, cardiac function and blood clotting.

In the healthy individual, calcium homeostasis is controlled by parathyroid hormone, vitamin D and the hormone calcitonin.

Hypocalcaemia is found in chronic renal failure where phosphate retention is present (calcium carbonate is given to alleviate this; see Ch. 9). Chronic hypocalcaemia causes an excess of parathyroid hormone to be excreted into the blood stream which in turn releases calcium from the bone, resulting in the renal bone disease often seen in conjunction with vitamin D deficiency in renal patients. In nephrotic syndrome low levels of calcium will be found due to albumin leaking into the urine, taking bound calcium with it. In the nephrotic patient the ratio of protein-bound and ionised calcium will remain the same. The acidosis of chronic renal failure is an added cause of loss of bone calcium. Hypercalcaemia may be an indication of hyperparathyroidism, sarcoidosis or malignancy. High levels of calcium can cause renal stones and renal tubular disease.

Phosphate

Phosphorus is found in the diet. Phosphate (normal value PO_4^{3-} 0.8–1.5 mmol L^{-1}) is mainly combined with calcium in the skeletal bone. It is controlled, with calcium, by parathyroid hormone and apart from its skeletal function has a part in the metabolism of glucose and lipids. Phosphates are excreted by the kidney. When phosphate is increased, calcium is lowered and vice versa.

Hypophosphataemia may be found in the patient with renal tubular disease who loses phosphate, possibly leading to osteomalacia. Hyperphosphataemia will often be found in conjunction with hypocalcaemia.

Other biochemical blood tests

Uric acid

Uric acid (normal value female 200–350 µmol L^{-1}, male 260–500 µmol L^{-1}) is an end-product of purine metabolism and is excreted mainly by the kidney, but in part by the bowel. In gout, excess uric acid crystallises in joints. Patients in renal failure have an impaired ability to excrete uric acid and a high serum level may be found in association with raised urea and creatinine. Increased serum uric acid is also found in pre-eclampsia of pregnancy, leukaemia, multiple myeloma, various cancers and in acute shock.

Bicarbonate

The normal value of HCO_3^- is 22–30 mmol L^{-1}. Low plasma HCO_3^- indicates metabolic acidosis caused by chronic renal failure with an inability to excrete hydrogen ions adequately.

Glucose

The normal value of fasting serum glucose is 3.5–5.9 mmol L^{-1}. Blood glucose levels are maintained by the liver, which absorbs and stores glucose as glycogen and releases it into the circulation in response to the demands of the body. Glucose is regulated by insulin which is synthesised by the beta cells in the islets of Langerhans in the pancreas.

Plasma total proteins

The normal value of plasma total proteins is 60–80 g L^{-1}.

Hypoproteinaemia associated with low albumin (normal value 35–55 g L^{-1}) levels may be found in the many conditions associated with nephrotic syndrome where protein leakage occurs from the kidney into the urine. Also, decreased total protein in conjunction with low albumin may be found in liver disease, burns and haemorrhage.

Hyperproteinaemia (increase of total plasma protein) with a normal albumin/globulin ratio may occur in dehydration. If total protein increases with albumin/globulin ratio falling (i.e. a raised globulin), this may indicate autoimmune disease such as systemic lupus erythematosus, or shock, chronic infection or myeloma.

Albumin
The normal value of albumin is 35–50 g L^{-1}.

Albumin levels can be elevated in patients with dehydration. Low albumin levels are common in renal patients due to protein loss through peritoneal dialysate, poor dietary intake and nephrotic syndrome. Other causes of low albumin levels are decreased absorption in liver disease and increased breakdown in malignancy.

Lipids
The normal values are: total cholesterol 3.5–5.7 mmol L^{-1}; triglycerides 0.45–2.0 mmol L^{-1}. A major cause of morbidity and mortality in renal patients can be attributed to cardiovascular events, one of the main risk factors of which is hyperlipidaemia. Hyperlipidaemia is often found in those with renal failure, especially those with nephrotic syndrome and in transplanted patients.

Parathyroid hormone
See below in the section on EPO.

Serology
Serological tests are frequently required as renal impairment is often only one manifestation of a systemic disease. Many renal disorders arise from immune dysfunction and serology will often, therefore, provide an exact diagnosis. Antineutrophil cytoplasmic antibodies (ANCA) are present in collagen or autoimmune diseases and they are an important diagnostic marker. The test itself will identify whether antibodies are present using the technique of immunofluorescence. A positive ANCA test is found in disease states such as systemic and renal vasculitis. Antiglomerular basement membrane (anti-GBM) is an antibody detected in Goodpasture's syndrome. Other tests include immunoglobulins that are found in auto-immune diseases.

Complement
The most common complement studies performed are for C3 and C4. These levels rise during an acute inflammatory state. However, there are many other specialised complement studies that can be undertaken in order to diagnose a particular disease process.

Haematology
Haematological tests give information about anaemia, haematological malignancies and clotting disorders. Infections, inflammatory disease and other conditions can be indicated by changes in total and differential white cell counts. Normal values are shown in Table 6.2 (there may be slight local variations, especially in the paediatric normal range).

Table 6.2 Normal values—haematological tests

Haemoglobin	Male 13.5–18 g dL^{-1} Female 11.5–16.5 g dL^{-1}
Haematocrit	Male 40–55% Female 35–45%
Platelets	150–350 × 10^9 L^{-1}
Leukocytes (white bloodcells)	5–10 g L^{-1}

Full blood count (FBC)

This test provides information regarding the platelets and the red and white blood cells, often providing evidence of renal anaemia in the patient with chronic renal failure. It may be appropriate to investigate further those values falling outside normal parameters (further information is given in the EPO section below).

Coagulation

In circulating blood a series of factors are present that provide the means for clot formation as appropriate when damage to a vessel occurs. Prior to many renal procedures, such as kidney biopsy, it is standard practice to ascertain that the patient has normal clotting function to avoid the risk of haemorrhage. Those with uraemia are more prone to bleeding as urea affects the clotting cascade.

Included in this group of tests are platelets (normally, 150–400 × 10^9 L^{-1} are included in the FBC). Platelets adhere to each other and initiate the clotting cascade when damaged endothelium is encountered. Platelet deficiency (thrombocytopenia) is a common cause of prolonged bleeding.

Other coagulation studies likely to be encountered in renal investigations include the bleeding time (normal <10 min); partial thromboplastin time (PTT); activated partial thromboplastin time (APTT); fibrinogen and international normalised ratio (INR). Most methods in current use require a very precise amount of blood in coagulation tests; the blood sample should exactly reach the marked line. Blood for coagulation studies during or immediately posthaemodialysis or from heparinised lines (e.g. temporary or permanent dialysis catheters) should not be taken from a central line as the result will be falsified—it is recommended to use a vein instead.

Erythropoietin

Tests to be performed before commencing therapy

Anaemia is a major complication of chronic renal failure and a contributory factor to cardiovascular disease in dialysis patients. The major cause is the lack of production of the hormone EPO which is produced by the kidney. Recombinant EPO is now recognised as the standard treatment for the patient who is suffering from renal anaemia—anaemia caused by endogenous EPO deficiency. Correction of renal anaemia has been shown to improve both cardiac function and the quality of life of dialysis patients (Macdougall 2000). The desired rate of increase in haemoglobin is 1 g dL^{-1} month^{-1} until the target haemoglobin is reached. Before starting EPO therapy, some basic investigations must be completed in order to correct any deficiencies which may prevent an adequate response to this very expensive therapy. EPO should be administered subcutaneously in pre-dialysis and peritoneal dialysis patients. Haemodialysis patients can have EPO administered either subcutaneously or intravenously; lower EPO dose requirements can be achieved via the subcutaneous route.

Symptoms of anaemia

- Lethargy
- Dyspnoea
- Pallor.

Before starting EPO therapy it is important to exclude or treat (if possible) underlying causes such as:

- iron deficiency
- blood loss
- infection or inflammatory disease
- hyperparathyroidism
- aluminium toxicity
- vitamin B$_{12}$ and folate deficiency
- haemolysis
- haemoglobinopathies.

The main adverse effect of EPO therapy is hypertension, and blood pressure should be closely monitored for the first 2–4 weeks of commencing therapy. A baseline blood pressure lower than 140/90 mmHg should be aimed for if possible, and treatment of hypertension may be necessary with fluid management and antihypertensives.

Other adverse events are:

- Vascular access thrombosis
- Occasionally, elevated potassium, phosphate and creatinine
- Influenza-type symptoms on administration of the first few injections.

Full blood count

Haemoglobin

Haemoglobin should be checked to ensure that anaemia is not present. Haemoglobin varies with age, gender and ethnicity. The level at which it is considered that EPO should justifiably be given varies from one centre to another, but a haemoglobin of less than 8 g dL^{-1} or haematocrit below 25% is commonly given as a guideline. The recommendations from The European Best Practice Guidelines (1999) is for haemoglobin to be >11 g dL^{-1} within 3 months of commencing therapy (1 g dL^{-1} month^{-1}). Normocytic erythrocytes are typical in the patient with renal anaemia. However, in the case of iron-deficiency anaemia, normocytic and hypochromic red blood cells will be seen.

Haematocrit

Haematocrit is the percentage of red cells in the whole blood volume, which will be low in the patient with renal anaemia, running in parallel with the low level of haemoglobin. When the patient responds to the effect of EPO, a rise in haematocrit will be seen in conjunction with a rise in haemoglobin and red blood cells.

Other tests

Having ascertained that the patient has renal anaemia, the next step is to carry out certain investigations to check that there is no condition present which may prevent or reduce the effect of EPO. These tests should be repeated if diminished or non-response to EPO occurs at a later date.

Haematinics

In order to maintain the haem component of the healthy red blood cell, an adequate amount of available and stored iron must be present. There are several tests which can be carried out to determine this very important factor—the main cause of non-response to EPO has been found to be low available iron.

Iron-deficiency anaemia is either absolute or functional.

Ferritin

The normal range in health is 15–300 ng/mL, but an individual with renal failure needs a minimum of 100 ng/mL. Ferritin is the main stored iron form found in all tissues, but especially in the liver, spleen and bone marrow. Ferritin found in the serum relates to the amount of stored iron, but is not necessarily an accurate assessment of available iron.

Unless ferritin levels are at least 100 ng L^{-1} before EPO therapy is started, the response will be short-lived. Ferritin levels should be kept in excess of this by infusing intravenous iron to allow adequate erythropoiesis, as oral iron supplementation is inadequate.

Transferrin

Iron is transported by the specific plasma protein transferrin (or sidero-philin). A useful test of available iron for red cell production is the transferrin saturation rate. Transferrin saturation indicates how much iron is circulating in the plasma relative to total iron-binding capacity.

Serum iron

Serum iron (normal value 14–28, μmol L^{-1}) in those with chronic renal failure is of no great significance (except in iron overload) but is necessary for calculating transferrin saturation rate.

Reticulocytes

Reticulocytes (normal range in men 0.5–1.5%, in women 0.5–2.5%) are immature red blood cells which have been newly released from the bone marrow, and can be recognised as such for about 48 h before reaching a mature state. Patients with renal anaemia have a depressed reticulocyte count before EPO therapy and a rise should be seen when stimulation of erythrocyte production occurs as a response to EPO. If no response occurs, further investigation should be considered.

The percentage of hypochromic red blood cells will assess how much iron is being incorporated into the red blood cell. This level should be <10%; greater levels indicate iron-deficiency anaemia.

Folic acid is absorbed from the duodenum and jejunum. It is necessary for normal DNA synthesis and affects the erythrocyte precursors. The stores last only a few months.

Vitamin B_{12} level

The normal range is 150–1000 ng L^{-1}. Vitamin B_{12} is absorbed in the ileum. The uptake is dependent on the production of acid and intrinsic factor in the stomach, adequate oral intake and production of transcobalamin (transport protein). Vitamin B_{12} is required for normal red cell production, although the body stores can last several years without oral intake.

Aluminium

The normal range is less than 20 μg L^{-1}. In dialysis patients who have been prescribed aluminium hydroxide as a phosphate binder, or who have used dialysate containing aluminium or water with high aluminium levels, a high serum aluminium level may be exhibited. Aluminium has been implicated in osteomalacic bone disease, dialysis dementia and, importantly, in EPO therapy which is unresponsive due to hypoplasia of the bone marrow (Rao et al 1993). Owing to the current acceptance that aluminium ingestion should be kept to a minimum, especially for the kidney patient, measures have been taken to provide purer water and dialysate. Aluminium hydroxide has mainly been discontinued as a phosphate binder in favour of calcium carbonate. However, serum aluminium levels should still be checked. Venous samples (10 mL) are collected in a plain plastic tube, as samples can become contaminated by the aluminium content of glass.

Parathyroid hormone

Normal values of parathyroid hormone vary according to the local assay method being used.

Parathyroid hormone is a hormone produced in the parathyroid gland and it is concerned with the regulation of extracellular calcium. This test is useful in establishing whether hypercalcaemia is due to an overactive parathyroid. Increased parathyroid hormone is found in chronic renal failure, vitamin D deficiency and osteomalacia. Hyperparathyroidism has been implicated in reduced response to EPO therapy, possibly due to inducing bone marrow fibrosis or suppressing the erythroid cell growth (Rao et al 1993).

Blood for parathyroid hormone analysis should be delivered immediately to the laboratory for analysis or, if this is impossible, kept on ice for a maximum of 30 min.

C-reactive protein is a globulin that is synthesised by the liver and is present in small amounts in a normal individual. An elevated C-reactive protein is indicative of infection, inflammation or malignancy.

Reasons for low or non-response to EPO therapy other than haematinic may be underlying infection or inflammation, occult malignancy, inadequate dialysis, immunosuppressive drugs and chronic blood loss (e.g. haemorrhoids, menorrhagia, gastrointestinal bleeding). These possibilities should be investigated.

URINE INVESTIGATIONS

Urinalysis plays an important part in the assessment of renal disease, as renal damage may allow increased concentrations of various chemicals through to the urine together with other signs of disease such as haematuria or proteinuria. The quantity of urine passed during the day together with its specific gravity also gives an indication of renal function.

Table 6.3 lists the normal volumes of urine passed per day.

Urine is composed of about 95% water and 5% solids, mainly urea and sodium chloride, it is slightly acidic (pH 6.0) and it has a specific gravity of 1.010–1.030 (specific gravity of water = 1.000).

Urinalysis

Measurement of specific gravity can be unreliable in the presence of water and electrolyte imbalance, low-protein diets, chronic liver disease and pregnancy.

Appearance

Urine can vary in colour from pale straw to dark amber:

- Pale urine is dilute because of:
  - heavy fluid intake

Table 6.3 Normal volumes of urine	
Healthy adult	1–1.5 L day^{-1}
Newborn baby	50–300 mL day^{-1}
Infant	350–550 mL day^{-1}
Child	500–1000 mL day^{-1}
Adolescent	700–1400 mL day^{-1}

- polyuria due to renal disease where the tubules fail to reabsorb water
- diabetes-insipidus or diabetes mellitus.
- Dark urine may indicate:
  - concentration due to fluid depletion
  - presence of bile.
- Haematuria can vary in appearance from 'smoky' to 'tea' to red, either bright or dark.
- Coloured urine can be caused by beetroot in the diet and other vegetable food dyes, porphyria and some drugs, for example, orange-coloured urine is caused by rifampicin.
- Frothy urine indicates heavy proteinuria.
- Smoky urine may indicate the presence of bleeding from the kidney.
- Deposits or turbid urine, which occurs when the urine sample is left to stand, may be crystals of phosphate, oxalate or urates, or due to pus in the presence of infection.

Dipstick tests

Dipstick tests can be carried out in the clinic or ward situation as well as in the laboratory. Dipsticks are available which accurately show the presence of a variety of substances which may occur in the urine (e.g. protein, glucose, ketones, blood) as well as giving the pH of the urine sample. The stick should be briefly dipped into a fresh sample of urine and read after 1 min or according to the manufacturer's instructions. The results are then compared with those supplied on the instruction sheet.

Caution

These kits are very reliable providing that the container is always kept dry and capped between use, the strips are only briefly dipped into the urine sample and the expiry date is not exceeded.

The majority of biochemical laboratory tests performed on blood samples can also be carried out on urine—usually taken from a mixed 24-h urine collection (see section on creatinine clearance, below).

Osmolality

Osmolality (normal 500–800 mOsmol kg^{-1}) measurement indicates the kidney's ability in concentration and dilution and is considered more reliable than measuring the specific gravity. Collection methods vary from one centre to another (Malarkey & McMorrow 2000).

Glucose

The presence of glucose may indicate diabetes mellitus, proximal tubular dysfunction, Fanconi's syndrome, glomerulonephritis or nephrotic syndrome.

Proteinuria

No more than a trace of protein should be found in the normal collection (i.e. less than 25 mg 24 h^{-1}, mainly albumin). However, proteinuria may be present up to 150 mg in 24 h before a dipstick test shows a positive reading.

(The procedure for collecting the 24-h sample is the same as is detailed for creatinine clearance.) The urine should be kept refrigerated during the collection period to minimise bacterial growth.

Persistent proteinuria is a common sign of many forms of renal disease. In nephrotic syndrome, proteinuria may be as high as 4--30 g 24 h^{-1}.

Bence Jones protein

This test consists of a sample of urine from the first specimen of the day. In the laboratory the urine is heated; if this protein is present, it will precipitate on heating and dissolve at 100°C; on cooling the protein will precipitate again. This test is now performed by electrophoresis and immunoelectrophoresis. It is most commonly (70–80% of positive results) found in multiple myeloma due to the proliferation of paraprotein-producing bone marrow. It is also occasionally seen in amyloidosis, cryoglobulinaemia and hyperparathyroidism.

Microalbuminuria

Microalbuminuria—persistent small amounts of albumin not determined by the usual dipstick test—is of importance as a predictor of renal involvement in patients with insulin-dependent diabetes mellitus. Whereas a normal sample of urine may contain albumin 2.5–25 mg 24 h^{-1}, microalbuminuria is in the range 30--150 mg 24 h^{-1} and macroalbuminuria is generally more than 150 mg 24 h^{-1}.

Those with type 2 diabetes mellitus who have an albumin excretion of between 50 and 250 mg 24 h^{-1} have a 20-fold greater risk of developing diabetic nephropathy than do patients with an excretion rate below this figure (Viberti & Walker 1992). Laboratory testing for microalbuminuria, therefore, is of importance in the care of those with diabetic nephropathy, although the cost-effectiveness of screening all those with diabetes for microalbuminuria has been questioned.

Myoglobin levels

Myoglobinuria may occur due to conditions such as rhabdomyolysis where there is a breakdown of muscle tissue, causing the release of myoglobin into the blood stream. This may occur due to trauma or crush injury to an area, seizures, immobility or severe exercise. The kidneys filter the blood and excrete the myoglobin in the urine. Myoglobin is nephrotoxic and large amounts of this protein can cause the occlusion of the renal tubules, leading to acute tubular necrosis and acute renal failure. This can be diagnosed by a sample of urine—usually the first sample of the day.

Urine microscopy and culture

Microscopy will reveal information from the sediment found in urine—casts, crystals, blood cells and bacteria. The site of origin of casts can often be determined, indicating the type and extent of damage to the kidney. It is normal to find red blood cells in urine at approximately 0.8–2 × 10^6 L^{-1} and these normally originate from the renal pelvis, ureter or bladder and are uniform in shape and size. Leukocytes are also present at approximately 2×10^6 L^{-1} but the presence of eosinophils can be indicative of an allergic interstitial nephritis.

Casts

Different types of casts can be found in the urine and these indicate underlying conditions. Hyaline casts known as Tamm–Horsfall proteins originate from the renal tubules. They may be present due to the use of diuretics, fever and exercise; however, they also present in renal disease. Granular or cellular casts may be seen in renal parenchymal disease. Red cell casts indicate bleeding and white cell casts indicate pyelonephritis.

If microorganisms are found to be present in the urine specimen—usually determined by the Gram staining method—the laboratory will provide information as to which antibiotic is most appropriate. It is important that the urine sample is collected before a broad-spectrum antibiotic is taken—this may be given in the interim period before specific sensitivity is ascertained.

A positive microscopy sample shows at least 10 000 organisms mL^{-1}; below this figure is not considered significant. However, with very dilute urine, a false-negative result may occur despite infection being present.

KIDNEY FUNCTION TESTS

In chronic renal disease a regular assessment of kidney function can be useful in monitoring renal decline and in predicting the time when renal replacement therapy is likely to be needed. Glomerular filtration rate tends to decrease in a linear fashion over time in progressive renal disease and so, by extrapolation, predictions can be made as to when end-stage renal failure may occur.

Knowledge of the amount of nephron damage is useful in assisting in making the choice of suitable drug regime. When there is more than 30% of nephron loss, certain drugs should be avoided or used with caution because of the slow excretion of the drug or its metabolites. Glomerular filtration rate declines with age at approximately 10 mL min^{-1} per decade, starting at the fourth decade.

Increased glomerular filtration rate

- Increased protein intake
- Diurnal variation
- Pregnancy.

Decreased glomerular filtration rate

- Exercise
- Age

- Low-protein diet
- Liver disease.

Many research studies and clinical trials of pharmaceuticals depend on regular glomerular filtration rate calculations to monitor the effect of treatments with regard to renal function.

Kidney function investigations discussed here include creatinine clearance, the [51] chromium ethylenediaminetetraacetic acid glomerular filtration rate, (^{51}Cr EDTA GFR).

Creatinine clearance

The principle of clearance is that an estimation of a known substance in the plasma is compared with the amount in the urine. This substance must only be excreted in the urine. The calculation by which the clearance of the substance occurs can be measured is thus:

$$\frac{\text{Urine concentration of substance } (U) \times \text{Volume of urine in 24 h } (V)}{\text{Plasma concentration of substance } (P)}$$

Because creatinine is believed to be manufactured at a fairly constant rate by the muscle mass, is circulating in the blood stream and is filtered by the glomeruli (although a very small amount is excreted by the tubules), this is the usual substance measured. When used in the above example, this is known as creatinine clearance.

About 50% of nephrons will have lost their function before an appreciable alteration occurs in the result of the creatinine clearance test. The normal value of creatinine clearance should be between 70 and 125 mL min^{-1}; the function lessens with age. A creatinine clearance result of less than 10 mL min^{-1} is an indication to start renal replacement therapy.

Procedure

A 24-h urine collection is made which will provide the urinary creatinine content (U) and volume (V). A blood sample should be taken to indicate the plasma creatinine (P).

Patient information for 24-h urine collection

Patients should be given an explanation of the reason for the test and what is expected of them. One (or more) 2-L collection bottles containing no additives or preservatives should be given to the patient. While male patients can usually void straight into the bottle, female patients should be provided with a suitable receptacle in which they can catch the urine. The patient must be instructed to discard the first urine of the day (on day 1) into the lavatory and then collect all urine passed for the next 24 h into the bottle provided. On the following morning (day 2), the first sample should be collected and then the collection is complete. The completed urine collection should be labelled with the date and time of start and completion of the collection as well as the usual details such as name, identity number and date of birth.

The urine collection and the blood sample should be delivered together to the laboratory with the request form, which should specify creatinine clearance test. The above formula is then applied and this will calculate the creatinine clearance.

Glomerular filtration rate

If the patient is stable and has chronic renal failure, and is not obese or fluid-overloaded, this calculation can be used as a rough guide for estimating glomerular filtration rate:

$$\text{Estimated glomerular filtration rate} = \frac{(140 - \text{age in years})(\text{weight in kg})}{72 \times \text{serum creatinine}}$$

Values for women are 85% predicted.

$$\text{Creatinine clearance (mL min}^{-1}\ 1.73\ \text{m}^{-2}) = \frac{(98 - 0.8)(\text{age} - 20)}{\text{Serum creatinine}}$$

Values for women are 90% predicted. (Wallach 1998)

^{51}Chromium EDTA GFR

A more accurate method of assessing renal function than the creatinine clearance test is the ^{51}Cr EDTA GFR. As with the creatinine clearance test, the normal range is a clearance of 70–125 mL min^{-1}.

Patient preparation

The patient should be informed of the reason for this test, the fact that a small dose of a radioisotope will be injected, and the necessity of a series of blood samples over a 4-h period, and consent should be sought.

Procedure

The radiolabelled substance is given by intravenous injection. The patient's weight and height must also be recorded to enable the result to be normalised for the individual patient's body surface area.

Over the 4 h following the injection the usual procedure is for four blood samples to be drawn from the opposite arm to the injection of the radioisotope. (This is to avoid contamination from any activity still lingering around the injection site, which will falsify the result.)

Whilst the ^{51}Cr EDTA GFR is considered to be very accurate, only personnel who have completed a radiation protection course in accordance with the Ionising Radiation (Medical Exposure) Regulations (Department of Health 2000) are permitted to administer radio-labelled substances.

RENAL BIOPSY

Patients who are referred to the nephrology outpatient clinic with proteinuria, haematuria or renal impairment with no obvious cause require a renal biopsy in order that the nephrologist can make a diagnosis and commence appropriate treatment. Patients referred in acute renal failure may also require a renal biopsy to provide a diagnosis. Whilst in experienced hands renal biopsy is a fairly safe procedure, there are risks which should be taken into consideration. Risks of renal biopsy, which are greater in the acute renal failure patient, are perirenal haematoma, prolonged and severe bleeding necessitating blood transfusion and possible surgery, irreparable damage to the kidney requiring a nephrectomy (1 in 1500), and, rarely, death (Baker et al 2000).

Renal biopsy is contraindicated in the following:

- Small kidneys
- A single kidney
- Gross obesity
- Uncontrolled hypertension
- Non-compliant patient
- Obvious diagnosis
- Severe anaemia
- Uncontrolled coagulopathy.

Patient preparation

Information regarding the benefits and risks attached to this procedure should be given to the patient, who should be allowed the opportunity to ask questions and time to consider the implications before consenting to the biopsy. Child patients under 16 years need written parental consent.

Patients are usually admitted to the ward on the day planned for biopsy and a further explanation of the exact procedure and what is expected of the patient should be given prior to signature of a consent form. Children are fasted for 4 h before the biopsy as they will be sedated with a preparation such as midazolam following a mild premedication. In order to gain full compliance, whilst still in the ward, it is helpful to ask the patient to practise deep breathing and breath-holding. Unless the patient can cooperate with breath-holding on demand, the procedure should not be attempted, as the danger of malplacement of the sharp biopsy needle causing laceration or haemorrhage becomes a possibility.

Blood samples should be taken for bleeding times, FBC, plasma viscosity, INR, group and save, full biochemical and immunology profile. Biopsies should not proceed if any bleeding disorder is present (platelets $<100 \times 10^9$ L^{-1}, INR >1.2, bleeding time >10 min), or if the blood pressure exceeds 160/95 mmHg, as the highly vascular kidney can haemorrhage even when clotting times are within normal limits.

Procedure

Patients will be asked to empty their bladder before the procedure. Percutaneous renal biopsy is usually done in a ward treatment or side room, or X-ray department, under local anaesthetic. The patient lies in a prone position, with a pillow under the upper abdomen to isolate the kidney, perhaps supported with sandbags to prevent movement. The kidney (usually left) is identified by ultrasound as to position and depth and the skin is marked as to where the needle should be inserted. After cleaning the ultrasound gel from the skin, using a full aseptic technique, the area is cleaned, the area infiltrated with lidocaine (lignocaine) as a local anaesthetic and a spinal needle is inserted into the lumbar muscle layer until the needle is noted to swing with the patient's respirations. The patient should be asked to hold the breath whilst the needle is advanced 5 mm at a time, leaving the needle to swing free when the patient breathes in and out. When the needle has located the kidney, more local anaesthetic should be injected.

The spinal needle is then withdrawn, a small incision is made at the needle exit site and a Tru-cut renal biopsy needle is inserted along the pathway made by the spinal needle in the same manner, making advances as the patient holds the breath. When the kidney is again located, the biopsy is taken with the patient holding a breath. The biopsy needle is withdrawn and the specimen obtained is immediately placed on a slide and viewed under a dissecting microscope to ascertain that cortex which has been obtained is large enough (about 5 mm length) to divide into three samples. If not enough cortex has been obtained, the biopsy needle will have to be inserted again until a suitable strip of cortex containing sufficient glomeruli has been identified. Samples are sent to the laboratory for histology (in a 10% formalin pot), for immunofluorescence (in sterile normal saline) and electron microscopy (in specific glutaraldehyde fixative, kept cold). These samples should be delivered immediately (within minutes, not hours) to the laboratory, which must have had advance warning of the biopsy.

Finally, after the needle has been withdrawn, a pressure dressing is applied and the patient is asked to remain flat in bed. The patient will need much encouragement and reassurance during the renal biopsy procedure as it can be painful, despite local anaesthetic. A friendly hand to hold and quiet encouragement to cooperate with breathing requirements from the attending nurse can be very reassuring.

Patient care following renal biopsy

It is usual practice to keep patients in the ward on bed-rest for 24 h following this procedure. Haemorrhage is the main complication following renal biopsy; the wound site should be frequently checked for surface bleeding and blood pressure and pulse observations should be carried out until stable, for example on the time scale of every 15 min for 2 h, then every 30 min for 2 h, and then hourly for 4 h. The signs and symptoms giving an indication of internal bleeding are a rise or fall in blood pressure and dull aching pain in the abdomen, back or shoulder. The patient should be warned that some degree of haematuria will occur initially, but only persisting or heavy haematuria is of significance. Small urine samples from each void should be retained in transparent specimen containers for observation of diminishing haematuria and dipstick testing. It is becoming common practice for suitable patients to be admitted to day-case units for this procedure. These patients must be carefully chosen and must fully understand instructions for aftercare at home. The patient should be advised not to do any strenuous activity for 2 weeks following renal biopsy.

Renal biopsy in the transplanted patient

Closed percutaneous biopsies of the transplanted kidney are undertaken to support evidence of rejection and also to confirm suspicion of recurrent or primary glomerular disease (see Ch. 11). The procedure is similar to the biopsy of the native kidney but more straightforward due to the superficial position of the transplanted kidney. The patient will be placed in a supine position with a pillow beneath the transplant side to move the intra-abdominal contents away from the site. The amount of tissue required in a transplant biopsy will be less than in a native kidney biopsy as fewer tests will be performed. The patient should remain resting in bed for 4–6 h and may be discharged home the same day, though it is important to ensure the patient has passed urine and a dipstick test has been performed to check for blood.

RADIOGRAPHIC INVESTIGATIONS

Investigations using various radiographic methods are often employed to assist diagnosis and to assess progression of renal disease and its attendant side-effects. The most common techniques are discussed here.

Patients should have received adequate explanations before entering the department in order to allay any fears they may have on finding themselves in a department full of strange machinery, hazard warnings and unfamiliar staff. If they are aware of the reasons for the investigation and what will be expected of them, the likelihood of an accurate result of the examination will be enhanced. The patient will be asked to sign a consent form for some invasive tests and early information will be of help for understanding the procedure.

All investigations involving X-rays must be performed according to the safety regulations in using a potentially hazardous substance, and these techniques must not be used unless the risk to the patient is outweighed by the benefit. Some departments follow the practice that women with reproductive capacity should only be subjected to X-rays and other procedures using ionising radiation during the 10 days following the commencement of the last menstrual period to avoid possible damage of a vulnerable fetus—the so called '10-day rule'. More recently, guidelines have indicated that minimal exposure to a possible fetus must be ensured with the use of shields, as developing fetal organs are at higher risk of radiation.

Plain abdominal X-ray

Plain abdominal X-rays incorporating the kidneys, ureters and bladder (KUB) indicate the size, shape, position and the presence or absence of one or both kidneys, and may be taken before other more complicated radio-logical procedures in order to provide an overall background picture. Most calculi may be seen as they are usually composed of radiopaque material. KUB X-rays are usually taken from the anterior aspect. A combination of KUB and ultrasound often forms the basic routine screening in those with renal failure.

Skeletal X-rays

Skeletal X-rays may be taken in the dialysis patient. This is to detect renal osteodystrophy, which may become apparent in association with impaired glomerular filtration and associated disturbed metabolism of calcium and phosphate. Those bones most likely to show the characteristic abnormalities are the phalanges, skull, pelvis and vertebrae. Pain and deformity will ultimately develop unless imbalances of calcium and phosphate can be corrected and inadequate metabolism of vitamin D can be halted (see Ch. 9).

Intravenous urogram (IVU)

This procedure is also known as the intravenous pyelogram (IVP). This examination indicates the size and position of the kidneys and the anatomy of the calyces and pelvis. The ureters are also outlined by the progression of the dye containing urine to the bladder and the subsequent use of sequential X-rays, enabling any deformities in these organs to be demonstrated.

Patient preparation

The patient should be told that the investigation will take about an hour to complete—longer if there is renal impairment.

It should be ascertained that the patient is not allergic to iodine or shellfish and caution should be observed with asthmatics and others who have allergic conditions, as the contrast medium is iodine-based. Therefore, it is standard procedure that injections of adrenaline (epinephrine) 0.5–1 mg (0.5–1 ml of 1:1000 solution = 1 mg mL^{-1}) i.m., antihistamine (e.g. chlor-phenamine (chlorpheniramine) 10–20 mg i.v.) and hydrocortisone should be immediately available to treat anaphylaxis should it occur.

Laxatives should be given to the constipated patient prior to this examination to clear the bowel so that there is no interruption to the view of the urinary system. Adult patients should fast for 3 h, but limited fluid is usually allowed until 1 h before the IVU. After an explanation of the procedure with adequate time to ask questions, the patient may be asked to sign a consent form. Emptying the bladder beforehand is important, or the contrast will become overdilute on reaching a full bladder and a poor picture will result.

Following this test, patients should be encouraged to drink fluids, as they may become dehydrated if fluids were restricted prior to the examination. Nurses should be aware that there is a possibility of acute renal failure following this investigation, so urinary output should be monitored.

The IVU gives little useful information in advanced chronic renal failure and consequently is not the investigation of choice if more than 50% of nephron loss is suspected. If impaired renal function is known and an IVU is indicated, a greater dose than usual of the radiopaque contrast medium may need to be given—this in itself is nephrotoxic and may exacerbate renal failure, at least temporarily.

Retrograde pyelogram

In this examination, radio–opaque dye is injected directly into the upper urinary tract via a catheter inserted through a cystoscope into the ureter. A series of X-rays are performed on one or both kidneys. This test is useful in outlining stones, calyceal defects and masses in the ureter or renal pelvis and in defining deformities such as hydronephrosis or hydroureter. This investigation is sometimes performed after an IVU or ultrasound (US) has demonstrated a hydronephrosis and more clarification is needed for a diagnosis. After the procedure the urine should be observed for haematuria and patients should be watched for signs and symptoms of infection. They should be encouraged to drink copiously to help avoid infection (antibiotics may be given as a prophylaxis).

Computed axial tomography or computed tomography (CAT/CT) scan

This investigation is reserved for the patient who needs staging of a renal mass or a diagnosis when other methods of detection have failed to provide a clear picture. CT is an X-ray technique which uses a computer to reconstruct cross-sectional images of 1-cm slices of the organ targeted. The dose of radiation is about the same as that for an IVU. A clear bowel is necessary so a suitable laxative may be given 2 days before the scan. A light diet should be taken for 2 days before the scan and nothing on the day of examination apart from clear fluids. Patients must be able to follow instructions such as when to hold the breath, to be able to lie motionless and not to talk.

Nuclear magnetic resonance or magnetic resonance imaging (MRI)

This form of scanning involves application of a strong external magnetic field along with a radiofrequency signal that produces a current in a receiving coil proportional to the density of protons in the body organ being scanned. This signal is processed by computer to create a tomographic slice of the organ similar to a CT scan. In renal medicine a clear picture of tumour invasion into blood vessels can be demonstrated as well as differentiation of tissue character.

The advantage of MRI over CT imaging is that no ionising radiation or contrast media is used and many planes can be visualised. However, this method is three times as expensive as CT imaging.

It is vitally important that the patient is not wearing any magnetic metal object, and it must be ascertained that no internal metal objects are present such as aneurysm clips, screws, pacemakers or shrapnel. Therefore, an X-ray may be taken before the procedure to ensure that no hidden metal objects are within the body.

Ultrasonography

US investigations have replaced some X-ray procedures (especially the IVU) to a large degree, and because this procedure does not carry the hazards associated with radiation this method can be used in women without consideration of the possibility of pregnancy. This is a non-invasive procedure where a transducer (sonar probe) is moved in close contact with the skin over the area of investigation and it can be repeated frequently if necessary, unlike X-ray. US is especially useful in examinations of the abdominal and pelvic organs. It is widely used to determine the size and shape of the kidney, its presence and position, and the composition of cysts or neoplasms if present, and also in the diagnosis of polycystic kidney disease. However, it is less useful in providing information about the ureters. US is also used to guide the operator in procedures such as renal biopsy.

Patients who are to have renal US scans are usually asked to fast for 6–8 h (in order to keep pockets of air in the gut to a minimum) except for drinks of clear fluids.

Ultrasound in renal transplantation

US scanning is an ideal method of examining the transplanted kidney, as it is a simple and non-invasive technique (Nicholson et al 1990a). The most important and common cause of early transplant dysfunction is acute rejection, which occurs in 10–20% of all patients. This is accompanied by inflammation, which leads to swelling of the kidney and an increase in pressure inside the organ. US is used to diagnose the increase in size using diameters relating to the local renal anatomy (Nicholson et al 1990a). This procedure should be used daily and two size increases on consecutive days would be strongly indicative of acute rejection. However, dysfunction attributed to other causes must be excluded. Infection may be associated with an increase in the kidney size, but this is easily diagnosed by routine testing of midstream specimens of urine.

Renal vein thrombosis is a serious complication and will cause a rapid increase in size, possibly resulting in a tear of the kidney substance. If this condition is quickly diagnosed with US, rapid surgical intervention is possible and the graft may be rescued. Renal artery thrombosis may be diagnosed ultrasonically by the observation of lack of vessel pulsation. For greater accuracy, duplex scanning using a combination of imaging and frequency waveform analysis is available.

Early complications following transplantation include urine leaks, usually from the site of the ureteric anastomosis. These are seen ultrasonically as a fluid collection around the graft site. Later complications are obstructive lesions, which are often insidious in onset and lead to deteriorating renal function. Routine scanning of outpatients is a simple and easy method of detecting dilatation and stenoses of the urinary tract, which are then treated surgically.

Needle core biopsy of the transplanted kidney remains the best method of detecting rejection (Nicholson et al 1990b). Using ultrasound guidance of the biopsy needle, a good core of the renal cortex may be safely obtained, carefully avoiding the structures of the renal medulla and damage to the graft.

Ultrasound is therefore a valuable tool in the detection and diagnosis of renal allograft dysfunction, allowing intervention and early treatment of problems.

Renograms

Renograms calculate percentages of renal function and indicate position of obstruction. This investigation can be used in place of IVU if the patient is allergic to iodine contrast medium, and it is also used in transplanted patients. In renal artery stenosis, a renogram may be performed and then repeated, incorporating an injection of captopril to outline any response induced.

Renal scanning

There are two types of radioisotope scan that can be performed to provide quantitative data on the function of the kidneys.

Firstly, the isotope, ^{99m}technetium-labelled diethylenetriaminepenta-acetic acid (^{99m}Tc DTPA), is rapidly excreted by the kidney and shows the blood flow through the kidneys, identifies obstructions, e.g. renal artery stenosis, and provides valuable information about the function and excretion capacity of the kidney. A diuretic may also be given intravenously and the patient should be well hydrated. The procedure takes about 1 h.

The other isotope is ^{99m}Technetium-labelled dimercaptosuccinic acid (^{99m}Tc DMSA) which is retained by the cells in the proximal tubules and parenchyma and enables the identification of areas of cortical scarring, contusions and solid lesions. This will provide quantification of relative renal function between kidneys and within a kidney.

MAG 3

MAG 3 is the isotope 99m technetium-labelled benzoylcaptoacetyltriglycerine which is a dynamic imaging scan that is rapidly excreted by the kidney via glomerular filtration or a combination of filtration and tubular secretion. The test enables visualisation of the aorta and renal perfusion. Quantification of renal blood flow can be calculated and it identifies the overall kidney function and presence of obstruction, thrombus, emboli and stenosis. When patients undergo radioisotopic scans they should empty their bladder immediately before scanning. Patients should be advised that they are radioactive for 24 h and nursing staff should ensure universal precautions when managing waste disposal.

Renal angiogram

This is performed through a catheter inserted via the femoral vein and fed to the renal artery. Contrast dye is radiopaque; this is injected and a series of X-rays performed. It identifies tumours, trauma and stenosis of vessels. Caution should be taken with patients who have some degree of renal insufficiency as the dye is nephrotoxic. If patients are able then they should drink plenty of fluids to flush through the contrast.

The most common complication of a femoral angiogram is haemorrhage and haematoma.

The patient should be fasting for 6–8 h and must be checked for any allergies to iodine and shellfish prior to the procedure.

After the procedure, observations of the puncture site and haemodynamic status should be performed every 15 min for 1 h, then half-hourly for 2 h for any signs of bleeding. It is also important to check the pedal pulses for any neurological or circulatory changes. The above observations may change depending on the hospital and usually the patient is required to lie flat for the first 2 h and remain resting in bed for 24 h.

SUMMARY

The investigations which have been discussed above are by no means exhaustive. Since those with renal disease usually have multifactorial disease processes, many other specific investigations may be indicated, especially cardiovascular tests such as electrocardiography and echocardiography. The gastrointestinal tract in the renal patient is frequently investigated for bleeding problems using techniques involving endoscopy (e.g. gastroscopy, colonoscoscopy).

Such is the commercial pressure to exploit the latest technology, it is inevitable that new methods and procedures will enter the renal field in the near future, condemning some present-day tests to redundancy. However, it is hoped that if nurses understand something of the current techniques used in renal investigations, they will be able to inform and reassure their patients reliably.

REFERENCES

Baker LRI, Hurst MJ, Rudge CJ et al. Practical procedures in nephrology. London: Arnold Publishers, 2000.

British Medical Association. A code of practice for the safe use and disposal of sharps. London: British Medical Association, 1990.

Department of Health. Guidance for clinical health care workers, protection against infection with blood-borne viruses—recommendations of the expert advisory group on AIDS and the advisory group on hepatitis. London: HMSO, 1998

Department of Health. The ionising radiation (medical exposure) regulations, London: HMSO, 2000.

European Best Practice Guidelines for the management of renal anaemia in patients with chronic renal failure. Nephrol Dialysis Transplant 1999; 14 (suppl. 5).

Greenhalgh Report. The interface between junior doctors and nurses. Macclesfield, UK: Greenhalgh, 1994.

Macdougall IC. Hematological problems and their management in hemodialysis and peritoneal dialysis patient. In: Lameire N, Mehta R, eds. Complications of dialysis. New York: Marcel Dekker 2000: 303–325.

Malarkey L, McMorrow ME. Nurse's manual of laboratory tests and diagnostic procedures. 2nd edn. Philadelphia: WB Saunders, 2000.

Nicholson ML, Williams PM, Bell A et al. Prospective study of the value of ultrasound measurements in the diagnosis of acute rejection following renal transplantation. Br J Surg 1990a; 77:656–658.

Nicholson ML, Attard AR, Bell A et al. Renal transplant biopsy using real time ultrasound guidance. Br J Urol 1990b; 65:564–565.

Rao SD, Shih M-S, Mohini R. Effect of serum parathyroid hormone and bone marrow fibrosis on the response to erythropoietin in uraemia. N Engl J Med 1993; 328:171–175.

United Kingdom Central Council for Nursing, Midwifery and Health Visiting. Scope of professional practice. London: UKCC, 1992.

Viberti GC, Walker JD. Pathogenesis of diabetic nephropathy. In: Raine AEG, ed., Advanced renal medicine. Oxford: Oxford University Press, 1992:83–91.

Wallach J. Handbook of interpretation of diagnostic tests. Philadelphia: Lippincott–Raven, 1998.

FURTHER READING

Andrew ER, Bydder G, Griffiths J et al. Clinical magnetic resonance—imaging and spectroscopy. Chichester: Wiley, 1990.

Fischbach F. A manual of laboratory and diagnostic tests. Philadelphia, USA: Lippincott, 1992.

Thorpe S. A practical guide to taking blood. London: Baillière Tindall, 1991.

Haemodialysis

Nicola Thomas

■ CONTENTS

■ LEARNING OUTCOMES FOR THIS CHAPTER

- To describe the physiological processes of dialysis
- To evaluate the nurse's role in care of vascular access
- To identify the components of the haemodialysis dialysis circuit
- To outline the principles of patient-centred predialysis assessment
- To recognise and prevent complications of haemodialysis.

INTRODUCTION

Haemodialysis is an area of renal nursing that has developed and continues to develop at a very fast rate. Expert practitioners in this field are constantly striving to promote excellence in the application of nursing care and are implementing evidence-based practice.

Terms and definitions

'Haemodialysis' is a term used to describe the removal of solutes and water from the blood across a semipermeable membrane (dialyser). Techniques have become increasingly sophisticated, resulting in a variety of highly efficient methods of clearing waste products that would normally be removed by the healthy kidney.

The process of dialysis depends on the physiological principles of diffusion and ultrafiltration. It is essential to have a clear understanding of how these physiological principles relate to dialysis to appreciate fully both the benefits and the limitations of this form of renal replacement therapy (RRT).

Diffusion

Diffusion is the term used to describe the movement of molecules from an area of high concentration (of solutes) to a region of low concentration (of solutes) until they are equal. For diffusion to take place, a concentration gradient is essential, and the rate of diffusion is greatest when the concentration gradient is highest. In RRT a physiological solution (dialysate) passes on the opposite side of the semipermeable membrane to the blood. The dialysate contains essential solutes in similar concentrations to normal serum. The dialysate, however, does not contain waste products such as urea and creatinine and so these substances will pass across the membrane from the region of high concentration (the patient's uraemic blood) to the region of low concentration (the dialysate).

Diffusion is also proportional to the temperature of the solution (increased temperature increases random molecular movements) and inversely proportional to the viscosity and size of the molecules (small molecules diffuse more quickly).

Hydrostatic pressure

As blood is pumped through a dialyser, a positive pressure will be exerted on the membrane. The pressure in the space on the opposite side of the membrane will be lower, whether or not the space is filled with dialysate. As a result, fluid and small solutes will move from the area of greater pressure to the area of lower pressure.

Ultrafiltration and convection

As a result of hydrostatic pressure, fluid will move across the semipermeable membrane, and this process is called ultrafiltration. The rate of ultrafiltration depends on the permeability of the membrane and the hydrostatic pressure exerted upon it. The sum of the positive pressure in the blood compartment and the negative pressure in the dialysate compartment equals the transmembrane pressure (TMP).

The removal of fluid by ultrafiltration also results in the removal of solute, or those molecules dissolved in the water; this process is known as convection or solvent drag. Again, the higher the permeability of the membrane, the higher the removed volume of fluid and contained solute will be.

Haemodialysis

Haemodialysis depends on diffusion for the efficient clearance of waste products. The patient's blood is pumped through the circuit (via blood tubing) on one side of the membrane whilst a physiological dialysis fluid (dialysate) is passed through the circuit (via dialysate tubing) on the opposite side of the membrane. To optimise the concentration gradient, the blood and the dialysate flow in opposite directions (countercurrent flow).

During conventional haemodialysis treatment, fluid will be removed by ultrafiltration, but this is usually a small amount (2–3 L) and will not provide significant removal of waste products by convection.

Haemodialysis has traditionally been the standard form of extracorporeal treatment: haemofiltration and haemodiafiltration are usually limited to use in acute renal failure and intensive care as continuous therapies (see Ch. 4). Some centres, however, now routinely use intermittent haemodiafiltration in place of conventional haemodialysis. For the purpose of this chapter, however, the reference is to standard haemodialysis unless otherwise stated.

ACCESS FOR HAEMODIALYSIS

The success of haemodialysis therapy depends almost entirely on the adequacy of the blood flow through the dialyser. Optimal clearance of waste products depends on dialysate flow rate, membrane permeability, membrane surface area, duration of dialysis and, most significantly, blood flow rate. Dysfunctional access will therefore adversely affect dialysis adequacy and consequently increase patient mortality and morbidity (Butterley & Schwab 1996).

The nurse has a responsibility to ensure that the prescribed blood flow is achieved. Poor access should be addressed as a priority.

Various types of access can be used for haemodialysis which fall broadly into two categories:

1. Percutaneous access, including jugular, subclavian and femoral lines which can be either temporary or permanent.
2. Arteriovenous fistulae (AVF) and arteriovenous grafts.

For those with end-stage renal failure the AVF is preferred, as there is evidence of long-term patency, improved flow rates and fewer complications than other methods. The creation and maintenance of long-term access remains one of the most challenging aspects of caring for those with renal failure, particularly patients with vascular disease such as older people and those with diabetes mellitus.

The arteriovenous fistula

The AVF is created during a surgical procedure to anastomose an artery and a vein (Fig. 7.1). Most commonly the radial artery and the cephalic vein are used in the patient's non-dominant forearm. Other sites include the upper arm—the brachial artery and cephalic vein or brachial artery and basilic vein.

As a result of the anastomosis, blood from the artery is forced into the vein where it flows in a retrograde direction. The increased blood flow and pressure cause the vein to thicken and dilate. Once established, blood flow of up to 800–1000 mL min^{-1} can be achieved.

Ideally the patient should have the fistula created at least 3–4 months before the need for dialysis arises. This will ensure that the operation is performed when the patient is well and will allow the fistula time to mature, preventing the need for insertion of temporary access and the associated risk of infection. Many renal centres have a policy that medical and nursing staff should avoid phlebotomy or cannulation into the forearms of patients with suspected renal disease. This precaution will help to prevent damage to vessels that may subsequently be required for fistula formation. Repeated use of subclavian central venous catheters prior to fistula formation can also

Before anastomosis

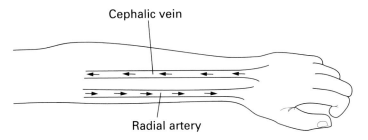

Cephalic vein

Radial artery

After anastomosis

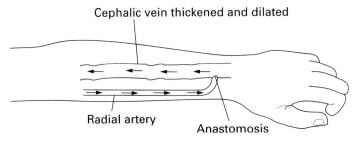

Cephalic vein thickened and dilated

Radial artery

Anastomosis

Figure 7.1 Arteriovenous fistula.

cause swollen arms and dilated chest veins following fistulae formation, so should be avoided.

Formation of the arteriovenous fistula

Preoperative care
Patients should be given every opportunity to participate in their plan of care and all aspects of treatment should be discussed with them. As part of the patient's predialysis preparation and education a full explanation of the surgical procedure and aftercare should be given to the patient. The patient may wish to visit and speak with someone who has a well-established functioning fistula to find out what it looks and feels like.

Information should include that the fistula will be cannulated each dialysis, often using a different site (see explanation of the rope ladder puncture, below), and the needles that will routinely be used should be available for the patient to see and examine. Patients should be well hydrated before surgery, and above their target weight if recently dialysed.

Postoperative care
In addition to routine postoperative care the nurse should ensure that the following specific postoperative care is carried out:

- The limb should be kept warm and well supported to help peripheral circulation.

- Blood pressure should be monitored closely and maintained at a minimum of 100 mmHg systolic. If the blood pressure falls below this, peripheral blood flow may be affected, with an increased risk of fistula thrombosis. It may be advisable to avoid antihypertensive therapy in the postoperative period.
- The wound site should be examined regularly for signs of excess bleeding or swelling.
- The blood flow through the fistula should be checked regularly by completing the following observations:
  — placing a stethoscope lightly over the incision, a 'whooshing' sound should be heard. This is called a bruit. The bruit should be loudest near the incision and it gradually becomes softer as the stethoscope is moved further up the vessel.
  — placing a hand lightly over the incision site, a buzzing sensation should be felt. This is called the thrill.
- The bruit and thrill should be checked regularly (half-hourly at first) and the patients should be taught how to perform these observations as soon as they are able.
- Before discharge the patient should be informed how to care for the fistula and advised to avoid using the fistula arm for carrying heavy loads and to avoid tight or restrictive clothing on the arm. Hand exercises (such as clenching and releasing pressure on a squash ball or small bandage) may promote fistula maturation. Additionally, the patient must be advised to inform non-renal doctors and nurses that the arm should never be used for phlebotomy, cannulation or for recording blood pressure, as all of these may result in permanent damage to the fistula.
- Patients should be advised to contact the hospital immediately if they notice bleeding, swelling or absence of bruit or thrill.

Complications of arteriovenous fistulae

Thrombosis
Thrombosis may occur in the immediate postoperative period or at a later date, sometimes following a hypotensive episode on dialysis. Surgical treatment (thrombectomy) may be indicated but salvage is often unsuccessful. Percutaneous angiopathy using a balloon catheter may be more successful (Rocek & Peregrin 2001). However, if reported promptly, permanent damage may be avoided by the use of thrombolytic agents.

Aneurysm
This can be caused by the repeated area puncture (Fig. 7.2). The skin eventually becomes much thinner as the aneurysms dilate. Cannulation in the aneurysm should be avoided.

Steal syndrome
The patient may complain of pain, oedema, coldness or 'pins and needles' as blood is 'stolen' from the hand as a result of the fistula (lower resistance

in the arteriovenous anastomosis). Surgical correction to restore blood supply to the hand is usually required, with subsequent loss to the fistula.

Cannulation of the arteriovenous fistulae

In the first instance the fistula should be allowed 2–3 months to mature before cannulation is attempted, to allow healing of the anastomosis and some development of the vessels. After this time the fistula can be safely cannulated but the procedure should only be undertaken by experienced practitioners.

New fistulae may be prone to extravasation and clotting which can be painful and distressing. Therefore, all attempts should be made to minimise trauma during the first few visits. If the patient is anxious, a local anaesthetic may be offered. Topical creams are a sensible choice (as subcutaneous injections rather defeat the object of painfree cannulation) but need to be applied at least 30 min before cannulation.

Prior to each cannulation a thorough physical examination of the fistula should be undertaken to check that there is no evidence of oedema, infection or bruising and that blood flow through the fistula is evident through the presence of the bruit and thrill.

The unit policy for strict asepsis and cleansing of the arm should be adhered to. Universal precautions should be employed, including wearing gloves, aprons and a face visor, as blood may splash into the face and eyes during cannulation. A tourniquet may be used prior to cannulation to help engorgement of the vessel but in well-established larger fistulae this is often unnecessary.

Cannulation protocols

Many units are now evaluating the use of planned protocols to insert fistula needles, with the aim of reducing complications and extending the longevity of the fistula. The effect of repeated puncture on fistulae was first described by Kronung (1984).

During each cannulation a small area of vessel tissue is displaced. When the needle is removed this area is filled with a thrombus. Scar tissue is then formed, resulting in increased tissue and subsequent elongation of the vessel wall. Over time this results in a loss of elasticity of the vessel and dilation results in aneurysm formation and adjacent stenosis.

Kronung (1984) described three methods of cannulation and the effects of each (Fig. 7.2). They are:

1. Rope ladder puncture: This describes the systematic use of the entire length of the vessel. Each needle is inserted at approximately 2 cm above the last site and back again, resulting in a uniform use of the vessel. This demonstrated less aneurysm formation as the punctures per area were reduced.
2. Area puncture: This describes the development and use of one or two areas of the fistula which are regularly used. This may result in increased aneurysm formation related to the number of repeated punctures over a small area causing increased tissue elongation and aneurysm formation.

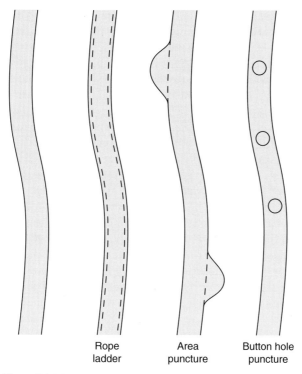

Rope ladder   Area puncture   Button hole puncture

Figure 7.2 Needle protocols. (Kronung 1984.)

3. Button hole puncture: This describes the repeated puncture of exactly the same site at exactly the same angle into exactly the same hole each dialysis. Over time cylindrical scar tissue develops, guiding the needle into the right place. It is suggested that the button hole technique results in less aneurysm formation.

Whilst the adoption of protocols may be beneficial and ensure high standards of uniform practice, it is acknowledged that additional evaluation is necessary to provide evidence for the long-term effects of any of these protocols on the longevity of fistulae. Hayes (1998) described the use of an access scoring system and staff cannulation programme to decrease access complications and increase staff competence. Both these initiatives are important in ensuring good standards of nephrology nursing practice.

Needle sets
The achievable blood flow for many patients is often underestimated. The careful selection of needles will ensure that optimum flows are obtained. Smaller needles (e.g. 16- and 17- gauge) produce high resistance as the blood pump is increased. This results in a 'sucking' effect of the needles and machine arterial alarms. Larger needles (14-g and 15-g) produce lower resistance and therefore avoid negative pressure as the blood pump speed is increased.

Needles should be inserted aseptically at 45° to the skin following appropriate skin preparation. The entire needle shaft should be inserted and the butterfly wing secured with tape. On insertion, a syringe should be attached to the end of the needle tubing and blood withdrawn. Any resistance to withdrawal may indicate that the needle position needs adjusting. Often the needle hole is occluded against the side of the vessel wall. This can be corrected by placing a small piece of sterile gauze under the butterfly: this will lift the needle externally and lower the needle tip internally. If flow still cannot be obtained the presence of a clot may be suspected or there may be complete misplacement of the needle. In this event the needle should be removed. Arterial and venous needles need to be placed at least 5 cm apart to avoid recirculation.

If the needle punctures the wall of the vessel extravasation will occur, resulting in a painful visible swelling around the site. The needle should be removed and firm pressure applied for about 10 min before further insertion is attempted. On no account should the nurse push and pull the needle blindly, hoping that the needle will finally find the vessel. This will result in much pain and discomfort for the patient and will bruise and damage the surrounding tissue, which may in turn cause permanent damage to the fistula.

It is also important that nurses, no matter how experienced, recognise their limitations in relation to cannulation. If a cannulation attempt has failed after more than two or three attempts, assistance should be sought from a colleague, as the increased anxiety of the nurse and patient may negatively influence further attempts at successfully siting the needle.

A review of arteriovenous fistula care can be found in Yang & Humphrey (2000).

Arteriovenous grafts (Fig. 7.3)

If the peripheral blood vessels are unsuitable for fistula formation the surgeon may decide to create a graft. Most grafts are created using synthetic materials such as polytetrafluoroethylene (PTFE). Grafts may be cannulated soon after insertion, preferably after 14 days.

The graft may be configured in a straight line or in a loop. Grafts are less compliant than fistulae, resulting in higher pressure through the vessels. Patients should be taught how to care for the graft in the same way as a fistula.

The nurse should perform the same predialysis physical examination prior to cannulation. Thorough skin preparation is vital and sterile gloves must be used for cannulation of grafts, as there is high infection risk. The arterial needle should be inserted at the arterial end of the graft at least 5 cm from the anastomosis site. The venous needle should be inserted in the venous end with the same considerations. For loop grafts it is important to identify the arterial and venous sides of the graft as incorrect needle placement will result in recirculation. Needles may be rotated through 90° following insertion (bevel of needle downwards), to reduce the risk of graft damage.

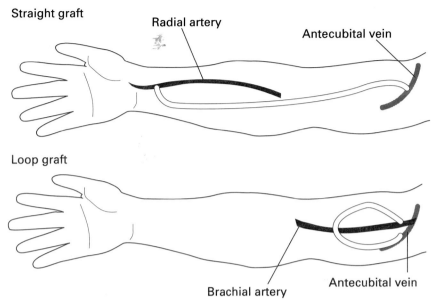

Figure 7.3 Arteriovenous graft configuration.

Vascular access standard

The Kidney Alliance (2001) has stated that the renal service in the UK should aim to have the percentage of new haemodialysis patients with natural AVF approach the European average of 66%. If this is to be achieved then there will be increasing pressure on nurses to care for AVF proactively and to ensure that only well-trained competent nurses carry out cannulation. Detailed ways in which the multiprofessional team can work together to achieve this aim are beyond the scope of this book, but Berkoben & Schwab (1995) provide a good review of how to prolong vascular access patency.

Percutaneous access (Fig. 7.4)

Percutaneous access is the term used to describe the insertion of a cannula or catheter into a major vein. Catheters may be inserted as a temporary measure, as in acute renal failure, or for temporary use whilst a fistula matures. Potential sites include the subclavian, femoral and internal jugular veins. The use of the subclavian vein is not recommended in patients with end-stage renal failure as this may adversely affect the success of the creation of an AVF due to central venous stenosis (Uldall 1996). Femoral catheters should only be used in those who are immobile and should be changed every 1–3 days.

More commonly, percutaneous catheters are being inserted as permanent access for patients whose fistulae have either failed or whose vessels are inadequate to attempt AVF creation in the first place. The permanent catheters are cuffed and inserted through the creation of a subcutaneous tunnel, as this ensures optimal placement of the catheter and helps reduce the rate of infection.

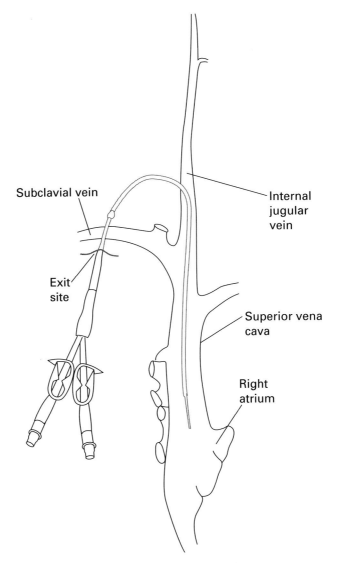

Figure 7.4 Permanent tunnelled percutaneous catheter.

Catheters may be single- or double-lumen depending on the unit's policy for single-needle or dual-needle dialysis. Catheters may be inserted under general or local anaesthetic and nursing care pre- and postoperatively will be the same as for any surgical procedure. Postinsertion it is essential that the correct placement of the catheter is checked by X-ray prior to dialysis as postinsertion complications may include pneumothorax and puncture of the adjacent vessels.

The nurse's responsibility includes the maintenance of catheter patency, patient education, prevention of infection and early intervention when infection occurs. Nurses caring for percutaneous access must demonstrate meticulous care, as defined by a strict unit policy. This policy should include the need for strict asepsis during any catheter intervention. The exit site should be examined before each dialysis and observed for signs of infection such as soreness, redness or the presence of exudate. Exit sites should be covered with a dressing that will maintain an optimum environment conducive to healing (not too wet and not too dry) and one that will repel *Staphylococcus aureus* (Wittich 2001). Many units use povidone-iodine to clean the exit site and then a non-occlusive dressing is applied. Ends of catheters should always be handled aseptically.

Patency

To maintain patency between dialysis treatments a bolus of heparin (usually 5000 iu mL^{-1}) equal to the volume of each catheter lumen is inserted. It is important that the exact volume of each respective lumen is ascertained to prevent giving a systemic dose of heparin to the patient.

Before the next dialysis treatment, the heparin lock should be removed by aspirating the catheter with a syringe and then flushing with 0.9% normal saline before connecting the dialysis lines. Nevertheless, clotting is a common complication. Several attempts may be needed to aspirate a clot in the catheter if resistance is felt. It is vital that any clot is removed and no attempt is made to flush a catheter which cannot be aspirated from either lumen. In permanent catheters, the administration of urokinase should dissolve the clot if all other methods have failed, and should be left for at least 30 min before or between dialysis sessions.

In dual-lumen catheters it is important to use the arterial and venous lumens appropriately. Occasionally, flow from the arterial lumen is partially occluded owing to poor positioning of the arterial holes against the side of the vessel wall. The lines may have to be reversed to achieve an acceptable blood flow, but it should be remembered that reversal of the lines will result in increased recirculation (Twardowski et al 1993).

Some authors are fearful that there is an increasing trend towards the use of central venous catheters, and Swartz et al (1997), whilst recognising this development, outline some ways in which these catheters can be best cared for.

Arteriovenous shunt (Fig. 7.5)

Until the early 1980s, the arteriovenous shunt was used as a method of access for both chronic and acute haemodialysis. Current use is rare and is generally limited to acute use for patients undergoing continuous renal replacement.

The creation of a shunt involves the surgical cut-down of the peripheral vessels of the forearm where the radial artery and cephalic vein are used, or the ankle where the posterior tibial artery and long saphenous vein are used (Uldall 1996). Teflon tips are inserted into the vessels and silicone tubing attached.

HAEMODIALYSIS EQUIPMENT

The dialyser

The dialyser is the functional unit of the extracorporeal circuit just as the nephron is the functional unit of the kidney, and some patients and nurses refer to the dialyser as the 'kidney'.

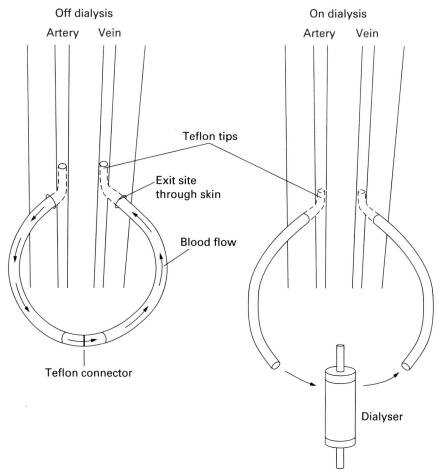

Figure 7.5 Arteriovenous shunt.

Manufacturers have made significant advances in the development of membranes which provide highly efficient clearance of waste products and which are biocompatible for the patient. There are two types of dialyser design: the hollow fibre and the parallel plate.

The hollow fibre dialyser (Fig. 7.6)
The hollow fibre dialyser is made up of thousands of hollow fibres or capillaries about the thickness of a human hair. The fibres are secured at each end of the cylindrically shaped dialyser in a polyurethane potting compound. Blood passes through the centre of each fibre like a straw, whilst the dialysate passes on the outside of the fibres in the opposite direction.

The parallel plate dialyser (Fig. 7.7)
The plate dialyser consists of sheets of membranes arranged in layers. Blood passes through the space between one set of layers whilst the dialysate passes through the adjacent layers in the opposite direction.

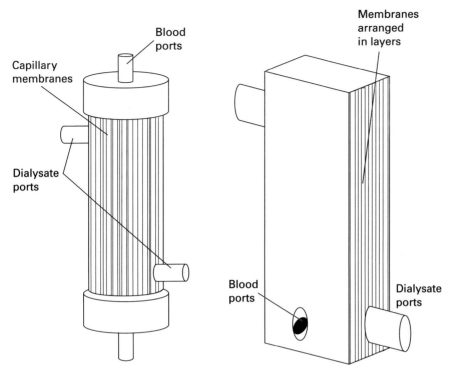

Figure 7.6 Hollow fibre dialyser.   **Figure 7.7** Parallel plate dialyser.

Plates have more compliance (stretch) than hollow fibre dialysers and therefore have higher priming volumes.

The membrane

The choice of membrane type is becoming increasingly important as part of the patient's individual dialysis prescription. In addition to selecting the membrane which provides the desired clearance and fluid removal, the nurse should also consider the issue of biocompatibility related to the patient's needs.

There exists a large and increasing variety of membrane types available, but these fall broadly into three categories, which are:

1. Cellulose membrane (e.g. Cuprophan): low flux
2. Modified cellulose membranes (e.g. cellulose acetate, cellulosynthetic such as Hemophan, cellulose triacetate): low or high flux
3. Synthetic membranes (e.g. polysulfone, polyacrilynitrile (PAN), polymethylmetacrylate (PMMA), polycarbonate (Gambrane) and polyamide): low or high flux

The efficiency with which a membrane clears water and solutes is described as its flux properties. Thin membranes with large pores are very permeable to water and large molecules and are called high-flux membranes as they have the ability to clear solutes with a molecular weight of up to 30 kDa. Low-flux membranes are less permeable to water and solutes but will provide adequate clearance of solutes up to molecular weight 10 kDa. The membrane's permeability to water is described as its ultra-filtration coefficient (KUf), and is measured in ml h^{-1} mmHg^{-1}—in other words, the number of millilitres per hour of fluid that is removed for every one unit of pressure across the membrane. The efficiency of solute clearance is measured by the mass transfer urea coefficient or KoA.

High-flux membranes have a high KUf (>10) and moderate-water-permeability membranes have a KUf of between 5 and 10 ml h^{-1} mmHg^{-1}. Details of the properties of each dialyser can be found on the dialyser specification sheet which is often provided with each box of dialysers.

Solute removal by modified cellulose and synthetic membranes is similar, although β_2-microglobulin clearance is greater with synthetic membranes, and this may translate into fewer amyloid dialysis deposits (Levy et al 2001).

Biocompatibility

The process of dialysis requires the repeated exposure of the patient's blood to foreign substances including the dialyser membrane, blood lines, dialysate, chemicals, drugs and water. These components of dialysis may initiate immunological responses which include activation of the complement system and release of cytokines involved in the inflammatory process and anaphylactic reactions. Improved biocompatibility may reduce amyloid deposition and give fewer hypersensitivity reactions and may give better long-term morbidity and mortality.

Haemodialysis is regarded as a sophisticated and safe procedure but the aim of correcting the patient's uraemia to improve quality of life may overshadow the fact that the procedure in itself may be a precipitating factor to many complications. In recognition of this, the issue of biocompatibility is becoming increasingly important. Major biocompatibility issues relate to dialyser membranes, methods of sterilisation and water purification.

Preparation of the dialyser

Priming and rinsing of the extracorporeal circuit is a crucial process in the preparation of the dialysis treatment. Manufacturers provide guidelines and recommendations for priming volume and rinsing time and these will vary depending on whether the dialyser is hollow fibre or parallel plate, the membrane type and the dialyser sterilising agent. There are two important aspects to consider:

1. The removal of air. Air must be removed from the blood lines and from all surfaces of the dialyser membranes. Pockets of air retained in the dialyser will result in less efficient dialysis and will promote clotting in the dialyser.
2. The removal of any chemicals or sterilising agents used during the dialyser manufacturing process. Of most concern is ethylene oxide (ETO), a gas which is a highly effective sterilant against all microorganisms. It may, however, have toxic effects and cause

hypersensitivity reactions in some patients (see section on first-use syndrome on p. 200). Alternative sterilising methods are now routinely used, including heat sterilisation and gamma radiation. Typically a minimum of 1L of saline is required to remove residual ETO.

Dialyser reuse

Most dialysers are packaged with a statement from the manufacturers indicating that the dialyser is for single use only. Many patient groups are very strongly against the practice of reuse of dialysers. Despite this, many centres reuse dialysers (up to 20 times) with no complications. The most significant advantage to reusing a dialyser is the cost saving achieved and this is often the driving force for commencing a reuse programme. The cost saving allows the selection and use of superior dialysers that are efficient and bio-compatible but these would be cost-prohibitive without a reuse programme. The Renal Association (1997) accepts that there are strong environmental arguments for reprocessing disposable medical equipment, and emphasises the importance of auditing the quality of the water, demonstrating that the dialyser has been washed free of the sterilant prior to use and confirming that the volume of the blood compartment has not been compromised.

The reprocessing of dialysers is a technical and time-consuming role. If a reuse programme is introduced, dedicated technicians should be employed and given training on all health and safety aspects of this procedure.

The dialysate

Dialysate is the term used to describe the fluid which is pumped through the dialyser on the opposite side of the semipermeable membrane to the patient's blood. The purpose of the dialysate is to create a concentration gradient to promote diffusion of waste products from the patient's blood.

Dialysate is produced by mixing a concentrated electrolyte solution (concentrate) with a buffer (bicarbonate) and purified water. Dialysate composition can be tailored to individual patient requirements (particularly potassium and calcium levels, and sodium levels if sodium profiling is being used to minimise hypotension) but on the whole the solution will be physiological, i.e. it will resemble normal serum biochemistry with specific deviations (Table 7.1).

Table 7.1 Concentration of substances in blood and a typical dialysate

Blood	Solute	Dialysate
133–144	Sodium (mmol L^{-1})	132–155
3.3–5.3	Potassium (mmol L^{-1})	0–3.0
2.5–6.5	Urea (mmol L^{-1})	0
60–120	Creatinine (mmol L^{-1})	0
2.2–2.6	Calcium (mmol L^{-1})	1.25–2.0
0.85	Magnesium (mmol L^{-1})	0.25–0.75
4.0–6.6	Glucose (g L^{-1})	0–10
22–30	Bicarbonate (mmol L^{-1})	30–40

Water

Patients on maintenance haemodialysis are exposed to approximately 400 L of dialysis water per week (Ismail et al 1996). Because of this level of exposure, water should be considered a drug (Schulman 1996). Water contains many contaminants that pose a potential risk to the patient. Examples of major contaminants include aluminium (with associated risks of dementia and osteomalacia), chloramines (haemolysis and anaemia), fluoride (osteomalacia, osteoporosis), calcium, magnesium (hard-water syndrome), copper (haemolysis and liver damage), zinc (anaemia) and endotoxins (pyrogenic reactions).

Methods of water treatment

1. A reverse osmosis unit uses a semipermeable membrane to filter water and works by rejecting 90–95% of univalent and divalent ions in addition to microbiological contaminants.
2. Water softeners remove calcium and magnesium by ion exchange.
3. Carbon filters adsorb chlorine, organic contaminants and chloramines.
4. Sediment filters remove particulate matter (Ismail et al 1996).

Standards for water quality have existed for many years, but in many countries in Europe there is no legal obligation to comply with the European Phamacopoeia and testing is not mandatory. Water should be regularly analysed to measure endotoxin levels and numbers of organisms to ensure that they do not exceed the standard for the dialysis unit. There is evidence however that many European dialysis facilities do not routinely check the quality of their water (Lindley et al 2000). Research by the European Dialysis and Transplant Nurses' Association/European Renal Care Association (EDTNA/ERCA) surveyed the treatment of water for dialysis in almost 70 participating centres in 14 countries, and as a result EDTNA/ERCA is working on best practice guidelines for microbiological monitoring. An excellent article by Lindley et al (2000) provides the reader with further information.

Dialysate composition

Sodium

Standard sodium concentrations are set at approximately 140 mmol L^{-1}. Below this level the patient may suffer symptoms such as hypotension, muscle cramps and disequilibrium. Levels higher than this may cause thirst and hypertension. Many machines now offer the option of programming a variable sodium concentration. This sodium profiling allows the nurse to tailor the sodium concentrations to the individual patient's needs. Protocols differ however, with some preferring high early concentrations of sodium when maximum fluid removal is taking place, whilst others prefer high late concentrations when symptoms are most severe. There do appear to be some benefits of sodium profiling for some patients, and Palmer (1999) provides further reading.

Potassium

Many renal patients present for dialysis with raised potassium levels. Standard dialysate concentration is 1.0–2.0 mmol L^{-1} which will allow for steady and efficient removal of potassium. Patients who routinely present with lower potassium levels or those who are dialysing for the first time should dialyse against a solution containing 3.0 mmol L^{-1}.

Calcium

Dialysate calcium should be lowered (1.25 mmol L^{-1}) if the patient has hypercalcaemia or uncontrollable hyperparathyroidism.

Buffers (acetate and bicarbonate)

Haemodialysis patients tend towards a moderate to severe acidosis. The aim of the buffer in dialysis is to normalise the patient's acid–base balance as far as possible. Bicarbonate is the body's major buffer and is the preferred choice to use in the dialysate.

The use of acetate is largely historical and there is no feasible argument for its use as a first choice. In the early days of dialysis bicarbonate was the buffer used but this caused many operational problems, largely due to dialysate preparation. In the 1960s acetate was used as an alternative to bicarbonate, so acetate dialysis became the norm and was convenient and cheap to use. Acetate is an organic ion which generates bicarbonate when metabolised. Metabolism in the body takes place in the muscle cells and the mitochondria of the liver. However, as dialysis techniques have become increasingly efficient, the disadvantages of acetate have become apparent. Symptomatic hypotension, nausea and vomiting and dialysis fatigue were shown to increase with acetate dialysis and to decrease or disappear with bicarbonate dialysis.

A patient's ability to metabolise acetate is considered critical. It is essential that patients are able to metabolise acetate at a rate equal to the rate at which they lose bicarbonate. Patients who are at risk of poor metabolism include those with reduced muscle mass and those with liver failure (Ledebo 1990).

The Renal Association (1997) has recommended that all units move towards the universal availability of bicarbonate dialysis, and bicarbonate cartridges are now widely used.

Anticoagulation

As blood comes into contact with the extracorporeal circuit the clotting cascade will be initiated. Optimal anticoagulation regimes, like all aspects of the dialysis prescription, should be tailored to the needs of the individual patient. Heparin is the most commonly used anticoagulant for haemodialysis: the average patient receives approximately 1.5 million units per year (Vienken & Bowry 1993). A baseline clotting time should be recorded before the anticoagulation regime is commenced. An activated clotting time is the most commonly used method of monitoring, and automated methods are available whereby the blood is added to an activating agent in an assay tube and the time taken for clotting to occur is recorded.

For standard heparinisation a value of 1.5–2.0 of the baseline (approximately 180–250 s) should be aimed for during dialysis, with a reducing value towards the end of dialysis. Usually a bolus dose of heparin is given at the start of dialysis and then a continuous infusion set at a rate to maintain the clotting times within predetermined limits.

Reduced heparin should be used for patients who are at risk of bleeding or who are dialysed preoperatively. Activated clotting times within the range of approximately 150–180 s are acceptable. The clotting time should be monitored every hour.

Heparin-free dialysis should be performed for patients who have a bleeding disorder or who are considered to be at risk from bleeding, i.e. postoperatively. Heparin-free dialysis requires excellent priming of lines and dialyser before dialysis to remove air, a rapid blood flow (at least 250 mL min^{-1}), frequent flushing (every 15–30 min) of the lines with normal saline (the additional saline must be accounted for in the total ultrafiltration volume) and close monitoring and observation of the blood lines and dialyser for clotting.

Further reading on anticoagulation can be found in a very good overview by Ouseph & Ward (2000). Other types of anticoagulation, such as low-molecular-weight heparin, are described in an overview by De Vos (2000).

The haemodialysis machine (the monitor)

The haemodialysis machine is simply a monitor to ensure the safe delivery of dialysis to the patient (Fig. 7.8). State-of-the-art machines offer impressive and sophisticated systems which can assist the nurse to deliver a wide range of treatment options. It is important that the nurse remembers that the patient, and not the machine, is the focal point in all nursing interventions. Despite the huge variances, machines are all broadly separated into two component parts—the blood monitor and the fluid monitor.

The blood monitor

Blood pump
Peristaltic blood pumps are integral to the machine. Blood pumps can be set to deliver blood flow rates of between 0 and 600 mL min^{-1}.

Air detector
An ultrasonic detector is situated at the venous chamber. The detector will detect air bubbles or the lowering of the level within the drip chamber. An audible alarm will sound and the venous line will clamp, preventing the risk of administering air to the patient.

Air detector   Venous drip chamber   Normal saline   Blood pump   Heparin

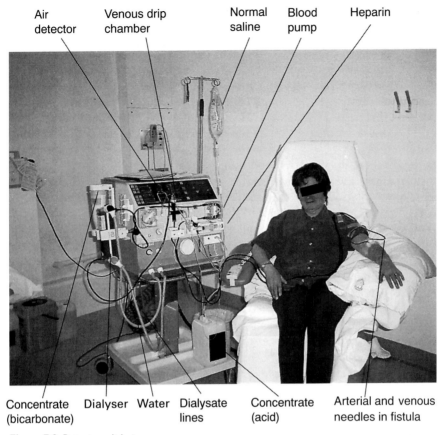

Concentrate (bicarbonate)   Dialyser   Water   Dialysate lines   Concentrate (acid)   Arterial and venous needles in fistula

Figure 7.8 Patient on dialysis.

Arterial and venous clamps

These clamps close the respective lines automatically if there is an alarm. They are also used to regulate the blood flow in single-needle dialysis.

Venous pressure monitor

Venous pressure is monitored continuously during treatment. A transducer monitors the venous pressure through an isolator attached to the venous chamber. Alarm limits can be set to alert the nurse to significant changes in venous pressure. High venous pressure can be caused by incorrect positioning of the fistula needle, a clot within the needle, vessel stenosis or occluded blood lines.

Arterial pressure monitor

This can be monitored either via a transducer which is the same as the venous pressure or with an arterial sac and a sensor plate. If the arterial flow is reduced the sac will collapse, causing the sensor plate to trigger an alarm. Low arterial pressure can be caused by incorrect positioning of the needle (against the wall of the vessel), a clot within the needle, vessel stenosis or a poorly developed fistula (source failure).

The fluid monitor

Temperature
The machine can provide dialysate temperature between 30 and 40°C. High temperatures increase the risk of haemolysis and hypotension due to vasodilation. Low temperatures result in less efficient dialysis and hypothermia. Within reason the patient can adjust the temperature for comfort. Low temperature dialysis is an efficient way of cooling the patient with pyrexia.

Conductivity
In the machine the correct proportion of concentrate electrolytes to water is measured by the electrical conductivity of the solution. Conductivity is usually set at between 13 and 14 mS. If the dialysis solution is more dilute or concentrated than the set standard the machine will alarm and the dialysate flow will be cut off. A pH meter will ensure that the correct acid and base concentrates are used; this is important for safety in bicarbonate haemodialysis.

Blood leak detector
A small leak or larger rupture of the dialyser membrane will result in blood escaping into the dialysate. A detector on the dialysate outflow line will sense this and the machine will alarm. The effluent dialysate should be tested for blood in this instance using a urine testing stick. Large leaks are serious, as there is a risk that the dialysate will enter the patient's blood. In this instance dialysis should be discontinued without returning the blood to the patient.

Bypass valve
If there is an alarm related to the dialysate, e.g. a blood leak, conductivity alarm or temperature alarm, the dialysate flow will be diverted from the dialyser via the bypass valve. This enables the patient to remain on the dialysis machine without risk whilst the problem is rectified.

Ultrafiltration control
Current machines achieve ultrafiltration by volume control or by flow sensors rather than by pressure control. With pressure control, the TMP is calculated by the machine as the difference between the pressure in the dialyser blood compartment and the dialysate compartment. For example, if the venous pressure is +50 mmHg and the dialysate pressure is –150 mmHg, the TMP will equal 200 mmHg (50 – (–150) = 200). With volume control, machines can respond to pressure drops in the dialyser and compensate for them with a resultant accuracy of around ± 50 mL h^{-1}.

Modern machines may also have the facility to monitor blood volume by optical or ultrasonic sensors (to assess risk of hypotension), to assess recirculation and to calculate delivered dialysis dose from the online measurement of urea removal.

Single-needle dialysis
When two needles are used for dialysis there are, in effect, two separate blood pathways—one removing blood from the patient and the second

returning blood to the patient. Single-needle dialysis is ideally used for those patients with good established access. The use of single-needle dialysis for patients with failing access should be discouraged (Aldridge 1991). If, however, access is a problem, single-needle dialysis can be considered as a temporary measure to enable the patient to dialyse (albeit inadequately) if only one needle can be inserted, if the patient has a single-lumen catheter, or if one lumen of a dual-lumen catheter is blocked.

To facilitate the treatment a Y-connector is attached to the single source of access. Once the blood flow has been established through the circuit, the single-needle mode is activated. This initiates the alternate clamping of the arterial and venous lines to control the blood flow through the dialyser. Blood is removed from the patient with the venous line on the machine clamped. This will cause the venous pressure to rise. When the pressure reaches a predetermined limit the pump will stop, the arterial clamp will close and the venous clamp will open, allowing the blood to return to the patient under pressure by gravity. During single-needle dialysis, some plate dialysers are compliant enough to accommodate the extra volume of blood in the extracorporeal circuit. Hollow fibre dialysers are not, and therefore a compliance chamber must be added to the circuit to prevent rupture of the dialyser membrane. During a 4-h treatment there will be a reduction in the total volume of blood processed through the dialyser in comparison with dual-needle dialysis. In addition, there will be recirculation of dialysed blood around the Y-connector and catheter, resulting in a further reduction of dialysed blood volume. The use of a second pump in the circuit increases the total volume of blood processed through the dialyser.

PRESCRIBING THE DIALYSIS DOSE

For many years patients were given dialysis treatments based entirely on the subjective evaluation of blood biochemistry along with a general assessment of perceived patient well-being. Patients themselves have been held responsible for the success of their treatment in relation to these parameters by being instructed to comply with restricted diets aimed at maintaining biochemistry within acceptable limits. Limited resources and lack of understanding have compounded this philosophy over time.

More recently there have been attempts to provide a more objective and scientific method of assessing dialysis adequacy. The aims of nursing care, utilising the dose of dialysis and nutritional parameters, should be to measure dialysis adequacy as well as encouraging patients to eat well.

Urea kinetic modelling

Many years ago the direct relationship between dialysis dose and long-term patient survival was demonstrated (Lowrie et al 1981). Today, the positive correlation between good dialysis adequacy and dialysis outcome also exists (Charra 2000). It is therefore essential that dialysis prescription is aimed at preventing or reducing the mortality and morbidity of patients receiving haemodialysis. High levels of urea clearance are correlated with improved patient outcomes.

One method of determining the dose is by the use of Kt/V. Kt/V is estimated by measuring pre- and postdialysis urea concentrations. K equals the dialyser clearance of urea, t equals the treatment time and V equals the amount of urea distributed in the body water.

To complete the equation it is necessary to know the clearance of urea through the dialyser. This is estimated by the pre- and postdialysis urea ratio. To ensure an accurate assessment of V the nutritional status of the patient must be optimised, ensuring that the patient has an adequate protein intake. The patient's weight, height and gender are included in the calculation to estimate the percentage of body weight that is water (usually 55% in women and 65% in men).

For accurate assessment of K it is essential to calculate the pre- and postdialysis urea ratio. The dialyser data sheet may be cautiously used to estimate the dialyser clearance but it is wise to assume a 10–20% reduction on the manufacturers' in vitro values. An approximate example is given but more precise information is essential (i.e. the patient's height, etc.) for accurate calculation. For example:

A woman weighs 60 kg, therefore, an approximate estimation of $V = 33$l

$$K = 150 \text{ ml min}^{-1}, t = 4 \text{ h (240 min)}, K \times t = 36 \text{ l } (150 \times 240 = 36\ 000 \text{ ml}),$$
$$\text{divided by } V = 36/33 = 1.09.$$

Therefore $Kt/V = 1.09$

Measuring the urea reduction ratio (URR) is possibly the simplest method of determining dialysis adequacy. This is expressed as a percentage reduction:

$$\text{URR} = 100 \times (1—Ct/Co)$$

where Ct = postdialysis urea and Co = predialysis urea.

These parameters can now provide an acceptable standard for dialysis dose. The Renal Association (1997) recommends the following: URR of 65% or a Kt/V of greater than 1.2 in patients dialysing three times per week. However, it should be noted that these recommendations are individual targets which each patient should reach or exceed, and if a patient is found to be receiving less than this amount, steps should be taken to increase the blood flow, the dialyser size or the duration of dialysis.

The Kidney Alliance (2001) states that haemodialysis adequacy should be assessed regularly and the above targets should be achieved in more than 90% of patients. Haemodialysis should be provided three times per week for >90% of patients (Case Study 7.1).

The mathematical concepts of urea kinetic modelling (UKM) can be complicated but there are many computer software packages available to complete the calculations and to advise on corrective measures to achieve the desired Kt/V. However, it is important to be aware that there is no internationally agreed method for measuring Kt/V in everyday practice (Renal Association 1997).

Some of these computer packages also measure protein catabolic rate, and this has been shown to be an increasingly important variable in patient morbidity and mortality, as it estimates daily protein intake (see Ch. 9).

■ CASE STUDY 7.1

An 85-year-old woman with renal failure secondary to diabetes mellitus was dialysing for 4 h twice a week. Following adequacy studies, the nurses found a Kt/V of 0.9 on two consecutive measurements taken 3 months apart. It was likely that the value of Kt/V had dropped because of recent blood flow difficulties with her permanent central venous catheter.

As increasing the blood pump speed was not possible, and a large dialyser was already in use, it was proposed that this patient should attend the dialysis unit three times a week to improve her dialysis dose. The patient was very reluctant to do this.
- What benefits of increasing the Kt/V could be explained to this patient?
- Is it the quantity or quality of dialysis that is important in this case?
- Who should be involved in making the final decision about dialysis treatment times?

What is vital is a clear understanding of the need for highly accurate sampling of pre- and postdialysis blood specimens and the comprehensive dietary support of the patient. Postdialysis samples are of particular importance and the method described by Priester Coary & Daugirdas (1997) is recommended by the Renal Association (1997). Another significant role of the nurse is to ensure the delivery of the prescribed dialysis and to understand the effect of deviations in treatment on the dialysis dose and the subsequent effect this may have on the patient's well-being:

- Prescribed dialysis dose versus delivered dialysis dose: the dialysis prescription may be affected by a number of events that will effectively reduce the dialysis dose.
- Errors of time (t): the patient starts dialysis late; the machine is in bypass due to concentrate running out; there is another machine fault or isolated ultrafiltration; the patient comes off dialysis early.
- Errors of clearance (K): blood flow is reduced; the wrong dialyser selected; there is recirculation.
- Errors of volume (V): residual renal function increases or decreases; there is excessive or inadequate protein intake; there is incorrect sampling.

High-flux/high-efficiency dialysis by Kt/V measurement and high-flux membrane dialysis treatment time can be shortened using rapid blood and dialysate flow rates. The benefits for the patient of less time on dialysis may be outweighed by the potential complications such as increased hypotensive episodes. The use of short high-efficiency treatments is controversial—the long-term survival of patients has been correlated with longer treatment times (Charra et al 1996).

PREPARATION FOR HAEMODIALYSIS

The period of time from diagnosis to commencement of RRT may be sudden, but often there is a period of time from a few months to several years when patients will have time to adjust their lifestyle and prepare for whichever form of dialysis is appropriate. The need for predialysis care, including psychological support as well as clinical monitoring of the progression of the renal failure, cannot be overemphasised (see Ch. 3 for further reading).

All patients with chronic renal failure and a plasma creatinine above 150 mmol L^{-1} and/or significant proteinuria (<1 g 24 h^{-1}) should be referred to a specialist nephrologist. Those with a creatinine above 300 μmol L^{-1} should be referred urgently. Structured education and counselling for those approaching end stage renal failure should be given by the multidisciplinary team (Kidney Alliance 2001). For further information regarding predialysis care, refer to Chapter 5.

For those requiring long-term haemodialysis there are a number of options to be considered in relation to the location of the haemodialysis treatment.

In-centre haemodialysis

Regional dialysis centres may provide both an acute and chronic haemodialysis service. In-centre haemodialysis may be offered, but the service may be overstretched in terms of available dialysis space. For this reason the options of home haemodialysis or satellite haemodialysis should be explored for those who choose haemodialysis.

Home haemodialysis

The patient who expresses a desire to take the home haemodialysis treatment option should receive support and encouragement from the multidisciplinary team. The patient, once established and familiar with the dialysis regime, may want to learn the technique quickly in order to be self-supporting at home at the earliest possible time. With support and cooperation a training programme can be completed in 6 weeks if the patient is well and has no other complications such as poor access, but most training programmes aim to get the patient home within 12 weeks.

To optimise training and learning opportunities the patient can be encouraged to come to the unit on non-dialysis days to practise lining and priming the machine. Partners should be encouraged to attend as often as they can, but will need to negotiate a minimum amount of time with the nurse to learn emergency procedures. It should be emphasised to the patient and partner that the overall management of the treatment (setting up, monitoring and discontinuing the treatment) is primarily the responsibility of the patient. The partner is there to provide support and help, not to accept complete responsibility for the procedure.

Although there is evidence that home haemodialysis is declining in popularity in the UK (Ansell & Feest 2000), Lunts (2001) believes that patients maintain independence and have better outcomes if they choose to dialyse at home.

Satellite haemodialysis

The availability of satellite dialysis is increasing within the UK. Satellite centres provide an ideal setting for patients on maintenance haemodialysis.

The centres are community-based, closer to the patient's home, making them more convenient and accessible. Satellite centres are essentially nurse-managed and led. A nephrologist will oversee patient dialysis prescription and consultation, but day-to-day dialysis management is the responsibility of the nurse.

ASSESSMENT OF THE PATIENT (Fig. 7.9)

Before dialysis, the nurse must carry out a comprehensive predialysis assessment. This includes discussing any concerns the patient may have in general or about the last dialysis session, reading the notes of the previous dialysis session and asking about any intradialytic problems. Measurement of blood pressure, fluid allowance and clinical assessment all contribute to the correct dry-weight assessment.

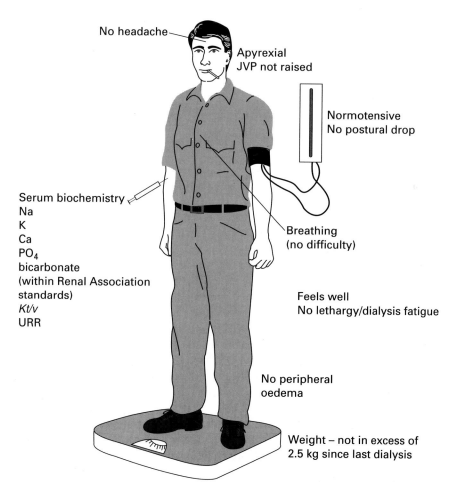

Figure 7.9 Predialysis assessment and postdialysis evaluation. JVP, jugular venous pressure; URR, urea reduction ratio.

Weight

Regular assessment of dry weight is essential to enable the nurse and patient to determine the amount of fluid removal required during dialysis. One kilogram is equal to 1 L of fluid, meaning that patient weight is a simple and accurate method of assessing fluid gain or loss between dialysis treatments. The term 'dry weight' refers to the weight at which there is no clinical evidence of oedema, shortness of breath, increased jugular venous pressure or hypo-/hypertension.

The initial determination of dry weight should involve the expertise of the nurse, doctor and dietitian. However, on a day-to-day basis this remains the responsibility of the nurse and many nurses are now trained in the routine clinical skills of fluid assessment.

The aim of dialysis is to remove the excess volume of fluid to ensure that the patient comes off dialysis at the dry weight. To calculate this, the following formula is used:

Actual weight	68.5 kg
Dry weight	66 kg
Weight gain	2.5 kg
Add any additional fluid intake during treatment	Washback of saline (300 mL) Two drinks (300 mL)
Total fluid to be removed	2.5 + 0.3 + 0.3 = 3.1 L

Blood pressure

Blood pressure should be recorded predialysis to provide a baseline from which to measure any significant changes during treatment. If a patient is overloaded prior to dialysis, blood pressure may be raised due to an increased circulating volume. Patients who are hypertensive as a result of their underlying renal disease may be prescribed antihypertensive medication. If these patients become hypotensive on dialysis it may be necessary to omit the dose before or nearest to the next dialysis session. Recommended target blood pressures should be <140/90 mmHg for those less than 60 years of age and <16/90 mmHg for those more than 60 years (Renal Association 1997). A good review article exploring hypertension in those in dialysis (Luik et al 1997) offers further reading.

Temperature and pulse

The patient's temperature should be routinely recorded predialysis, particularly if a temporary central line is being used. Pyrexia prior to dialysis should be investigated immediately. Pulse should be recorded on all patients.

Serum biochemistry and haematology

Blood tests are routinely carried out monthly but more frequent tests may be ordered as necessary. Target predialysis values recommended by the Renal Association (1997) are:

- Potassium: 3.5–6.5 mmol L^{-1}
- Phosphate: 1.2–1.7 mmol

- Calcium: total calcium within the normal range quoted by the local pathology laboratory, corrected for serum albumin concentration
- Haemoglobin: >10 g dL^{-1}, although at the time of writing there is evidence that >11 g dL^{-1} should be aimed for.

Anaemia management is an increasingly important issue for those caring for patients with renal disease, and many renal units are now employing specialist anaemia coordinators. Further reading on anaemia management can be found in Lewis et al (2000) and Macdougall (1999).

Infection control

The Rosenheim report (1972) set standards for infection control in relation to hepatitis B in renal units. Now patients and staff within renal units must acknowledge daily the risks associated, not just with hepatitis B, but with other blood-borne viruses (BBV) such as hepatitis C and human immuno-deficiency virus (HIV). A review of the Rosenheim report is currently in progress. It is generally accepted that carriers of hepatitis B should be dialysed separately on dedicated machinery, and carriers of hepatitis C should be dialysed in separate or single shifts, on dedicated machines but not necessarily isolated in separate rooms.

The practicalities of providing isolation for every patient with BBV will need to be explored along with the desired philosophy of care towards patients with BBV. Whilst the identification of patients with hepatitis is, on the whole, accepted, the screening of patients for HIV is controversial and nurses must ensure that they advocate for patients and are satisfied that the rationale for testing is in the patient's interests and is only carried out with informed consent. The Renal Association (1997) recommends testing every 3 months for hepatitis B surface antigen (HbsAg), every 6 months for hepatitis C and annually for HIV. Some units only screen for HIV for those awaiting transplantation. An annual test for HbsAg is sufficient for those who have demonstrated immunity, and all long-term patients on dialysis should be immunised against HBV.

Facilities and policies for the containment of methicillin-resistant staphylococcus aureus (MRSA) in renal units must be available and should be drawn up with the local infection control team. Patients colonised with MRSA must be isolated form other patients (Renal Association 1997). Universal precautions should be used as standard practice in the haemodialysis unit for the protection of the patients and the staff. Universal precautions require that body fluids of all patients are treated as potentially infectious and therefore protocols for hand-washing, protective clothing, eyewear and disinfection of machinery should be strictly adhered to prior to nursing interventions with all patients. When universal precautions are used effectively the isolation of patients should be unnecessary unless it is to protect the immunocompromised patient from opportunistic infections.

Commencing dialysis

On completion of the pre-dialysis assessment and preparation of the access, the nurse should complete an additional machine check before connecting the patient to the machine. It is also necessary to ensure that the priming and rinsing have been optimal and that additional rinsing is completed if the machine has been left to stand. On connection, careful attention must be paid to both the patient and the extracorporeal circuit at this vital time. As the blood passes through the lines the nurse ensures that there are no obstructions to flow, no air is visible in the line and that all connections are secure. Those dialysing for the first time may be alarmed at the sight of their blood travelling through the circuit and should be reassured.

Blood flow through the extracorporeal circuit

Blood is pulled from the patient by the blood pump through the arterial line by negative pressure. Once the blood has passed the occluding pump rollers, the pressure then becomes positive and the blood is pushed through the circuit. Heparin is infused on the positive-pressure side to prevent heparin, or air, or both, being sucked into the circuit.

The blood is pumped through the arterial end (top) of the dialyser and leaves the dialyser at the venous end (bottom). The blood then passes through the venous chamber and returns to the patient via the venous needle.

Flow through the fluid monitor

Purified water is taken into the machine via the water inlet port at the back of the machine. It is then heated, degassed and mixed with the concentrated electrolyte solution to make the dialysate. The machine will measure the correct proportioning of the solution through the conductivity meter. Dialysate enters the dialyser at the venous end (bottom) and leaves the dialyser at the arterial end (top) to maintain countercurrent flow between the blood and the dialysate. The dialysate is pulled through the circuit by a pump situated at the outflow line, resulting in negative pressure in the machine dialysate circuit.

Completing dialysis

Before completing dialysis the nurse must make sure that the prescribed dose has been delivered and that time has been added for any lost dialysis when the machine has been in bypass. The total ultrafiltrate volume should be checked. Postdialysis blood samples should be taken if required from the arterial access with the venous line clamped prior to washback with saline. The blood pump should be stopped and the arterial and venous lines clamped. The arterial line is then disconnected from the arterial needle and connected to a bag of 0.9% normal saline. Once connected, the clamps on both lines are removed and the pump is restored, allowing the saline to push the blood through the circuit back to the patient. When the lines are clear (rosé wine colour in the venous chamber) the pump can be stopped and the lines clamped. The lines can be disconnected and the machine stripped and put into disinfect mode. The needles can then be removed or, if there is percutaneous access, the catheter flushed and the heparin lock installed.

Postdialysis clinical observations of blood pressure and weight are completed to check that the patient has lost the desired weight and is not hypo-/hypertensive. It is important that patients are advised to wait until blood pressure is normalised, particularly if they are travelling home alone.

HAEMODIALYSIS COMPLICATIONS

Continuous and progressive development of equipment and expertise has ensured that haemodialysis is a safe procedure and, if prescribed and monitored correctly, serious complications should be rare. The treatment should only be carried out under the supervision of an expert practitioner. The aim of nursing care should be to prevent the occurrence of complications through comprehensive assessment and planning.

Hypotension

Hypotension will occur if the rate of fluid removal in the dialyser exceeds the plasma refilling rate in the patient. Some measures can help to limit the risk of hypotension, including advising the patient to ensure that interdialytic weight gains are not excessive. Intake of fluid remains a difficult aspect of treatment for patients to control. In addition to beverages, fluid contained in food will need to be accounted for. Time and patience must be afforded to patients when they are attempting to grasp the principles and realise the consequences of poor fluid control.

Sodium profiling (discussed previously in this chapter) may assist in reducing the risk of hypotension. Another method of potentially reducing the risk of hypotension related to slow plasma refilling is the use of the haematocrit and blood volume monitor. Some machines have this device as an integral part of the machine, but a separate monitor can be used. Changes in blood volume are measured through the haematocrit and oxygen saturation of the blood. The monitor will alarm when the patient is at risk of hypotension.

Nausea and vomiting

Nausea and vomiting may be associated with hypotension. This may either be before a hypotensive episode, i.e. the patient has nausea, vomits and then becomes hypotensive, or, conversely, the patient is hypotensive first, is revived with intravenous saline and then vomits subsequently. It may be helpful for some patients if they refrain from eating a meal until dialysis is complete.

Cramp

Cramp is another common side-effect of haemodialysis. Cramps, as with hypotension, may be caused by the ultrafiltration rate being set too high, causing rapid fluid shifts. Patients with cramp in the leg or foot may wish to stand up and push the foot against the floor to help relieve the pain. This should be avoided where possible as simultaneous hypotension will result in the patient falling to the floor. Pressure can be applied to the foot by allowing the patient to push the foot against the nurse. The use of a heat pad and/or vigorously rubbing the painful area may also help.

Disequilibrium

Dialysis relies upon the diffusion of solute across the semipermeable membrane of the dialyser. At the same time diffusion will be taking place across the semipermeable membranes between all body compartments from the intracellular, interstitial and intravascular compartments. The rate of diffusion should be equal to maintain equilibrium. If diffusion in the dialyser is highly efficient, the result will be disequilibrium in the body compartments. Rapid urea removal will result in the plasma in the intravascular compartment being hypotonic to the fluid in the cells. This will result in osmotic shifts of fluid from a region of low concentration to a region of high concentration. This is particularly significant in the cerebrospinal fluid and brain cells. Additionally, rapid changes in the pH of the cerebrospinal fluid may predispose to disequilibrium (Bregman et al 1994).

Symptoms of disequilibrium can be mild or severe. Mild symptoms may include headache, dizziness, nausea and vomiting, or disorientation. Severe symptoms include fits, coma and potentially death.

Patients who are acutely ill, have a very high urea predialysis or who are dialysed for the first time, are considered most at risk of disequilibrium. For those considered at risk the nurse undertakes the following dialysis prescription to ensure that the blood urea level is only reduced by a maximum of 30%.

- Blood flow rates should not exceed 150–200 mL min^{-1}.
- Dialysers with low surface area should be used.
- Treatment time is limited to approximately 2 h.

This type of prescription may need to be performed daily until the patient is considered stable and risk of disequilibrium is reduced. If disequilibrium is suspected the dialysis should be discontinued: infusion of hypertonic solutions such as mannitol may help to correct the fluid shifts.

Dialyser reactions (membrane reaction/first-use syndrome)

Allergic responses may occur as the patient's blood is exposed to foreign materials. Some examples include the dialyser membrane, the chemical sterilising agents such as ETO, and bacteria or endotoxin (Hoenich & van Holder 1993). Allergic reactions can be type A or type B (Daugirdas 2000). Type A is a severe anaphylactic reaction usually occurring within the first 5 min of dialysis. Symptoms can begin with an itchy rash and become severe, including dyspnoea and a burning sensation throughout the body. There may be laryngeal oedema and possibly cardiac arrest.

Treatment necessitates the immediate discontinuation of dialysis; the blood should not be returned to the patient. Maintenance of the airway is paramount and the administration of oxygen is required. The administration of adrenaline (epinephrine), chlorphenamine (chlorpheniramine) and hydrocortisone may be necessary.

Patients who have suffered this type of reaction should be dialysed against membranes which have been steam-sterilised. Extra rinsing of the dialysis circuit may also be advised.

Type B reactions are less severe and include chest pain, and may occur up to 1 h after dialysis is commenced. The cause is unknown but it is suggested that the use of synthetic membrane and/or reuse is beneficial (Bregman et al 1994).

Haemolysis

Haemolysis is the damage or rupture of red blood cells. As most of the body's potassium is contained within the cells, massive haemolysis can quickly lead to hyperkalaemia and cardiac arrest. Haemolysis may be caused by dialysing against dialysate that is too hot or dialysing against water or hypotonic dialysate.

Modern blood pumps have low shearing stresses and should not cause haemolysis but, if wrongly adjusted, the rollers of the blood pump may cause damage to cells. The high venous pressure resulting from occluded or obstructed (kinked) venous access or blood lines may also damage red blood cells. The patient will complain of chest pain and dyspnoea and may be in a state of collapse. If haemolysis is suspected the dialysis should immediately be discontinued and the blood should not be returned to the patient. Another machine should be prepared as a standby, as emergency dialysis may be needed to treat hyperkalaemia.

Air embolism

Modern monitoring equipment with integral ultrasonic air detectors provides some assurance to patients and nurses for the prevention of air embolism. But the equipment is only as good as its user and strict adherence to alarm and safety checks prior to initiating each treatment is essential.

Extreme care should be taken during the priming procedure and when connecting the patient to the extracorporeal circuit. The air detector should be activated during the priming procedure, and any problems with false alarms resolved prior to the patient commencing dialysis. An air detector which persistently or intermittently alarms with no obvious cause should not be accepted as troublesome or oversensitive. The machine should not be used, and should be sent to the technicians for service.

In the event of a patient receiving an air embolus the nurse must stop dialysis and lay the patient on the left side with the head lower than the rest of the body. This will force air in the circulation into the ventricle which is said to act as a bubble trap (Daugirdas et al 2001). Immediate medical assistance must be sought and emergency resuscitative measures commenced. Outcome may be related to the volume of air infused.

Clotting of the blood lines and dialyser

Clotting of the circuit will occur if anticoagulation is inadequate, if blood flow is inadequate or not continuous and if there is air in the circuit. A change in the pressure of the circuit will occur as a result of clotting. If the dialyser has clotted there will be a decrease in the venous pressure and possibly a rise in the arterial pressure. Clotting of the venous chamber will result in a raised venous pressure. If clotting occurs the treatment should be discontinued without returning the blood to the patient. The cause should be investigated, i.e. anticoagulation regime, access or dialyser preparation.

Table 7.2 summarises the complications of haemodialysis.

SPECIAL CARE ON HAEMODIALYSIS

An increasing number of those requiring haemodialysis have very special nursing needs, and although a detailed analysis of the care required is beyond the scope of this book, an outline of the care required and some useful further reading now follows.

Diabetes mellitus

Diabetes is the leading cause of end-stage renal failure in the western world, and approximately 20–30% of those with type 1 or type 2 diabetes will develop overt nephropathy (American Diabetes Association 1999). The prevention of end-stage renal failure in those with diabetes has been discussed in Chapter 5; many renal programmes in the UK have up to 25% of their dialysis population with diabetes as their underlying renal disease.

The following points should be considered when caring for those with diabetes on dialysis:

- Care of those with diabetes and renal failure should be through joint renal–diabetes management (Renal Association 1997), e.g. joint clinics.
- Those with diabetes should continue to attend specialist diabetes centres or specialist practice nurse clinics for annual review, to monitor complications of retinopathy, neuropathy and cardiac disease.
- Glucose monitoring should be invidualised according to patient requirements—tight glycaemic control is preferable to avoid further complications of diabetes. Insulin requirements may either be reduced (dialysis reverses insulin resistance) or increased (dialysis may reverse anorexia and may increase dietary intake). Dialysate should contain glucose to avoid hypoglycaemia.
- Tight blood pressure control is recommended (<140/80 mmHg), although it is recognised that hypotension on dialysis may be common. Sodium profiling may be helpful.
- Good nutrition is important as patients may suffer gastroparesis and subsequent nausea and vomiting.
- Dialysis nurses should carry out foot examination at least once per month as foot lesions are the most commonly mismanaged problem (De Francisco 1999). Patient teaching on foot care is vital.

De Francisco (1999) has written a useful review article on diabetes and renal failure and it is recommended for further reading. Kimmel et al (2000) have identified that those with diabetes have a decreased survival rate associated with increased interdialytic weight gain, so the importance of good patient education in this group is warranted. The poor survival rate

Table 7.2 Complications of haemodialysis (summary)

Complication	Cause	Prevention	Treatment
Hypotension	Dry weight too low Excessive UFR Antihypertensive drugs Acetate	Regular assessment of dry weight Correct UFR calculation Bicarbonate dialysis	0.9% NaCl Lay patient flat Reduce UFR and recalculate fluid loss
Cramp	Excessive UFR	Correct UFR calculations Quinine sulphate 2 h prior to HD	0.9% NaCl or hypertonic solution Heat pad/massage
Disequilibration	Too efficient dialysis	Small surface area dialyser <1.0 m^2 Reduce blood flow rate <150 mL min^{-1} Reduce time <2 h maximum Daily dialysis until biochemistry satisfactory Bicarbonate dialysis	Discontinue dialysis Mannitol i.v.
Arrhythmias	Underlying hypertension Coronary artery disease Excessive potassium shifts Digoxin	Dialyse against dialysate with minimum 3.0 mmol potassium	Monitor
Membrane reaction	Complement activation on exposure to membrane and/or ETO	Use synthetic membranes that have not been sterilised with ETO for patients who are at risk or with known allergies Correct rinsing and Preparation of dialyser	Stop dialysis Do not return blood to patient Treat as anaphylaxis Adrenaline (epinephrine)/ hydrocortisone/piriton i.v.
Air embolus	Air entry to venous end of extracorporeal circuit	Ensure all lines secure Ensure correct use of air detector Observe lines	Stop treatment Lay patient on left side Give 100% oxygen
Haemolysis	Damage to red blood cells through pump or kinked lines Dialysate temperature too high	Low shearing pumps Ensure venous pressure is not high Set temperature gauge	Give oxygen ?Give blood Test for high potassium from damaged red cells Dialysis
Clotting of blood lines	Inadequate anticoagulation Air in the dialyser	Review anticoagulation regime Review priming procedure Ensure air-tight connections	Stop treatment Discard dialyser and lines Review anticoagulation before resuming treatment
Blood leak	A tear or rupture in the membrane within the dialyser	Careful handling of the dialyser Keep pressures within limits	Stop dialysis Discard extracorporeal blood

ETO, ethylene oxide, HD, haemodialysis, UFR, ultrafiltration rate.

for older people with diabetes on dialysis has been highlighted by Khan et al (2000), and the importance of reducing or preventing the cardiovascular complications that cause high mortality rates is described.

Older people

Almost 50% of those requiring renal replacement are aged 65 or more (Ansell & Feest 2000), and it is becoming more recognised that this group requires special nursing care. Williams (2001) has emphasised how the occupational therapist can make a valuable contribution to the multiprofessional team in rehabilitating those who are elderly and frail. Bevan (2000) describes the implications of the increasing numbers of older people on dialysis, whilst Ashwanden (2000) has shown that the renal health care team is not fully conversant with the physiological or mental changes that old age makes to the body. The conclusion is that, because the renal population is growing older, the renal team needs to be more aware of the changes which occur as people grow older and to deliver care acknowledging these changes. The medical, ethical and psychosocial considerations of caring for older people on renal replacement are reviewed by Stack & Messana (2000).

Another important issue that is often overlooked by the renal care team is that of fatigue, and McCann & Boore (2000) have explained how it is a phenomenon that is poorly understood by healthcare professionals. They found that fatigue was significantly associated with the presence of symptoms such as sleep problems, poor physical health status and depression. Painter et al (2000) found that an individually prescribed exercise programme and exercise (cycling) whilst on dialysis showed an improvement in physical functioning, which may in turn have an effect on health outcome.

SUMMARY

Those requiring haemodialysis should have a named nurse who is responsible for the planning, delivery and evaluation of the highest standards of individual care. Patients should have the opportunity to participate in decision making related to all aspects of their care and have a right to be cared for by nurses who are competent in all aspects of haemodialysis treatments. Ideally this competence should be assessed in a formal and structured training programme. Finally, the skills needed to provide comprehensive nursing care to patients on haemodialysis cannot be measured solely by a nurse's competence to set up and use a haemodialysis machine or by the ability to insert a pair of fistula needles first time. The haemodialysis nurse is constantly demanding access to the skills and knowledge which tacitly underlie the rapidly expanding scope of professional practice. There is a professional expectation of all nurses to ensure continuous learning and development in order to keep abreast of new research findings, new technology and the ever-increasing needs and demands of the patient.

The nurse working within the haemodialysis unit is faced on a day-to-day basis with a practical dichotomy. On the one hand, the working environment is highly technical and the delivery of optimal treatment is a cognitive challenge. On the other hand, the nursing focus must acknowledge the very special affective skills required in providing support, counselling and rehabilitative interventions to patients with chronic ill health. Although units will function with nurses whose strength or preference lies in one or other domain, it is the careful combination of the skills, knowledge and attitudes of both aspects that results in the advanced and expert practice of the nurse on the haemodialysis unit.

REFERENCES

Aldridge C. The use and management of arterio venous fistulae: fact and fiction. EDTNA/ERCA 1991; 17:29–35.

American Diabetes Association. Position statement on diabetic nephropathy. Diabetes Care 1991; 22(suppl. 1).

Ansell D, Feest T. Third annual report of the UK Renal Registry. Bristol: UK Renal Registry, 2000.

Ashwanden C. The care of the elderly renal patient. EDTNA/ERCA 2000; XXVI:3.

Berkoben M, Schwab SJ. Maintenance of permanent haemodialysis vascular access patency. Am Nephrol Nurses Assoc J 1995; 22:17–24.

Bevan M. The older person with renal failure. Nurs Standard, 2000; 14:48–54.

Bregman H, Daugirdas JT, Ing TS. Complications during haemodialysis. In: Daugirdas JT, Ing TS (eds), Handboook of dialysis. 2nd edn. New York: Little Brown: 149–168.

Butterley DW, Schwab, SJ. (1996) Haemodialysis vascular access. Effect on urea kinetics and the dialysis prescription. Am J Nephrol 1996; 16:45–51.

Charra B. Improving adequacy improves haemodialysis outcome. EDTNA/ERCA J 2000; XXVI:6–10.

Charra B, Calemard E, Laurent G. Importance of treatment time and blood pressure control in achieving long term survival on dialysis. Am J Nephrol 1996; 16:35–44.

Daugirdas JT, Blake PG, Ing TS. (eds) Handbook of Dialysis. 3rd edn. Philadelphia: Lippincott Williams, 2001.

De Francisco ALM. Clinical outcomes for patients with diabetic nephropathy. EDTNA/ERCA 1999; XXV:23–26.

De Vos, JY. A nursing view of future haemodialysis anticoagulation treatments. EDTNA/ERCA 2000; XXVI:10–12.

Hayes J. Prolonging access function and survival—the nurse's role. EDTNA/ERCA J 1998; XXIV:7–10.

Hoenich N, Van Holder R. Allergic reactions associated with haemodialysis: biocompatibility monograph. EDTNA/ERCA J 1993 (suppl):3–6.

Ismail N, Becker BN, Hakim RM. Water treatment for haemodialysis. Am J Nephrol 1996; 16:60–72.

Khan MA, Collins MA, Keane WF. Diabetes in the elderly population. Adv Renal Replace Ther 2000; 7:32–51.

Kidney Alliance. End-stage renal failure—a framework for planning and service delivery. Kidney Alliance 2001

Kimmel PL, Varela MP, Peterson RA et al. Interdialytic weight gain and survival in hemodialysis patients: effects of duration of ESRD and diabetes mellitus. Kidney Int 2000; 57:1141–1151.

Kronung G. Plastic deformation of Cimino fistulae by repeated puncture. Dialysis Transplant, 1984; 13:635.

Ledebo I. Acetate vs. bicarbonate in everyday dialysis. Lund: Gambro, 1990.

Levy J, Morgan J and Brown E. Oxford handbook of dialysis. Oxford: Oxford University Press, 2001.

Lewis M, Wick GS, Foret J. Anemia management: recognizing opportunities and improving outcomes through nurse interventions. Nephrol Nurse J 2000; 27:507–512.

Lindley L, Lopot F, Harrington M et al. Treatment of water for dialysis: European survey. EDTNA/ERCA 2000; XXVI:22–27.

Lowrie EG, Lew NL. The urea reduction ratio (URR). Contemp Dialysis Nephrol 1991; Feb:11–20.

Lowrie EG, Laird NM, Paker TF et al. Effect of the haemodialysis prescription of patient morbidity. Report from the National Co-operative Dialysis study. N Engl J Med 1981; 305:1176–1181.

Luik AJ, Kooman JP, Leunissen KML. Hypertension on haemodialysis patients: is it only hypervolaemia? Nephrol Dialysis Transplant, 1997; 12:1557–1560.

Lunts P. 21st century home haemodialysis: a new approach to an old treatment. EDTNA/ERCA J 2001; XXVII:77–80.

McCann K, and Boore JRP. Fatigue in persons with renal failure who require maintenance haemodialysis. J Adv Nurs 2000; 32:1132–1142.

Macdougall I. Management of anaemia in renal failure. EDTNA/ERCA J 1999; XXV:19–22.

Ouseph R, Ward R. Anticoagulation for intermittent haemodialysis. Semin Dialysis 2000; 13:181–187.

Painter P, Carlson L, Carey S et al. Physical functioning and health-related quality of life changes with exercise training in haemodialysis patients. Am J Kidney Dis 2000; 35:482–492.

Palmer B. Dialysate composition in haemodialysis and peritoneal dialysis. In: Henrich WL, ed. Principles and practice of dialysis. Baltimore: Williams & Wilkins, 1999: 22–40.

Priester Coary A, Daugirdas JT. A recommended technique for obtaining the post dialysis BUN. Semin Dialysis 1997; 10:23–25.

Renal Association. Treatment of adult patients with renal failure. Recommended standards and audit measures. 2nd edn. London: Royal College of Physicians 1997.

Rocek M, Peregrin J. Percutaneous intervention for vascular dialysis access. EDTNA/ERCA J 2001; XXVIII:83–87.

Rosenheim M. Working party report. Hepatitis and the treatment of chronic failure. London: DHSS, 1972.

Schulman G. Dialysis prescription: introduction. Am J Nephrol 1996; 16:5–6.

Stack AG, Messana JM. Renal replacement therapy in the elderly: medical, ethical and psychosocial considerations. Adv Renal Replace Ther 2000; 7:52–62.

Swartz RD, Boyer CL, Messana JM. Central venous catheters for maintenance haemodialysis: a cautionary approach. Adv Renal Replace Ther 1997; 4:275–284.

Twardowski ZJ, Van Stone JC, Jones MRE et al. Blood recirculation in intravenous catheters for haemodialysis. J Am Soc Nephrol, 1993; 3:218–221.

Uldall R. Vascular access for continuous renal replacement therapy. Semin Dialysis 1996; 9:93–97.

Vienken J, Bowry S. Optimisation in anti coagulation. EDTNA/ERCA J, 1993; 19:12–17.

Williams M. Rehabilitating the frail and elderly on renal replacement. EDTNA/ERCA J 2001; XXVII:64–65.

Wittich E. Maintaining an optimum haemocatheter exit site. EDTNA/ERCA J 2001; XXVII:81–82.

Yang R, and Humphrey S. Review of arteriovenous fistula care. EDTNA/ERCA J 2000; XXVI:11–14.

Peritoneal dialysis

8

Janet Wild

■ CONTENTS

■ LEARNING OUTCOMES FOR THIS CHAPTER

- To recognise the importance of individualised care for those on peritoneal dialysis (PD)
- To review the anatomy and physiology of the peritoneum
- To identify best practice for the care of the PD catheter and exit site and the best use of each PD therapy option
- To understand the criteria for good patient selection for PD
- To review all factors required to dialyse a patient with PD adequately
- To review the complications of PD
- To understand the importance of good ongoing education for those on PD.

INTRODUCTION

PD as a treatment for end-stage renal disease (ESRD) is a relatively simple and very effective technique. As such, it has been successfully developed as the preferred first option of home dialysis.

From its introduction in the late 1970s, PD has been refined and developed into a flexible and adaptable therapy that is the treatment of choice for many patients. It has been found to be most effective if performed as a continuous treatment, either by the patient during the day (continuous ambulatory peritoneal dialysis or CAPD) or by a machine, usually whilst the patient sleeps (automated peritoneal dialysis or APD). Owing to its continuous nature, patients who are treated by this therapy tend to have a more stable biochemical and fluid profile. Its flexible nature makes it suitable for almost all ESRD patients.

This chapter discusses the importance of having an individualised treatment for each patient, which is structured around both clinical and lifestyle needs. The chapter starts with an overview of the anatomy and physiology of the peritoneum and practical aspects of the therapy, and different therapy options on PD; complications and patient education and training are also discussed. It should be noted here that the role of the nurse working within the field of PD has changed markedly over the last decade (Bender & Swartz 1999, Jacobs et al 1997, Kelman 1995). As the therapy is performed by the patients themselves, in the community, the main focus is on providing patients with not only an individualised treatment, but also adequate psychological and nursing care which are essential elements for the successful treatment of those needing PD and their families.

PHYSIOLOGY OF PERITONEAL DIALYSIS

The peritoneal membrane, so called because it covers the abdominal cavity and is derived from the Greek word *peritonaion* meaning to stretch around, has a surface area of up to 2 m^2. The peritoneal cavity is the potential space between the parietal membrane (which lines the abdominal cavity) and the visceral membrane (the inner layer which closely covers the organs and includes the mesenteries). Under normal circumstances this cavity contains between 50 and 100 mL of fluid which acts as a lubricant (Fig. 8.1).

During PD, physiological solution or dialysis fluid is instilled into the peritoneal cavity. Uraemic toxins and solutes move across the membrane by the process of diffusion, from the blood stream into the dialysis fluid, or vice versa, depending on the concentration gradient. The composition of the dialysis fluid is near to that of normal extracellular fluid.

Fluid removal takes place by osmosis. The dialysis fluid is made hypertonic to plasma by the addition of osmotic agent, usually glucose. Other osmotic solutions are discussed later in this chapter.

The membrane is made up of three layers (Fig. 8.2):

- The mesothelium. Underneath this lies the connective tissue. The luminal side of the mesothelium is covered with numerous microvilli that are believed to increase the surface area of the peritoneum to up to 40 m^2 in a healthy individual. During PD the density of these microvilli appears to be reduced (Dobbie 1989).
- The peritoneal interstitium. This is composed of fibres and bundles of collagen.
- The capillary endothelium. This forms a complex branching system.

Blood supply

The visceral peritoneum is supplied by the superior mesenteric artery. The parietal peritoneum is supplied by the intercostal, epigastric and lumbar arteries. Venous return from the visceral peritoneum is to the portal circulation whereas that from the parietal peritoneum goes into the caval circulation. This is important because it means that any drugs administered via the peritoneum will be transported to the liver, the normal route.

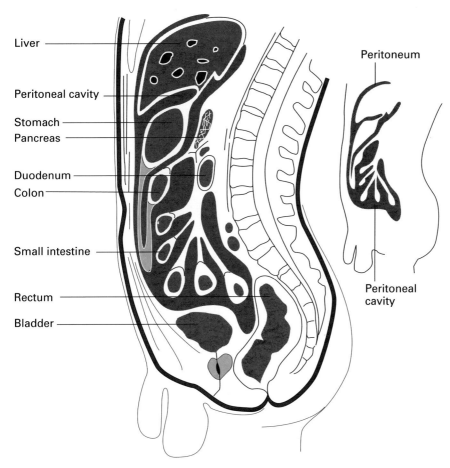

Liver

Peritoneal cavity

Stomach

Pancreas

Duodenum

Colon

Small intestine

Rectum

Bladder

Peritoneum

Peritoneal cavity

Figure 8.1 Location of the peritoneal cavity.

Lymphatic drainage

Lymphatic drainage from the peritoneal cavity returns excess fluid and proteins into the systemic circulation. Its other function is to remove foreign bodies from the peritoneal cavity. Lymphatic drainage is a one-way system, the flow rate of which may be affected by respiratory rate, intraperitoneal hydrostatic pressure, posture or peritonitis.

Peritoneal membrane transport characteristics

The peritoneal membrane is semipermeable and allows the passage of both water and solutes.

During PD three processes are involved in removing fluid and wastes from the blood stream and balancing electrolytes. These are osmosis, diffusion and convection.

Osmosis

This is the movement of water through a semipermeable membrane from a solution of low concentration into a solution with a higher concentration.

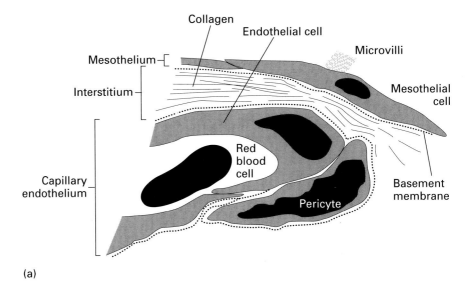

(a)

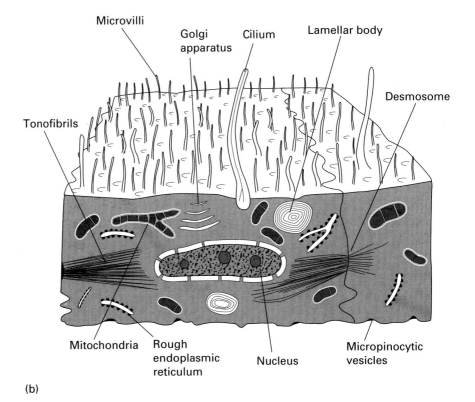

(b)

Figure 8.2 (a) The three layers of the peritoneal membrane. (b) Diagrammatic representation of a normal mesothelial cell.

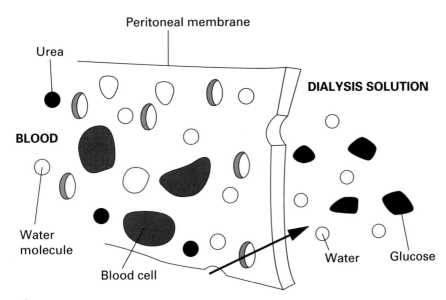

Figure 8.3 Osmotic ultrafiltration across the peritoneal membrane with a glucose dialysis solution in the peritoneal cavity.

The solution into which the water moves in PD contains an osmotic agent, usually glucose (other osmotic agents are discussed later in this chapter). The higher the glucose concentration, the greater the osmotic effect will be, so removing more water from the patient's blood stream (Fig. 8.3).

Diffusion

This is solute exchange between two solutions, usually separated by a semipermeable membrane. The solutes will travel in either direction across the membrane until equilibrium is achieved. The direction and speed at which the solutes flow depend on the concentration gradient. Solutes will flow from the stronger solution into the weaker solution (Fig. 8.4). Therefore, solutes can pass in either direction across the peritoneal membrane.

Other factors that affect diffusion rate are molecular weight and membrane resistance.

Molecular weight

Diffusion is a spontaneous process whereby solutes move randomly. Lighter, smaller molecules will move quicker than larger, heavier molecules. Urea (which has a molecular weight of 60 Da) diffuses from blood to dialysate more rapidly than creatinine (molecular weight 113 Da) or vitamin B_{12} (molecular weight 1352 Da). Unlike haemodialysis, where the membrane pore size is controlled, the peritoneal membrane allows transport of large molecules and even proteins. Protein transport into the dialysate is unfortunate as this is an essential nutrient, particularly in dialysis patients who may be catabolic.

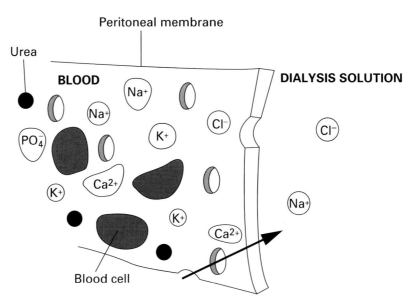

Figure 8.4 The peritoneum acts as a semipermeable membrane, allowing small solutes and water to diffuse through, but retaining large particles such as blood cells.

Membrane resistance

The permeability of the individual's membrane is an important factor controlling diffusion of solutes. Measurement of this is discussed later in this section.

A patient's peritoneal permeability may be changed during illness. Acute episodes of peritonitis appear to greatly increase the membrane permeability to both solutes and water. However, fibrotic thickening of the membrane, also due to peritonitis, may lead to a severe reduction in its permeability (Davies et al 1993).

Convection

Owing to the large amount of osmotic ultrafiltration that takes place during PD, convective flow transports or 'drags' water and solutes across the membrane. This occurs at a much faster rate than that which may be accounted for by diffusion alone.

The ability of glucose to exert an effective osmotic pressure depends on its ability to stay in solution in the dialysate. If the peritoneal membrane were perfectly semipermeable (i.e. only permeable to water), the osmotic pressure would be maximised. However, the peritoneum is permeable to solutes as well as water, and therefore allows the glucose through. The osmotic gradient is therefore maximal at the beginning of the exchange. The ultrafiltration will decrease during the dwell time as glucose is absorbed into the blood stream. It is estimated (Diaz-Buxo 1984) that the ultrafiltration volume peaks at a dwell time of around 2–3 h, when the ultrafiltration equals reabsorption. The total dialysate and ultrafiltrate volume continues to decrease after this point due to lymphatic absorption.

Measurement of peritoneal permeability

The peritoneal equilibration test (PET)

Twardowski et al (1987) and Twardowski (1989) developed a standardised test to measure the equilibration rates of various solutes during a 4-h dwell of PD. Based on their findings, an individual's peritoneal equilibration rate can be categorised as low, low-average, high-average or high. Twardowski standardised the tests to measure the equilibration rates of creatinine and glucose, therefore allowing measurement of the membranes solute and fluid transport rates.

A patient with a membrane of low transport characteristics (low transporter) will equilibrate creatinine and glucose slowly. Although solutes take a long time to cross this type of membrane, glucose also travels across slowly. This means that the glucose will stay in solution in the peritoneal cavity for longer, enabling the osmotic pressure gradient to be maintained, hence there is greater ultrafiltration. Patients whose membranes have very low transport characteristics therefore obtain maximum dialysis with long dwells of dialysis fluid.

A patient with a membrane that, on the other hand, shows high transport characteristics (high transporter) will optimise the amount of dialysis with short dwells. This is because both creatinine and glucose cross the membrane quickly, resulting in rapid clearance of solutes and rapid absorption of glucose. This glucose absorption results in a decrease in osmotic pressure and therefore poor ultrafiltration.

Performing a PET

The test has been standardised so that the results can easily be compared over time and between patients.

Sampling

This should be performed following a dwell of at least 8 h.

1. Prepare a 2000-mL medium-glucose-strength (2.27% or 2.5%) bag of dialysis fluid by warming to body temperature.
2. Drain out the patient's overnight dwell of dialysate over 20 min. The patient must be vertical, either sitting or standing. Measure and record the drained fluid volume.
3. Infuse the new solution at a rate of 400 mL min^{-1} (i.e. total infusion time = 10 min). The patient must be supine and should roll from side to side every 2 min to ensure solution mixing. Zero dwell time is the time at completion of infusion.
4. Collect dialysate samples at zero and 2 h dwell time:
   (a) Drain approximately 200 mL into the drainage bag and invert the bag to mix the solution.
   (b) Disinfect the sample port.
   (c) Withdraw 10 mL via the sample port and reinfuse the remaining 190 mL.
   (d) Transfer the sample to the appropriately labelled collection tube.

N.B. For the 0-h sample, 200 mL should be drained immediately follow-ing the fill period for sampling.

5. Draw a venous blood sample at 2 h dwell time. Transfer to an appropriately labelled collection tube.
6. At 4 h dwell time, drain dialysate over 20 min with the patient vertical.
7. Mix the sample by inverting the bag. Withdraw 10 mL. Transfer to the appropriately labelled tube.
8. Weigh and record drain volume, adding sample volumes to give total drain volume.

Calculating results

Creatinine and glucose values should be obtained on the three dialysate samples and the serum sample.

The dialysate-to-plasma (D/P) ratio for creatinine and dialysate-to-dialysate (D/DO) at 0 h ratio for glucose can be calculated by using the worksheet (Fig. 8.5). When the results have been calculated, they should be plotted on the PET curve graph shown in more detail in Figure 8.6, enabling membrane characteristic categorisation (Fig. 8.6). For a quick guide to the membrane transport characteristics it is possible to look at the D/P ratio at 4 h. The closer this number is to 1, the higher the patient's membrane transport characteristics.

Corrected creatinine

Owing to glucose interference with creatinine assays, corrected creatinine values may need to be determined. A corrected creatinine result may be provided by individual laboratories, depending on the type of laboratory test used. Enzymatic tests do not require correction. Analysis of samples must always be carried out on the same analyser to avoid erroneous results. If corrected creatinine is not available, the standard creatinine results should be used throughout (Baxter Healthcare 1992).

Analysis of results

The numbers themselves are not necessarily the most important feature of the test. Some significance can be attached to the shape of the curves on the graph and the position of individual patients within each of the bands.

It has been suggested (Davies et al 1993) that repeat tests should be rou-tinely performed once a year or if problems arise such as an apparent loss of ultrafiltration. Changes over time in the test results can then be related to clinical performance and treatment regimens may be altered accordingly.

Recommendations for optimal use of the PET

Patients should be in optimum health when the PET is performed. The catheter should be functioning well; the patient should not be constipated and should have no infection. Ideally the patient should not be fluid-overloaded.

Patients who normally have overnight APD should start their pro-gramme earlier in the evening before the day of the test. Their treatment should finish earlier in the morning with a last bag fill of 2000 mL. This can

Peritoneal Equilibration Test (PET)

1. Collect patient samples

Name patient:
Date:
Completed by:

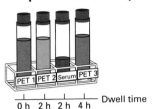

Dwell time
0 h   2 h   2 h   4 h

2. Calculations

a. Creatinine (D/P)

$$D/P = \frac{\text{dialysate concentration of corrected creatinine}}{\text{serum concentration of corrected creatinine}}$$

$$\frac{\text{PET 1} \dots}{\text{Serum} \dots} = A \dots \text{value (0 h)}$$

$$\frac{\text{PET 2} \dots}{\text{Serum} \dots} = B \dots \text{value (2 h)}$$

$$\frac{\text{PET 3} \dots}{\text{Serum} \dots} = C \dots \text{value (4 h)}$$

b. Glucose (D/DO)

$$D/O = \frac{\text{dialysate concentration of glucose at 2/4 h}}{\text{dialysate concentration of glucose at 0 h}}$$

$$\frac{\text{PET 2} \dots}{\text{PET 1} \dots} = D \dots \text{value (2 h)}$$

$$\frac{\text{PET 3} \dots}{\text{PET 1} \dots} = E \dots \text{value (4 h)}$$

3. Plot to graph

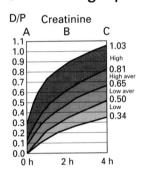

D/P   Creatinine
A   B   C
1.03
High
0.81
High aver
0.65
Low aver
0.50
Low
0.34

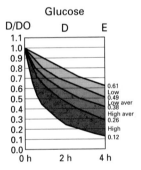

Glucose
D/DO   D   E
0.61
Low
0.49
Low aver
0.38
High aver
0.26
High
0.12

4. Diagnosis

Baseline PET prognostic value			
Solute transport	Predicted response to CAPD		Preferred dialysis
	UF	Dialysis	
High	Poor	Adequate	CCPD dry day CAPD dry night
High average	Poor-medium	Adequate	Standard CAPD or APD
Low average	Good	Adequate Inadequate	StandardCAPD High dose PD APD
Low	Very good	Inadequate	High dose PD Haemodialysis

Figure 8.5 Peritoneal equilibration test (PET). CAPD, continuous ambulatory peritoneal dialysis; UF, ultrafiltration; APD, automated peritoneal dialysis; PD, peritoneal dialysis.

Glucose

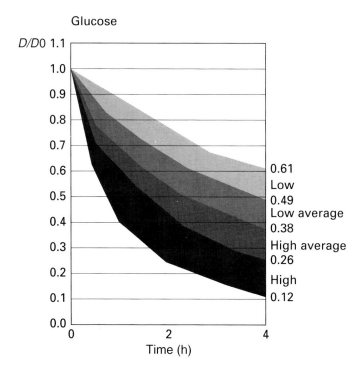

Corrected creatinine

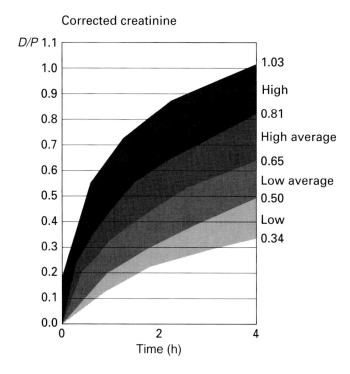

Figure 8.6 Peritoneal equilibration test (PET) curves.

then be drained at lunch time (following an 8-h dwell) for a test that afternoon. In this way a CAPD situation can be mimicked.

When interpreting the results, an abnormal PET curve on the graph may be due to an error in the way the test was performed or a clinical problem with the patient. It may also be due to a mathematical or laboratory error.

PERITONEAL DIALYSIS ACCESS AND EXIT-SITE CARE

It is widely agreed that the key to successful PD is good, permanent and safe access to the peritoneal cavity. Despite the reduction of catheter-related infection rates in patients undergoing PD, these infections remain major sources of morbidity and transfer to haemodialysis (Gokal, 2000). It is therefore essential that good catheter and exit-site practices are maintained by all those involved in the care of PD patients.

Types of catheters

The design of a peritoneal catheter needs to be such that it gives the patient the maximum inflow and outflow rates as well as discouraging infection.

The very early peritoneal catheters which were used in the 1960s for acute PD were rigid and made from polyvinyl chloride. Developments in the late 1960s led to the introduction of a flexible silicone rubber (Silastic) catheter, which is much more suited to chronic PD. There are currently five main types of permanent PD catheter in use:

- straight Tenckhoff (Fig. 8.7)
- curled Tenckhoff (Fig. 8.8)
- Toronto western (Fig. 8.9)
- swan-neck (Missouri; Fig. 8.10)
- T-fluted (Fig. 8.11).

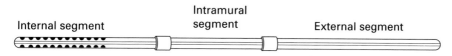

Figure 8.7 Straight Tenckhoff catheter.

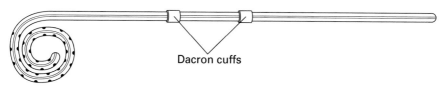

Figure 8.8 Curled Tenckhoff catheter.

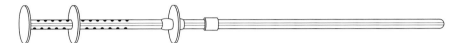

Figure 8.9 Toronto western catheter.

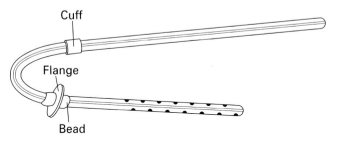

Figure 8.10 Swan-neck (Missouri) catheter.

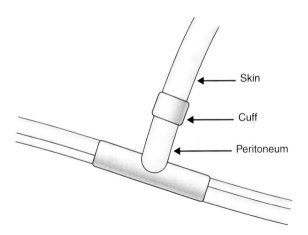

Figure 8.11 T-fluted catheter.

When implanted, the catheter has three functioning segments (Fig. 8.12):

- The outer part which connects via an adapter (usually titanium metal) to the solution transfer set.
- An intramural part which has either one or two Dacron cuffs. These cuffs are spaced about 8 cm apart. They create an inflammatory response which then progresses to form thick fibrous tissue which fixes the catheter cuff in position. This anchors the catheter, helps to minimise leakage of dialysate and acts as a barrier to infection by preventing bacteria entering the catheter 'tunnel'.
- The intraperitoneal part, which has many small holes up the side, is situated inside the peritoneal cavity for the in- and outflow of the solution.

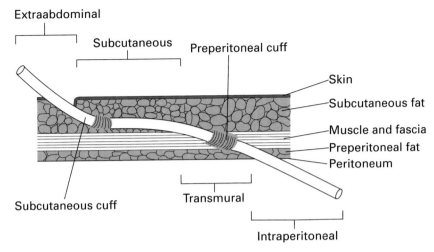

Figure 8.12 Functional parts of the peritoneal catheter.

The choice of catheter used is generally of local preference. The most widely used catheters are the straight and curled Tenckhoff catheters. They are easily inserted under local or general anaesthetic. The swan-neck, curled and Toronto western catheters were all developed to aid outflow of the dialysate. The swan-neck, because of its two downward-pointing segments, serves to aid outflow, as migration of this type of catheter is rare. It is also thought to prevent infections at the exit site as this segment of the catheter also points downwards, thus preventing accumulation of sweat and pus. The coil catheter also aids outflow as it too may be less prone to migration. It may also reduce patient discomfort during inflow because of reduction of the 'jet effect'. The two discs at the intraperitoneal part of the Toronto western catheter help it to prevent migration. This catheter also has a Dacron flange and bead at the deep cuff, which is sewn in position by a pursestring suture, helping to reduce leaks at the exit site. The T-fluted catheter is shaped like a T. The intraperitoneal portion lies against the parietal peritoneum. Instead of side holes, the intraperitoneal portion has eight, 1 mm wide longitudinal flutes or grooves. This design allows better flow and prevents migration (Ash & Janle 1993).

Moncrief et al (1996) described a catheter with a cuff made from a microporous material which passes through the exit site and allows microvascular ingrowth into the pores of the material. This has been shown to create a bacteriological barrier which may prevent infections at the exit site. The silver-coated catheter which was thought to contribute to a 50% reduction in exit-site infection rates (Vas 1996) has so far proved ineffective, possibly due to manufacturing difficulties.

Preinsertion preparation of the patient

The catheter exit site should be determined before the catheter is inserted. The preferred site should first be discussed with the patient to help promote participation in and an understanding of the therapy. The following points should be followed when determining the exit site of the patient's catheter:

- The site should be determined whilst the patient is in a relaxed sitting or standing position.
- It should be either above or below the belt line, whichever the patient prefers.
- Skin folds and abdominal scars should be avoided.
- The catheter exit site should be located where the patient can effectively carry out exit-site care.
- Once the exit site has been determined, it should be marked clearly with a permanent skin marker.

Preoperative care of the patient

On the morning of the operation, the patient should bathe or have a shower. If necessary, abdominal hair should be clipped. The bowel should be empty before the catheter is inserted. This may need to be achieved by administration of an enema. It is also important that the patient has an empty bladder before the insertion procedure takes place.

Staphylococcus aureus screening

There is recent evidence (Coles et al unpublished work) that patients who have nasal carriage of *Staphylococcus aureus* have an increased risk of exit site infection and peritonitis. Patients' nares may therefore be swabbed to determine nasal carriage of *S. aureus*. Eradication of nasal carriage has shown a significant improvement in exit-site infections but has a cost implication (Dryden et al 1991, Mupirocin Study Group 1996). Results of a multicentre trial on the use of mupirocin nasal cream to prevent such infections show that using it amongst *S. aureus* nasal carriers reduced exit-site infections from one episode in 28 patient-months to one episode in 99 patient-months (Coles et al 1994). It was concluded from this trial that intermittent use of intranasal mupirocin is effective in significantly reducing *S. aureus* infection in CAPD patients. There have been fears, however, that the use of such antibiotics may cause the emergence of resistant strains of bacterium.

Prophylactic antibiotics

There is now some evidence that prophylactic antibiotics may prevent catheter infections and peritonitis (Golper & Tranae 1996). In a controlled study using cefuroxime (1.5 g intravenously (i.v.) 1–2 h preoperatively, and 250 mg intraperitoneally (i.p.) perioperatively), the prophylactic group had fewer peritonitis episodes than controls (Wikdahl et al 1997). However, other reports differ (Lye et al 1992). US Renal Data System (USRDS) 1992 data in 3366 patients showed no difference between patients who had had antibiotic prophylaxis compared to those who did not.

Psychological preparation of the patient

This is of absolute importance for someone who is new to PD and it is discussed in detail in Chapter 3.

Insertion techniques

PD is a life-maintaining therapy. Access to the peritoneal cavity, via the PD catheter, is therefore particularly important in ensuring its success (Fig. 8.13). The insertion technique should be treated as a skill acquired by experienced surgeons and physicians only, rather like implantation of a pacemaker or similar device. A team approach is essential and nurse involvement is most important. The nurse's role in insertion of PD catheters starts with the preoperative preparation described above, all of which can be carried out by the nurse. In many centres the PD nurse accompanies the patient to the operating theatre to ensure correct procedures are carried out and that the catheter is functioning well before final wound closure is made.

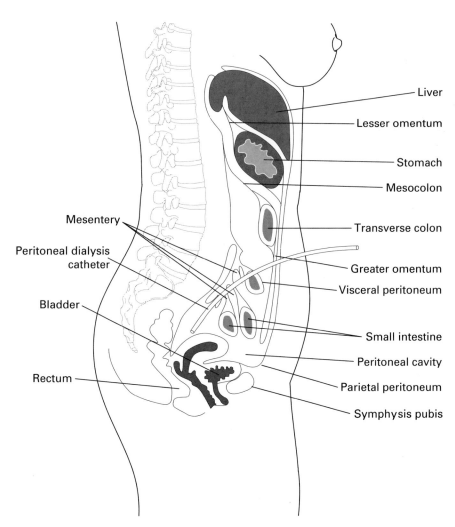

Figure 8.13 The position of a peritoneal dialysis catheter in the abdomen.

The four most frequently performed methods of catheter insertion include:

1. surgical placement by dissection (Ash & Daugirdas 1994, Ash & Nichols 1994)
2. blind placement using Tenckhoff trocar (Ash & Daugirdas 1994, Gokal et al 1998)
3. blind placement using guidewire (Seldinger technique: Ash & Daugirdas 1994, Ash & Nichols 1994)
4. minitrocar placement using peritoneoscopy (Ash & Daugirdas 1994, Ash & Nichols 1994).

Another implantation technique which has recently been described was the prolonged subcutaneous implantation of the catheter for up to 6 weeks before being brought to the surface and used. This technique has been shown in preliminary studies to reduce the rate of infection (Park et al 1996).

Postoperative care of the patient

The goals of postoperative catheter care are to:

1. minimise any bacterial colonisation of the exit and tunnel during the early healing period
2. prevent trauma to the exit site and traction on the cuffs by immobilisation of the catheter
3. minimise intraabdominal pressure to prevent leakage.

Ideally, the exit site should be undisturbed for 7–10 days following insertion of the catheter. The patient may be discharged home during this period. If, during the first 10 days, the dressing becomes soiled, it should be redressed by a nurse. If it merely becomes dislodged, it should simply be replaced with a fresh sterile dressing. During this period, the catheter tubing must be immobilised by securely taping it to the patient's abdomen.

Before discharge from hospital, during this resting of the patient's catheter, clear instructions must be given as to the correct procedures for caring for the catheter at home. It may be appropriate to involve the community district nursing team if no specific community PD nurse is available. In this case, adequate training and support must be provided for the nursing team.

Directly following insertion of the catheter, it may be flushed with 500–1500 mL of PD fluid to check patency. It may then be 'capped off' using a small locking cap on the catheter adapter (this adapter is usually made of titanium metal) and left covered until PD commences. Ideally, PD should not be started until healing of the exit site and tissue ingrowth into the catheter's Dacron cuffs have taken place, usually after 10 days. If dialysis is necessary before this time, and if haemodialysis is inappropriate or unavailable, automated PD would be the preferred method. This is because this treatment will help to minimise the risk of leakage of PD fluid by allowing the patient to be treated using small fill volumes of fluid in a supine position. It is worth noting that patient healing mechanisms may be altered in those patients who are uraemic or who have diabetes mellitus.

It appears that there are many different practices in postoperative catheter care across Europe, and the European Dialysis and Transplant Nurses' Association/European Renal Care Association (EDTNA/ERCA) Research Board is collecting data and analysing findings during 2001–2002.

Long-term care of the exit site

As with any wound, care is aimed at keeping the site clear of exudate or debris that could encourage bacterial growth (Prowant & Twardowski 1996). A method of exit-site care which best fits in with the patient's lifestyle is most likely to encourage full participation in the treatment, and therefore reduce the risk of complications. A number of studies have been undertaken to attempt to ascertain which particular method of exit-site care is preferred. Various protocols do exist, for example cleansing with soap and water (Khanna & Twardowski 1989, Prowant et al 1988) or cleaning with povidone-iodine (Piraino et al 1986, Starzomski 1984) or cleaning with chlorhexidine gluconate (Fuchs et al 1990); however, there is to date no consensus on which method will reduce the incidence of infection. Research suggests that chlorhexidine may be the agent of choice (Maki 1991).

Whichever solution is chosen, the following points should be considered:

- Harsh solutions should be avoided as they have the potential to cause skin damage, which may predispose to bacterial colonisation.
- Different agents may be preferred in different circumstances. In an immunosuppressed patient the normal skin flora may represent an infection risk; in this case an antiseptic solution may be preferred.
- Whichever method is used, it is important to ensure that the exit site is carefully dried to avoid skin maceration which could predispose the site to bacterial colonisation.

There is also some debate as to whether it is necessary to keep the catheter exit-site covered. The use of no dressing and a simple exit-site care routine for a well-healed exit site would appeal to many; however, most centres do use some kind of cover (Prowant & Twardowski 1996).

Catheter immobilisation

From the moment the catheter is inserted, it should always be securely anchored to the patient's skin to avoid torque movements at the exit-site. This has been shown to reduce the risk of exit-site infection (Gokal et al 1998) and can be achieved by using tape or a commercially available immobilisation device or tube holder.

Swimming and bathing

According to a consensus of opinions of leading nephrologists (Gokal et al 1998), PD patients may swim following healing of the catheter, usually 4–8 weeks following insertion. Swimming in rivers and lakes is not recommended. The exit site may be covered with either clear occlusive dressing or a colostomy bag. Diving should be avoided as this may put tension on the catheter at the exit site. Following swimming, the patient should shower, clean and dry the exit site and cover it with the usual dressing. Soaking the exit site, for example in a tub bath, is not recommended (Gokal et al 1998).

Indications for catheter removal

A PD catheter is designed to be a permanent access device, and its removal should not be routine. However, catheters may have to be removed under the following conditions:

- if they are no longer needed
- in recurrent peritonitis without an identifiable cause
- in peritonitis due to an exit-site and/or tunnel infection
- with an unusual causative organism of peritonitis, e.g. fungus, tuberculosis
- in bowel perforation accompanied by peritonitis
- with persistent and severe pain due either to the catheter impinging on internal organs or during solution inflow
- when there is Dacron cuff erosion and infection.

PERITONEAL DIALYSIS THERAPY OPTIONS

Dialysis should be prescribed according to each individual patient's need. The dose of PD can be increased or decreased by adjusting any one of the following parameters:

- dialysis fluid fill volume per exchange
- number of dialysis fluid exchanges
- length of dialysis fluid dwell time
- osmotic strength or type of dialysis fluid.

By using the PET each patient's membrane characteristics can be determined, therefore allowing optimisation of the therapy according to each patient's clinical and lifestyle needs.

There are two general methods of performing peritoneal dialysis: CAPD and APD.

Continuous ambulatory peritoneal dialysis

CAPD (Fig. 8.14) is carried out during the day time, manually by patients themselves or sometimes by a carer. Dialysis fluid is infused into the peritoneal cavity and left to dwell for between 3 and 10 h. After this time the dialysate is drained from the cavity, fresh solution is infused and the whole process starts again. Patients usually perform four exchanges of PD fluid each day (some patients may perform five, depending on the prescription), fitting them in as appropriately as possible with their normal lifestyle. For example, exchanges may be performed at breakfast, lunch and supper time with the last exchange of the day being carried out at bedtime. Each exchange takes about 20-30 min to complete.

CAPD is most suited to those patients whose membranes transport solutes at a slow to average rate (i.e. low, low-average and high-average

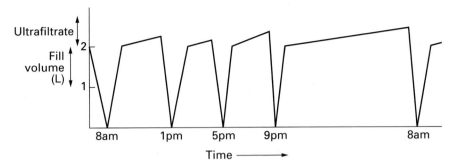

Figure 8.14 Continuous ambulatory peritoneal dialysis.

'transporters') as it provides the opportunity for longer dwell times. This long dwell period is best achieved during the night time whilst the patient sleeps. Those patients whose membranes transport solutes quickly ('high transporters') may need to use a polyglucose solution for the longest dwell overnight. This will avoid dialysate absorption that could occur in these patients during long dwell periods.

Automated peritoneal dialysis

APD has many advantages for patients, both clinical and lifestyle, mainly due to its flexibility. An APD machine automatically controls the fill volume, dwell time and length of treatment the patient receives. APD is most often carried out at home whilst the patient sleeps, but it may also be carried out in the hospital dialysis unit. The dose of dialysis can easily be increased during APD as it is easy and convenient to alter any of the parameters of the treatment. Dialysis fluid fill volumes can be safely increased due to the reduction in intraabdominal pressure achieved whilst the patient is supine. This not only decreases the risk of problems associated with high intraabdominal pressure such as leaks around the catheter exit site, abdominal hernias and back pain, but it also increases the amount of dialysis the patient can achieve, particularly in patients whose membranes transport solutes quickly.

The length of the dwell time and the number of exchanges can effectively be altered without disruption to the patient's lifestyle. This is a major advantage to 'high transporters'. Performing frequent exchanges is essential for these patients to achieve adequate dialysis but this can be inconvenient if the patient is on CAPD. APD provides an effective and convenient alternative by enabling rapid exchanges of dialysis fluid whilst the patient sleeps. This increases clearances of solutes whilst maintaining maximum ultrafiltration. As with CAPD, the osmotic strength of the fluid can be altered according to each patient's need. The reduction in intraabdominal pressure achieved during APD may also aid an increase in appetite.

APD is particularly suitable for those patients needing to be free from day-time CAPD exchanges. Patients who work or who are studying can benefit from this treatment, as the preparation time for the treatment is short and the dialysis takes place whilst they sleep, leaving them free during the day. APD is also suitable for those patients who rely on a carer to perform their dialysis, for example children, older people or those with disabilities. The carer simply prepares the machine, connects the patient to the machine at bedtime and disconnects them the following morning. APD is therefore an effective therapy option for those patients who require more dialysis and/or freedom during the day time. However, in order to achieve adequate dialysis many patients will also need to perform an exchange in the early evening.

Some APD machines have the facility to store information regarding the patient's therapy on a data card that is fitted inside the machine. This data card also stores the patient's individual prescription, enabling the prescription to be altered by a healthcare professional, without the need for the patient's intervention.

There are four different types of APD (APD being the term used to describe PD performed by a machine):

- continuous cycling peritoneal dialysis (CCPD)
- tidal peritoneal dialysis (TPD)
- optimised cycling peritoneal dialysis (OCPD)
- intermittent peritoneal dialysis (IPD).

Continuous cycling peritoneal dialysis (Fig. 8.15)

CCPD is performed overnight whilst the patient is asleep supine in bed. The 'continuous' part of the acronym is derived from the fact that the patient has dialysis fluid in constant contact with the peritoneal membrane. There are typically between five and seven exchanges of fluid with relatively short dwell periods, so maximizing the ultrafiltration and clearance capabilities of those patients whose membrane transports solutes quickly. The treatment regime can be programmed to end with a 'fill', giving the patient a 'wet day' (the fluid would be left inside the peritoneal cavity during the day and drained when the patient next starts treatment on the machine at bedtime).

The treatment may end following the 'drain', giving the patient a 'dry day'. This may help to prevent absorption of the PD fluid in 'high transporters'. It should be noted, though, that utilising a 'dry day' will result in reduced clearances and possibly underdialysis. Polyglucose solution, designed for long dwells, should be used in these circumstances.

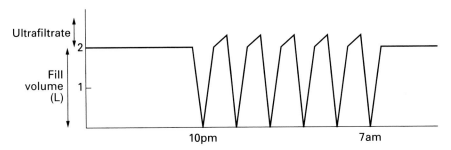

Figure 8.15 Continuous cycling peritoneal dialysis.

Tidal peritoneal dialysis (Fig. 8.16)

This regime is usually performed by a machine in the patient's own home at night. It can also be performed in the dialysis centre incorporated within an IPD regime (see section on IPD, below). The dialysis fluid fill volume is only partly drained, so leaving a designated reserve volume in contact with the peritoneal membrane at all times. The tidal fill volume brings fresh fluid to mix with part of the reserve volume on each cycle. As a result of dialysis fluid constantly being in contact with the membrane, some patients achieve improved clearance of up to 20%, compared to standard PD (Twardowski 1990). This means that patients can achieve the same clearances as CCPD in less time, or more clearance in the same time. Tidal PD can be used with a 'wet day' or a 'dry day', as discussed above. An additional benefit of tidal PD is that some patients experience less pain whilst draining out, since the peritoneal cavity is not totally emptied after each exchange. For a patient dialysing at night this may be extremely important in terms of comfortable, unbroken sleep.

Optimised cycling peritoneal dialysis (OCPD) (Fig. 8.17)

OCPD provides another way to individualise the patient's treatment. It allows the delivery of more dialysis as residual renal function declines. During OCPD the patient performs overnight CCPD or TPD as well as adding up to nine day-time exchanges of PD fluid. Some APD machines are designed so that the patient can perform both the night and day exchanges using the same disposable equipment and solution bags. The longer dwell

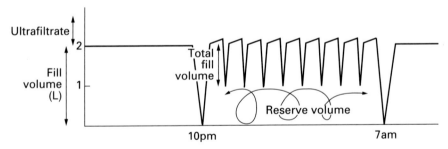

Figure 8.16 Tidal peritoneal dialysis.

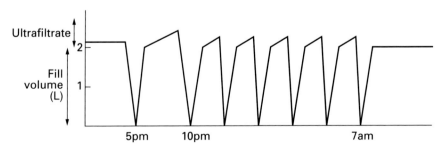

Figure 8.17 Optimised cycling peritoneal dialysis.

of fluid during the day time will optimise clearance opportunities and the shorter dwells of the night-time dialysis will help to achieve ultrafiltration goals.

Intermittent peritoneal dialysis (IPD) (Fig. 8.18)

This form of APD is now rarely carried out as it is difficult to achieve adequate dialysis with this technique. It is performed with the patient in a supine position. It is generally carried out in the dialysis centre in sessions of between 12 and 20 h, two or three times each week. Large volumes (20–40 L) of dialysis fluid are cycled each session with short dwell times and fill volumes of between 2 and 3 L per cycle. For patients with little or no residual renal function, IPD often fails to provide adequate dialysis in the long term.

This treatment is most appropriate for older people who are unable to dialyse at home and who are unsuitable for other therapies (i.e. haemodialysis or transplantation). These patients may gain from the regular social occasion, particularly if several people are treated in the same centre at the same time. IPD may also be used to treat acute patients or for catheter conditioning (following the insertion of the catheter) when dialysis fill volumes can be gradually increased.

Whichever method of PD is chosen for the patient at any particular time, it should provide a balance between both their clinical and lifestyle needs.

Figure 8.19 shows an example of an APD machine.

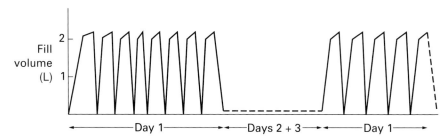

Figure 8.18 Intermittent peritoneal dialysis.

PATIENT SELECTION

An important consideration when developing a successful PD programme is good patient selection. Treating the most appropriate patients with PD will avoid the patient being subjected to increased risk of morbidity and mortality. In the early years of PD, selection was mainly based on the patient's inability to have haemodialysis—for example, those patients with poor or no vascular access, poor biochemical control on haemodialysis with high predialysis serum levels of creatinine, those patients with severe anaemia (i.e. haemoglobin of <5 g dL^{-1}) with a need for frequent blood transfusions, those patients with poorly controlled hypertension, those

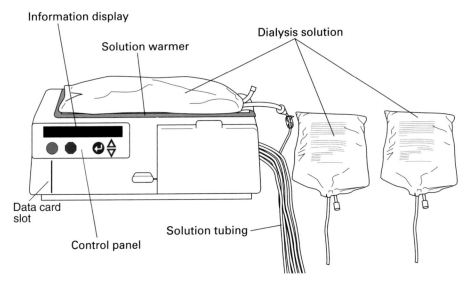

Figure 8.19 Baxter Healthcare Ltd HomeChoice Pro automated peritoneal dialysis machine (with permission).

with excessive fluid gain between dialysis sessions and those who had progressive metabolic and neurological complications. Although these criteria do recommend patients for PD, positive selection criteria are now preferred as PD has proven to be a successful viable alternative to haemodialysis as a treatment for chronic renal disease.

As there are two different therapy modes within the broad title of PD (i.e. CAPD and APD), the selection criteria for each are seen to be slightly different with many overlaps. Tables 8.1 and 8.2 indicate which patients are more suited to APD and those who are more suited to CAPD.

Table 8.1 Patients who are suited to continuous ambulatory peritoneal dialysis (CAPD) or automated peritoneal dialysis (APD)

Suited to CAPD	Suited to either CAPD or APD	Suited to APD
Patients whose membranes transport solutes slowly or at an average speed	Promotion of home dialysis Patients with complicating cardiovascular disease Children with small body size Patients with poor vascular access Patients with diabetes mellitus Patients with severe hypertension Patients with anaemia Patients who wish to travel	Patients who seek day-time freedom to attend work or school Patients at risk of complications associated with raised intraabdominal pressure Patients who require a carer to perform their dialysis Patients with chronic backache Patients who require enhanced dialysis, i.e those without residual renal function

Table 8.2 Patients who are unsuitable for continuous ambulatory peritoneal dialysis (CAPD) or automated peritoneal dialysis (APD)

Unsuitable for CAPD	Unsuitable for either CAPD or APD	Unsuitable for APD
Patients with chronic back pain Patients at risk of complications associated with raised intraabdominal pressure	Patients with chronic obstructive lung disease Patients with diverticular disease Patients who are unable to care for themselves and do not have the assistance of a full-time carer	

PERITONEAL DIALYSIS FOR THOSE WITH DIABETES

Diabetes mellitus can cause damage to many organs. The eyes, bladder, bowel, nervous system and kidneys can all be affected. If those with diabetes are given an intermittent form of dialysis, such as haemodialysis, rapid fluctuations occur in their blood chemistry and fluid status. This may cause episodes of hypertension, thereby increasing the risk of cardiac or cerebrovascular events. Hypertension may worsen peripheral vascular disease.

Access required for haemodialysis may prove difficult to achieve for those with diabetes due to poor vascular condition, whereas PD access is much easier to establish. Before using PD in diabetic patients, the following considerations should be taken into account:

- blood glucose control
- blood pressure control
- fluid and electrolyte control
- access.

Blood glucose control

Although glucose is used as an osmotic agent in PD, this does not deter from the therapy's ability to achieve good results for those with diabetes. An average PD patient will absorb between 100 and 150 g of glucose per day from the dialysis fluid and this has led to some problems in the past, such as hyperinsulinaemia and premature arteriosclerosis. Searches for alternative osmotic agents are promising. A solution which utilises larger molecules of glucose or polyglucose (icodextrin) is an advantage to diabetics as there is a marked reduction in the amount of glucose absorbed by the patient. Other solutions that use amino acids as the osmotic agent are glucose-free as well as having the advantage of providing the patient with a nutritional supplement.

There are a number of alternative methods of blood sugar control for the diabetic PD patient. These include subcutaneous or intraperitoneal insulin, oral agents or dietary control. Any combination of these methods can be used. No single method has been shown to be more suitable than another for all patients.

Intraperitoneal insulin

The normal route for insulin from the pancreas is via the portal vein to the liver, before it reaches the systemic circulation. Insulin administered i.p. is partly absorbed by diffusion across the peritoneum into the portal venous circulation. This closely mimics the physiological secretion of insulin.

If insulin is administered via the peritoneum it promotes blood sugar control throughout the dwell time—i.p. insulin is absorbed along with the glucose from the dialysis fluid. Approximately 50% of insulin injected i.p. is absorbed after an 8-h dwell time.

Insulin which is administered through the peritoneal membrane has a similar effect to physiologically administered insulin. This means that glycaemic control during PD is more physiological than during haemodialysis. Such an advantage should impact on the overall long-term progression of diabetic complications in patients on dialysis.

Insulin should be added to the bag of dialysis fluid before it is connected to the patient. In this way, the bag may be discarded if accidentally contaminated or punctured by the needle. Strict aseptic technique must be followed when adding the insulin, which is usually done through the specially designed medication port. Those with diabetes who also have poor eyesight due to retinopathy may need a community nurse to add the insulin to each bag of dialysis fluid. This will involve a daily visit when the nurse injects insulin into the dialysis fluid in the normal way but through a small hole made in the overpouch of the bags. All bags should be inverted several times before the fluid is drained into the patient to ensure thorough mixing of the insulin.

Several protocols of blood sugar control with i.p. insulin have been published (Khanna et al 1986, Lameire et al 1993, Routtembourg 1988, Scarpioni et al 1994). There appear to be no studies that compare the effectiveness of different methods; however, they all appear to be effective in achieving metabolic control of blood sugar. Most patients require more than 100% of their usual pre-CAPD subcutaneous insulin dose divided between four exchanges. A reduced dose should be added to the overnight dwell to prevent hypoglycaemia during the night. Higher levels of insulin may need to be added to hypertonic glucose dialysis fluid. The exact amount varies between patients but may be assessed at onset by using a sliding scale of insulin with capillary blood glucose monitoring.

Intraperitoneal insulin in automated peritoneal dialysis

Good blood sugar control can be achieved in APD patients with insulin being administered either subcutaneously or i.p., or both subcutaneously and i.p. The amount of insulin administered needs to be adjusted according to individual requirements. During the day, patients are given the daily dose of insulin, usually long-acting, by subcutaneous injection. Additional insulin can also be administered either i.p. or subcutaneously at the start of the APD therapy.

Blood pressure control

For those with diabetes, blood pressure can be well controlled by PD due to the continuous fluid and sodium removal during dialysis (Young et al 1984).

Fluid and electrolyte control

This is achieved by the continuous nature of PD and has advantages for diabetic patients in prevention of cardiovascular stress due to fluid overload or hyperkalaemia.

Access

One of the advantages of PD in those with diabetes is the ease with which the peritoneum can be accessed. The techniques involved in PD catheter insertion in the diabetic are similar to those for other patients. There does not seem to be any higher incidence of either infectious or non-infectious catheter complications for the diabetic patient treated with PD (Linbald et al 1989).

SOLUTION FORMULATION

The most commonly prescribed and, up until the early 1990s, the most widely available osmotic agent used in PD is glucose. Dialysis fluid comes in three glucose strengths (1.36%, 2.27% and 3.86% or 1.5%, 2.5% and 4.25% monohydrate glucose). The strong (hypertonic) solutions provide the greater osmotic strength. Patients would use 1.36% glucose most often whilst their weight is within 0.5 kg of their 'dry' or 'target' weight. Hypertonic solutions should be used when the patient has fluid overload. Most patients ultrafiltrate an extra 200–600 mL by using a 2000-mL medium (2.27%) glucose solution bag and an extra 400–1000 mL by using a 2000-mL strong (3.86%) glucose solution bag. Patients should be taught to record their body weight on a daily basis and choose the appropriate solution strengths for that day.

Ultrafiltration by hypertonic solutions is maintained for approximately 8 h in most patients (Fig. 8.20). After this time some reabsorption of fluid may occur. In those patients whose membranes transport solutes quickly (high transporters), reabsorption may occur sooner than 8 h, giving rise to the need to use other solution formulation exchanges for the longer dwell times (i.e. the overnight dwell in CAPD or the day-time dwell in APD).

The solution is presented in sterile plastic bags with a protective over-pouch in volumes of 500, 750, 1000, 1500, 2000, 2500 and 3000 mL. Bags of 5000 mL are available for use with APD machines.

The electrolyte concentration of dialysis fluid is similar to that of normal serum, with lactate acting as a bicarbonate-generating agent to combat metabolic acidosis, which is common amongst ESRD patients.

Electrolyte composition of the dialysis fluid has been changed several times over the years. A major challenge when treating ESRD patients has been effective phosphate control. Consequently, dialysis fluid does not

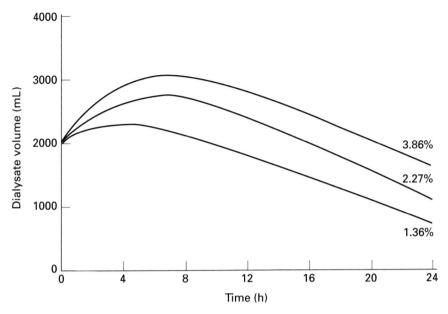

Figure 8.20 Dialysate volume versus time (approximate averages).

contain any phosphate, and patients are given oral phosphate-binding agents to help eliminate dietary phosphate intake from the body. In the past, these phosphate-binding agents were aluminium-based. However, these were implicated in aluminium-related bone disease which many patients experienced (Armstrong & Cunningham 1994). Aluminium toxicity may also cause microcytic anaemia and encephalopathy and so its use as a phosphate-binding agent in the present day has been reduced (Armstrong & Cunningham 1994). The alternative ingredient for an effective phosphate binder is calcium given in the form of calcium carbonate or calcium acetate. These binders have their problems too, leading in some patients to raised serum calcium levels, particularly if the patient is also having vitamin D therapy. This relatively recent complication of PD has led to the manufacture of a dialysis fluid containing physiological levels of ionised calcium and this solution (a) is compared to the original solution (b) in Table 8.3.

Table 8.3 Comparison of dialysis fluid containing ionised calcium (a) with original solution (b)

	a (mmol L^{-1})	b (mmol L^{-1})
Sodium (Na)	132	132
Chloride (Cl)	95	95
Lactate	40	35
Magnesium (Mg)	0.25	0.75
Calcium (Ca)	1.25	1.75

Bicarbonate/lactate-based peritoneal dialysis solutions

Bicarbonate/lactate has several advantages as a buffer for PD solutions. Bicarbonate is the natural buffer of the body. As a result of the metabolism of ingested foods, our body produces hydrogen ions (protons). This acid must be excreted or neutralised in order to maintain the body's acid–base balance. The kidneys play a key role in maintaining the acid–base balance. Not only do they excrete hydrogen ions, but they also regenerate bicarbonate. In people with renal failure this function is impaired or lost. Therefore it is important to replace the lost bicarbonate to maintain the acid–base balance and prevent the occurrence of acidosis. Using bicarbonate in the PD solution is the most natural way of restoring the bicarbonate level in renal patients. Alternative buffers, like lactate, need some conversion (metabolism) before they result in bicarbonate.

The biocompatibility of a PD solution has been defined as the ability of a solution formulation to permit adequate long-term dialysis without a clinically significant undesirable host response (Consensus Conference on Biocompatibility 1994). Di Paolo et al (1995) have defined biocompatibility of a PD solution as its capacity to leave the anatomical and functional characteristics of the peritoneum unmodified in time. These objectives will best be met by solutions whose composition is identical to the composition of extracellular fluid in the body, in particular to the composition of blood. A PD solution has been developed that contains an alternative buffer component, bicarbonate and lactate.

A clinical study on the treatment of pain on infusion (Mactier et al 1998) compared a bicarbonate/lactate solution and another experimental solution based on 38 mmol L^{-1} of bicarbonate (without lactate). The experimental solution and the bicarbonate/lactate solution both reduced the infusion pain, but the bicarbonate/lactate mix appeared the most effective.

The commercially available solution comes in a double-chambered bag because some of the compounds of the bicarbonate/lactate solution are not stable during the steam sterilisation process. Glucose needs to be in acidic conditions (low pH) in order to prevent caramelisation. Since the bicarbonate/lactate solution is neutral, the glucose has to be separated from the other compounds. The glucose sits in the upper, smaller chamber, together with calcium and magnesium salts, under acidic conditions. The bicarbonate, lactate and sodium salt sit in the lower, larger chamber. The two solutions are mixed just before infusion (usually whilst the patient is draining used fluid).

This solution, with a combination of bicarbonate 25 mmol and lactate 15 mmol as the buffer, is intended for all exchanges. The solution has a physiological buffer system, with a physiological pH of 7.4, and reduced glucose degradation product levels. It allows a significant reduction of inflow pain and/or discomfort in sensitive patients and has a high potential for improved long-term preservation of the peritoneal membrane (McEnzie et al 1998).

The composition of the most widely available bicarbonate /lactate-based solution is:

- glucose monohydrate: 1.36%, 2.27% or 3.86%
- sodium chloride: 5.38 g L^{-1}
- calcium chloride: 0.184 g L^{-1}
- magnesium chloride hexahydrate: 0.051 g L^{-1}
- sodium bicarbonate: 2.10 g L^{-1}
- sodium lactate: 1.68 g L^{-1}.

Using glucose polymer as an osmotic agent

Problems associated with the use of glucose as an osmotic agent, such as hyperglycaemia and hyperlipidaemia, may prove to be an issue in the management of PD patients. Patients who have poor ultrafiltration provide the greatest challenge in this area, and efforts have concentrated so far on developing a solution with prolonged ultrafiltration properties.

Icodextrin 7.5% is a formulation of a large-molecular-weight glucose polymer which is a more biocompatible solution as it is approximately iso-osmolar with serum. The use of this larger molecule means that less glucose is available for absorption through the peritoneal membrane. Its long-acting ultrafiltration performance (up to 12 h) is combined with low carbohydrate absorption. Its formulation is presented as a 7.5% solution of icodextrin. Icodextrin produces less than 50% of the calorie load of glucose per unit volume of ultrafiltrate and appears to be an effective osmotic agent (Mistry et al 1987, Peers & Gokal 1997).

The large multicentre MIDAS study (Gokal and the MIDAS Group 1994) demonstrated that icodextrin solution is well tolerated and is as effective as 3.86% glucose over long dwell exchanges. Peers et al (1995) demonstrated that in patients who are failing on glucose-based CAPD, icodextrin can extend technique survival by an average of at least 1 year when included in the dialysis prescription.

Cooper et al (1995) agreed that overnight APD could be further improved by a prolonged day-time dwell using icodextrin. To achieve this, icodextrin was compared with an empty peritoneum during the day in 8 patients and the authors suggested that icodextrin can be useful to increase clearances in APD.

Icodextrin solution (7.5%) is of particular value in patients with ultrafiltration failure, defined by Mactier in 1991 as 'Clinical evidence of fluid overload which persists despite restriction of fluid intake and the use of three or more hypertonic exchanges per day' (Stein et al 1994, Peers & Gokal 1997).

In summary, this solution has been demonstrated to be effective as a long-dwell solution for both CAPD and APD patients, resulting in more effective ultrafiltration and improved clearances.

Using amino acids as an osmotic agent

Forty per cent of PD patients suffer from protein malnutrition (Young et al 1991) and so it is important to be able to provide additional nutritional supplement to the patient's normal daily intake. There are a number of different methods of administering these supplements, namely oral, enteral, parenteral and i.p. These are discussed further in Chapter 9.

The traditional forms of supplementing these patients' diets all have shortcomings with regard to compliance, palatability and formulation. Administering amino acids via the peritoneal membrane has many advantages for PD patients in that the solution is specifically formulated for ESRD patients:

- There is no increased phosphate load.
- There is no increased fluid load.
- It reduces the daily glucose load PD patients receive.
- As it is used as a normal dialysis exchange, there are no extra responsibilities for the patient.

Intraperitoneal amino acid (IPAA) solution contains 15 amino acids. Eight are essential amino acids, two are considered essential to ESRD patients and five are non-essential. The electrolyte formulation is shown in Table 8.4. The osmotic agent glucose is replaced by 1.1% amino acids, which have the comparative ultrafiltration capability of 1.36% glucose solution. After a 4–6 h dwell, 65–95% of the amino acids are absorbed, the equivalent to about 18 g (from a 2000-mL bag containing 22 g of amino acids) or 0.3 g kg^{-1} day^{-1} in a 70-kg patient. This is approximately 25% of the daily protein requirement for a PD patient.

IPAA is administered in the same way as other PD solutions. It is prescribed for one exchange per day, replacing one of the usual glucose dialysis solution bags. It should be given either at a main meal or with a high-calorie snack, as this will ensure that the amino acids are used in the anabolic process to generate protein rather than being expended as an energy source. Its optimal dwell time is 4–6 h as described above. It is important to note that the solution should only be administered if the patient is receiving adequate dialysis, acidosis has been corrected and the energy intake of the patient is at least 35 kcal kg^{-1}. These conditions optimise protein synthesis.

A study by Kennedy et al (1999) showed that the use of amino acid solutions in adequately dialysed, malnourished PD patients does not increase acidosis or phosphate levels compared to malnourished PD patient receiving oral supplements. Along with this study there have been several other papers published showing the efficacy of this solution (Chen 1998, Faller 1996, Jones et al 1998, Randerson et al 1989).

Table 8.4 The electrolyte formulation of intraperitoneal amino acid solution

Sodium	132 mmol L^{-1}
Chloride	95 mmol L^{-1}
Lactate	40 mmol L^{-1}
Magnesium	0.25 mmol L^{-1}
Calcium	1.25 mmol L^{-1}

The 'perfect' peritoneal dialysis solution

Hutchison (1992) described the characteristics of the ideal PD solution as being:

- predictable, with sustained solute clearance and ultrafiltration capability
- able to supply deficient solutes and remove uraemic toxins
- able to supply part of the patient's nutritional needs without promoting metabolic complications
- an iso-osmolar solution at physiological pH, and containing a bicarbonate buffer to correct acidosis
- having minimal absorption of a non-toxic osmotic agent and providing an ultrafiltration of around 2000 mL daily
- able to inhibit bacterial and fungal growth, but without toxicity to the peritoneal membrane or host defences.

It now seems obvious that patients will benefit from using a combination of all the available solutions formulations, including amino acid, polyglucose, bicarbonate/lactate and glucose.

The effect of peritoneal dialysis on the peritoneal membrane

The use of the peritoneal membrane for dialysis may give rise to changes in its function and structure. However, despite this, the peritoneal membrane has proven to be remarkably resilient. There are a number of studies that have shown the peritoneal membrane to be stable (Davies et al 1996, Krediet et al 1996, Selgas et al 1998). 'Membrane failure' in PD is not yet well defined. However, if patients suffer from poor ultrafiltration and poor removal of solutes, they may well be said to have membrane failure. Also, failure of local host defence mechanisms and the development of peritoneal sclerosis are signs of failure of the peritoneal membrane.

Impaired transport of water and solutes has been reported as the reason for dropout in 16% of patients from three dialysis populations (CANUSA Peritoneal Dialysis Study Group 1996, Genestier et al 1995, Gokal et al 1987). Ultrafiltration failure was reported in half of these patients and inadequate clearances in the other half. However, the peritoneal clearances of low-molecular-weight solutes are mainly determined by the drained volume (Krediet et al 1998). Therefore, patients with the highest D/P ratios of creatinine may have the lowest peritoneal mass transfer of urea due to small drained volumes (Wang et al 1998).

Because of the strong relationships between the drained volume and solute transfer, it is likely that ultrafiltration failure as a reason for therapy transfer has been underestimated.

It follows from the above studies that poor ultrafiltration is the most frequent membrane problem in PD patients. Its occurrence may be dependent on the length of time the patient had been having PD. Using a clinical definition, Heimbürger et al (1990) estimated it to be present in 3% of patients after 1 year on PD, but in 31% of patients after 6 years on PD. It should also be noted that ultrafiltration failure is often difficult to diagnose because patients may be fluid-overloaded due to excessive fluid intake or reduced urine production.

There are four main causes of ultrafiltration failure (Krediet et al 2000):

- the presence of a large vascular surface area
- a decreased osmotic effect of glucose
- high lymphatic absorption
- an extremely small peritoneal surface area (e.g. due to multiple adhesions).

It is possible for patients to have more than one of the above causes of ultrafiltration failure. In severe cases of ultrafiltration failure, transfer to haemodialysis may be recommended.

ASSESSING PERITONEAL DIALYSIS ADEQUACY

Dialysis has shown over the years to be able to prolong the lives of many patients with ESRD. It would therefore follow that dialysis patients should not die from 'uraemia' (Burkart 1993).

Unfortunately, there is increasing evidence that inadequacies in dialysis dose or underdelivery of a prescribed dose of dialysis are contributing to high mortality rates amongst dialysis patients. Data compiled by the US Health Care Financing Administration (HCFA) and analysed by the US Renal Data System (USRDS) have shown that the gross mortality rate for the US ESRD population in 2000 was 20%. This means that, whilst the average US citizen aged 40 years has an additional added life expectancy of 37.4 years, the average 40-year-old ESRD patient has an additional added life expectancy of only 7.2 years (USRDS 2000).

Prolonged periods of inadequate dialysis can result in irreversible or slow reversible uraemia which can influence morbidity and mortality. Inadequate dialysis can be defined as the inadequate removal of waste material, clinical symptoms of which include itching, nausea, anorexia and uraemic smell, and inadequate ultrafiltration, clinical symptoms of which include weight gain, oedema and hypertension.

The goals of PD are to prolong life, reverse the symptoms of uraemia, maintain patients in positive nitrogen balance, have an adequate energy intake and have their maximum level of quality of life in a way that is least disruptive to their lifestyle. This can be summarised by saying that well-dialysed patients feel well enough to eat a sufficient diet rich in protein and experience a minimum of complications to their treatment.

There are a number of ways in which dialysis adequacy can be measured and all parameters must be taken into consideration:

- creatinine clearance—a solute-removal test based on body surface area
- Kt/V—a urea index relating urea clearance to the volume of urea distributed in the body (see below)
- protein nutrition
- general well-being.

A number of studies have linked a decrease in creatinine clearance and Kt/V to an increased risk of morbidity and mortality. Teehan et al (1990) found that Kt/V was linked to clinical outcome. For example, both death on CAPD and transfusion requirements are partially predicted by the level of Kt/V. Blake et al (1992) came to the same conclusion using creatinine clearance as a predictor of outcome.

The largest study of PD patients was conducted in 14 centres across the USA and Canada. The CANUSA study (Churchill et al 1996) investigated the impact of demographic, nutritional and adequacy parameters on morbidity and mortality and defined adequate PD according to estimates of solute clearance (e.g. urea and creatinine). The USRDS data show that there is no difference in survival between non-diabetic patients (all age groups) and diabetic patients under 58 years. The CANUSA study shows that estimates of patients' nutritional status and dialysis adequacy had clinically important and statistically significant associations with patients' survival, technique survival and hospitalisation. This study also indicated that increasing creatinine clearance and Kt/V will lead to higher survival rates. Churchill et al (1996) also stated that total creatinine clearance and Kt/V decreased during the trial period because loss of residual renal function was not compensated for by increasing the dialysis dose. Churchill et al (1996) also defined 'optimum dialysis' as the dialysis dose at which the clinical gain is not worth the increased patient effort or cost. The adequate dialysis dose should be the minimum target.

In summary, what the CANUSA study tells us is that more dialysis is better. Giving the patient a dialysis prescription which increases Kt/V and creatinine clearance will make the patient feel better and increase survival rate. It is also important to monitor nutritional status since this will influence survival. The risk of death increases with increased age, the presence of type 2 diabetes and a past history of cardiovascular disease.

Targets for adequate dialysis continue to be re-evaluated. Currently, a weekly creatinine clearance of >70 L per week per 1.73 m^2 body surface area (Dubois & Dubois 1916) and a Kt/V of >2.1 week^{-1} are deemed satisfactory so long as the patient's nutritional status and general well-being are also assessed as being satisfactory (Churchill et al 1996).

There are a number of computer programs available on the market that will calculate the patient's Kt/V, creatinine clearance and nutritional status. Some of these programs will also model the patient's treatment, allowing the nurse or physician to look at a wide range of PD therapy options for the optimal regime that meets the adequacy needs of each individual patient. This enables the clinician to eliminate the trial-and-error process of prescribing PD, takes away the need to perform manual calculations, and provides the renal unit with a database of their patients' quality of dialysis.

Creatinine as a measure of dialysis adequacy

Creatinine is a metabolic product from the breakdown of muscle. Patients who have a larger muscle mass therefore tend to have higher serum creatinine levels. Creatinine, with a molecular weight of 113 Da, will equilibrate more slowly across the peritoneal membrane than urea (molecular weight 60 Da).

When calculating creatinine clearance three values must be considered:

- solute generation rate
- residual renal clearance
- dialysis efficiency.

The consensus amongst dialysis care professionals suggests a minimum target of 70 L week^{-1} 1.73 m^{-2} BSA. A normalised BSA of 1.73 m^2 is used to enable an assumption of the creatinine generation rate based on a patient's size, provided that the patient is infection free and in nitrogen balance. Creatinine clearance for both the patient's dialysis regime and residual renal function can be calculated by using the worksheet (Fig. 8.21).

Urea as a measure of dialysis adequacy

Urea is a metabolic product of the protein we eat. As more protein is eaten, more urea is generated. It therefore follows that when examining a patient's serum urea levels it is important to take into consideration recent protein intake. A low serum urea in a patient with ESRD may simply be due to a low protein intake, rather than adequate dialysis. A high serum urea on the other hand may indicate increased catabolism, a deterioration in residual renal function or inadequate dialysis. Urea is a small molecule (molecular weight 60 Da) which is distributed in body water. It diffuses readily and is therefore easily removed from the blood.

The prescription index Kt/V was developed by Gotch et al (1983) and Gotch & Sargent (1985) in the National Co-operative Dialysis Study of haemodialysis patients. Kt/V is an index of urea removal, which is patient-specific as it looks at urea removal achieved over time ($K \times t$) and measurement of urea in the body water (V) for each patient. Therefore: K = clearance; t = time; V = volume of body water in which urea is distributed (Figs 8.22 and 8.23).

The index does not account for dietary protein intake, protein catabolic rate or urea generation rate. It is just as important to measure residual renal Kt/V as it is to measure dialysis Kt/V. The two should be added together to give a total weekly Kt/V value. Kt/V for both the patient's dialysis regime and residual renal function can be calculated using the worksheet shown in Figure 8.24.

Currently, a weekly Kt/V of at least 2 is deemed adequate for PD patients, providing their nutrition and general well-being are also assessed as satisfactory. The weekly goal for Kt/V for haemodialysis patients is 3.0–4.2 a week (1–1.4 per session). The reason that this level is higher than for PD patients is explained by the peak concentration hypothesis proposed by Keshaviah et al (1989) (Fig. 8.25). Kt/V for haemodialysis patients has to be increased to equate the peak urea concentrations reached between dialysis sessions.

Protein nutrition

'Over 40% of peritoneal dialysis patients are undernourished': Young et al (1991). Various terms have been used to identify a patient's nutritional

Name patient:
Date:

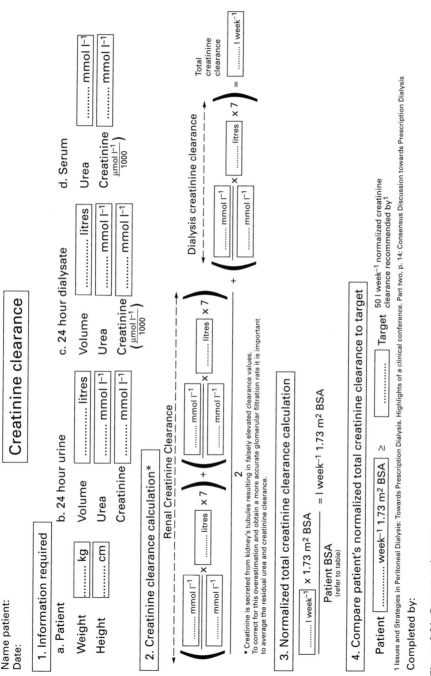

Figure 8.21 Creatinine clearance.

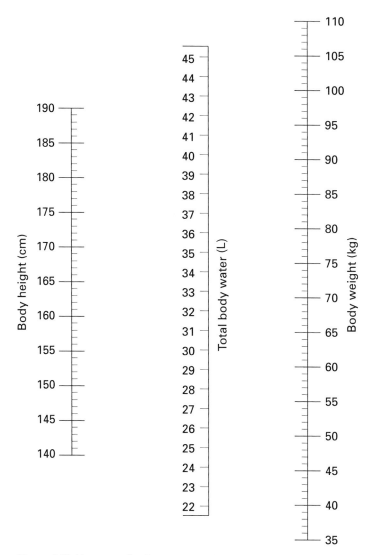

Figure 8.22 Nomogram for the estimation of total body water in females.

status; these include serum albumin level, dietary protein intake (DPI), protein catabolic rate (PCR) and subjective global assessment (SGA); Detsky et al (1987). A patient's nutritional status is an important factor in assessing a patient's dialysis adequacy but, as with all measures, it should not be taken in isolation.

Protein intake and PCR are important issues to be considered for those on PD. It is vital that the PD nurse and dietitian and the patient work closely together to avoid the complications associated with malnutrition.

SGA is a simple and reliable tool which is increasingly being used in the diagnosis of malnutrition amongst ESRD patients: see Chapter 9 for further details. A study performed by Enia et al (1993) showed that SGA of nutrition

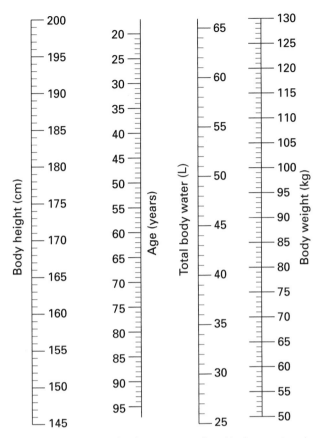

Figure 8.23 Nomogram for the estimation of total body water in males.

is a clinically adequate method of assessing nutritional status in dialysis patients. The CANUSA study (Keshaviah et al unpublished work) found that a lower SGA score was associated with an increased relative risk of death.

General well-being

Despite the efficacy of a combination of the above physical parameters for measuring adequacy of dialysis, there can be no doubt that the ultimate gauge of treatment success must increasingly become the overall quality of life of the patient. There is now widespread agreement that in assessing the effects of a treatment it is essential to assess both the quality and quantity of life. Healthcare purchasers are increasingly under pressure to demonstrate cost-effective utilisation of the limited resources available to them. Quality-of-life assessment is a key outcome measure in determining this cost-effectiveness, but its multidimensional and subjective nature means that it is problematic to measure.

There are a number of tools available for the measurement of quality of life amongst renal patients; however, to date there is no consensus on which measure is best to use. Welch (1994) describes a number of measures which have been used previously and may be of use in the clinical setting to

Name patient:
Date:

Kt/V*

1. Information required

a. Patient

Weight .... kg
Height .... cm

b. 24 hour urine

Volume .... litres
Urea .... mmol l^{-1}
Creatinine .... mmol l^{-1}

c. 24 hour dialysate

Volume .... litres
Urea .... mmol l^{-1}
Creatinine $\left(\dfrac{\mu mol\ l^{-1}}{1000}\right)$ .... mmol l^{-1}

d. Serum

Urea .... mmol l^{-1}
Creatinine $\left(\dfrac{\mu mol\ l^{-1}}{1000}\right)$ .... mmol l^{-1}

2. Kt/V calculation

a. Residual renal Kt/V

Step 1: $\dfrac{\text{......... mmol l}^{-1}}{\text{......... mmol l}^{-1}} \times$ .... litres $\times 1000$ $\overset{1440}{\underset{\text{min. in 24 h}}{\longleftrightarrow}}$ = ... ml min^{-1} Residual renal clearance

Step 2: $\dfrac{\text{......... mmol l}^{-1} \times 1440 \times 7}{\text{......... kg} \times \begin{array}{l}\text{♂ 0.6}\\\text{♀ 0.55}\end{array} \times 1000}$ = Weekly residual Kt/V

b. Dialysate Kt/V

$\dfrac{\text{......... mmol l}^{-1}}{\text{......... mmol l}^{-1}} \times$ .... litres $\times 7$ / $\text{......... kg} \times \begin{array}{l}\text{♂ 0.6}\\\text{♀ 0.55}\end{array}$ = Weekly dialysate Kt/V

3. Total Kt/V

Weekly residual Kt/V + Weekly dialysate Kt/V = Weekly total Kt/V

4. Compare patient's weekly Kt/V with target

Patient Weekly total Kt/V ≥ .... Target

* K = Urea clearance (l week^{-1}) · T = Number of days per week the patient dialyses
V = Volume of urea distribution

Figure 8.24 *Kt/V* worksheet.

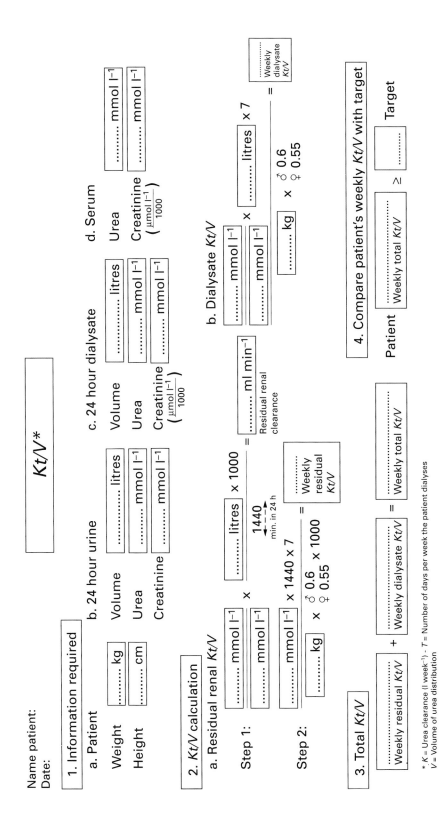

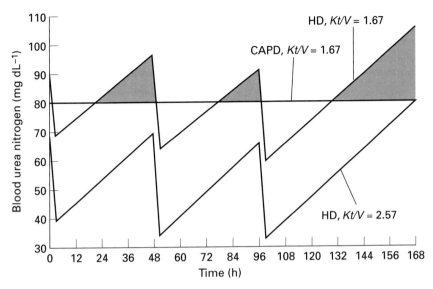

Figure 8.25 Keshaviah's peak concentration hypothesis. HD, haemodialysis; CAPD, continuous ambulatory peritoneal dialysis.

measure quality of life and general well-being. These include the Sickness Impact Profile (Bergner et al 1976), the Nottingham Health Profile (Hunt & McEwan 1983), the SF36 (Ware & Shelbourne 1992), the Dialysis Stress Scale (Burton et al 1986) and the Index of Well-being (Campbell 1976).

What most healthcare professionals do agree upon, however, is that assessment should become a routine that is systematically incorporated into the ongoing evaluation of patients (Renal Association 1997).

PROBLEM-SOLVING IN PERITONEAL DIALYSIS

Complications of PD can be divided into two main groups—those related to ESRD, and those problems directly associated with PD itself.

Anaemia and hypertension are discussed in Chapter 5. Many PD patients have evidence of some bone disease when they start dialysis. In order to prevent this problem worsening and to correct bone abnormalities it is important to maintain serum ionised calcium levels within the normal range. Many PD patients (up to 30%) experience hypercalcaemia partly due to the use of calcium carbonate or acetate as a phosphate-binding agent (Armstrong & Cunningham 1994). This can be corrected by using physiological calcium PD solutions (i.e. 1.25 mmol L^{-1}). Phosphate-binding agents are essential as PD alone cannot normalise serum phosphate levels (Armstrong & Cunningham 1994).

High levels of prolactin are often found in PD patients and this has been identified as one of the many causes of infertility and sexual dysfunction amongst these patients. Some male PD patients have lower than normal levels of testosterone. Women can have normal menstruation with ovulating cycles and some have become pregnant whilst on PD (Hou 1990).

Dialysis-related problems of PD patients

Protein loss

Protein is lost through the peritoneal membrane at a rate of $6-12$ g day^{-1} in stable patients. To compensate for this loss, PD patients need to eat between 1.0 and 1.2 g kg^{-1} of body weight day^{-1} of dietary protein.

This loss is increased during peritonitis, when a patient can lose up to 20 g day^{-1}. An alternative method of compensating for this loss is with IPAA solution.

Cardiovascular and lipid problems

Many patients reach ESRD with established left ventricular hypertrophy, coronary ischaemia and vascular disease. However, despite the fact that there have been many advances in the technology and analysis of adequacy of dialysis, cardiovascular morbidity and mortality remain very high in patients on dialysis, and this is the most common cause of death (Fried et al 1999).

Patients experience raised levels of cholesterol and triglycerides within the first year on PD. This is mainly due to the glucose absorbed from PD fluid. Several studies have shown that these changes are not long-lasting and peak levels are usually reached within $3-12$ months of starting dialysis. The levels often fall after this period back to pretreatment levels (Khanna et al 1983, Lindholm et al 1983, Ramos et al 1983). In fact, serum lipid levels in patients after 1 year on PD appear to be the same as in haemodialysis patients (Norbeck & Lindholm 1982). Guidelines on the treatment of lipid disorders were published by Fried et al (1999).

Raised intraabdominal pressure problems in PD patients

Raised intraabdominal pressure is caused by the pressure of high volumes of fluid in the peritoneal cavity. This pressure is further increased when the patient carries out strenuous exercise or suffers excessive coughing. Continuous raised intraabdominal pressure can increase the risk of abdominal hernias such as inguinal, incisional, diaphragmatic or umbilical, and of dialysate leakage around the catheter exit site.

Oedema of the labia in females and the scrotum and penis in males is a distressing complication caused by dialysate leakage through soft tissues. It is usually easily rectified by stopping PD for a short period (usually up to 1 week). Hernias and persistent leaks require surgical repair, while stopping PD for a time to allow the site to heal. If haemodialysis is not an alternative form of treatment for the patient during this temporary interruption to treatment, PD may be continued so long as the patient is lying down, therefore decreasing the intraabdominal pressure (i.e. by using some form of APD).

In the event of dialysate leakage at the exit site, PD must be ceased immediately as the presence of a glucose-rich solution at a wound site gives rise to a markedly increased risk of infection. Leakage can be identified by using urine test sticks or blood glucose reagent strips at the exit site. The normal healing time for dialysate leakage is 1 week, but this may be increased in diabetic, severely uraemic or malnourished patients.

CAPD patients with previous vertebral disease may experience back pain due to the raised intraabdominal pressure incurred in an upright position. In this situation APD may be the preferred therapy.

Drainage problems

These usually have a minor cause which, with proper patient training and education, can be rectified by the patients themselves at home. Reasons for poor inflow or outflow of dialysis fluid and their treatment are outlined below.

Kinks in the tubing

The most common cause of poor drainage or inflow of PD fluid is tubing kinks or closed clamps. Patients should be taught to check the tubing for kinks and closed clamps as a first line of action in the event of poor in- or outflow of dialysis fluid. Catheter kinks sometimes occur due to malpositioning during surgical insertion. This will become apparent shortly after insertion, if not during the insertion procedure, and can be confirmed by X-ray (the PD catheter has a radiopaque stripe along its length). This problem is usually rectified by surgical intervention; however, it can occasionally be improved if the patient has a bowel motion.

Constipation

Constipation should be avoided in PD patients, not only because it causes problems with dialysate outflow but also because diverticulosis of the colon increases the risk of peritonitis. Constipation prevention is achieved by encouraging the patient to take a diet high in fibre along with a mild laxative if appropriate. Regular exercise is also recommended. If constipation does occur, treatment can be with laxatives, glycerine suppositories or a saline enema. The use of phosphate-containing enemas should be avoided due to the absorption of phosphate through the bowel during their administration. For the same reason the use of magnesium-containing laxatives should also be avoided.

Fibrin formation

Fibrin strands or plugs (a protein formed from fibrinogen in blood plasma in the process of clotting) in dialysate effluent are a common cause of poor drainage. The blockage, usually in the catheter or tubing, can normally be removed by 'milking' the tubing. Heparin may be added to the dialysis fluid (200–500 units L^{-1}) as a prophylactic measure, as it prevents the formation of fibrin.

If 'milking' the tubing does not remove the obstruction a fibrolytic agent can be used. Both streptokinase (250 000 i.u.) and urokinase (5000 i.u.) in 2–3 mL sodium chloride 0.9% for i.v. injection are available and should be infused into the catheter under aseptic conditions; the catheter should then be clamped and the drug left to infuse for 2 h. The catheter can then be checked for patency.

Malpositioned catheter

If catheter obstruction is not relieved by any of the above techniques, the problem may be due to obstruction caused by omentum attached to the catheter tip. The omental attachment usually causes the catheter to migrate out of the pelvic cavity. In such cases it often proves difficult to resolve this problem without surgery.

It is possible to remove omentum from the catheter whilst leaving it in place during surgical procedure. It is common for the surgeon to perform a local omentectomy at the same time to prevent further obstructions by omentum. If it proves impossible to rectify the obstruction or position of the catheter by surgical methods the final option is to remove the catheter completely and replace it with a new one.

Shoulder pain

Occasionally, patients complain of shoulder pain following the infusion of fresh dialysis solution. This is thought to be a referred pain caused by intraabdominal pressure or air under the diaphragm (Uttley & Prowant 1986). Although it usually resolves within 10–20 min from onset, the patient may find relief by taking a mild analgesia such as paracetamol 1 g. Bicarbonate/lactate-containing PD solutions have also been shown to reduce pain on infusion of dialysis (Tranaeus et al 1998). This solution is discussed above.

Blood-stained effluent

This is a comparatively rare complication occurring most commonly in menstruating females. It may be due to endometriosis or retrograde bleeding through the fallopian tubes. The bleeding is usually mild and self-rectifies within a day or two without specific intervention.

More severe i.p. bleeding causing darkly blood-stained fluid can be caused by haemorrhage. This could be due to the patient straining whilst lifting a heavy object or suffering trauma to the abdomen.

INFECTIOUS COMPLICATIONS OF PERITONEAL DIALYSIS

Peritonitis

Peritonitis is a common clinical problem that occurs in patients with ESRD treated by PD (Keane et al 2000). The incidence of peritonitis varies widely; however, since the 1980s it has become less frequent and during the 1990s approximately one episode every 24 patient-treatment-months was routinely seen (Keane et al 1993). In some PD units, one episode every 60 patient-treatment-months has been achieved (King et al 1992). This is most likely to be due to very high quality patient education, as well as new bag connector and catheter technologies (Keane et al 2000).

There are many different protocols for the treatment of PD peritonitis. An ad hoc advisory committee has reviewed experiences reported in the literature and devised recommendations based upon these assessments. These recommendations were published in *Peritoneal Dialysis International* most recently in 2000 (Keane et al 2000). Antibiotics have been administered i.p. or i.v. or orally, and a number of different dosing regimes have been utilised. Unfortunately, to date there is no clear recommendation of the best single way to treat PD peritonitis. As always, individual clinical situations and variability in patient populations may necessitate modification of these recommendations.

The recent emergence of vancomycin resistance has created a big international problem in the treatment of peritonitis (Keane et al 1996). However, it is recognised that there are some clinical situations where the use of vancomycin may be the most appropriate antibiotic. The ad hoc advisory committee on peritonitis management therefore made further recommendations at the end of 1996. These can be found in Keane et al (1996).

Causes of peritonitis

Most episodes of peritonitis are caused by organisms which are normal skin and nasal flora, for example *Staphylococcus epidermidis* and *S. aureus*. Occasionally, water-borne organisms such as *Pseudomonas* may also cause this infection.

The development of disconnect systems has had an important effect on the overall reduction of the incidence of peritonitis episodes, particularly those due to skin organisms such as *S. epidermidis*. A variety of microorganisms may cause PD peritonitis. Gram-positive organisms, particularly *S. aureus* and *S. epidermidis*, are most commonly seen. However, in patients utilizing the disconnect systems, with the reduction in the incidence of Gram-positive staphylococcus peritonitis, the relative incidence of Gram-negative infection has increased (Keane et al 2000).

There are five main routes of infection causing peritonitis, each one giving rise to common organisms.

Intraluminal (contamination at the solution bag and transfer set connection site)

This contamination occurs most frequently when poor techniques have been used to make the connection. Good patient training and education regarding bag exchange procedure techniques and hand-washing are essential. The incidence of this cause of infection has reduced in recent years due to the use of disconnect systems. These systems incorporate a 'flush before fill' into the procedure, which has been shown to remove organisms caused by touch contamination (Verger & Luzar 1986).

Periluminal (infection introduced via the catheter tunnel from the exit site)

Bacteria present on the skin surface can enter the peritoneal cavity via the catheter tunnel. This infection can occur if there is infection present at the exit site or in the subcutaneous tunnel which has migrated into the peritoneal cavity. The most common organisms seen when periluminal contamination has occurred are *S. epidermidis*, *S. aureus*, *Pseudomonas*, *Proteus* and yeast. *S. aureus* nasal carriage is known to cause an increased risk of

S. aureus exit-site infections, tunnel infections, peritonitis and catheter loss. Prophylaxis with intranasal mupirocin exit-site mupirocin, or oral rifampin has been shown to be effective in reducing *S. aureus* exit site infections (Bernardini et al 1996; Zimmerman et al 1991). These studies recommend that a small amount of mupirocin ointment should be applied to the exit site every day after routine exit-site care, using a cotton swab. This has been shown to be as effective as oral rifampicin in reducing exit-site infection rates. Mupirocin is preferred to rifampicin for prophylactic use because toxicity from mupirocin is negligible. The use of mupirocin ointment at the exit site, however, should be avoided in patients with polyurethane catheters (Cruz catheters) as structural damage to the catheter has been reported. All patients at an increased risk for *S. aureus* infections, including *S. aureus* carriers, diabetics and immunocompromised patients, should be provided with prophylaxis. A practical approach is to prescribe exit-site mupirocin for all at-risk PD patients and so routine nasal swab tests are therefore not necessarily required in these patients.

Transmural (infection through the gut wall)
This infection occurs most commonly in patients with diverticular disease or bowel perforation, but can occur in other patients due to bacteria of intestinal origin entering the peritoneal cavity by migrating through the bowel wall. The most common organism seen as a transmural cause of peritonitis is *Escherichia coli*, although multiple contamination with anaerobes and fungi may also be isolated.

Haematogenous (infection via the blood stream)
This is a rare cause of peritonitis and it may be the peritonitis itself which causes septicaemia. The most common organisms associated with this cause of peritonitis are *Streptococcus* and *Mycobacterium*.

Vaginal (ascending through the vagina)
This is thought to be from bacteria entering the peritoneum via the fallopian tubes. The most common causative organisms seen here are *Candida* and *Pseudomonas*.

Diagnosis of peritonitis
Early diagnosis allowing prompt treatment of peritonitis is essential in minimising damage to the peritoneal membrane. Diagnosis is when two or more of the following conditions are present:

- cloudy PD effluent containing >100 white blood cells uL^{-1} (more than 50% of which are neutrophils)
- abdominal pain and tenderness and pyrexia
- identification of micro-organisms in the PD effluent by positive Gram stain or culture.

The process of diagnosis of peritonitis is summarised in Fig. 8.26.

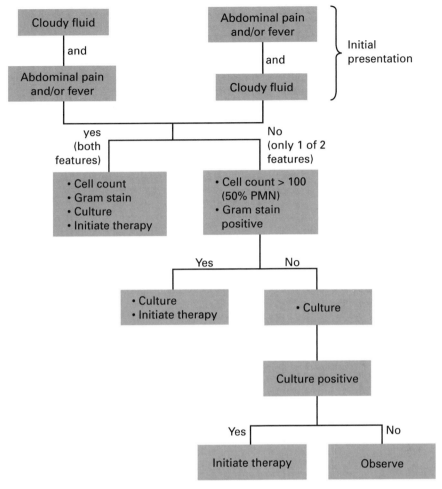

Figure 8.26 Initial clinical and laboratory assessment of a patient for peritonitis. PMN, polymorphic neutrophils.

Obtaining a PD effluent specimen

CAPD

After disconnecting the drainage bag containing the effluent from the patient's transfer set, the bag should be inverted several times to mix the contents. Using strict aseptic technique a sample is taken by sterile needle and syringe from the sample port on the bag (Fig. 8.27).

APD

A sample may either be taken from the day-time dwell, if the patient utilises a 'wet day' (i.e. dialysate in the peritoneum during the day), by attaching a drainage set and bag to the patient's extension set. The sample is then taken in the same way as for a CAPD patient. Alternatively, if the patient is usually 'dry' during the day (i.e. no dialysate in the peritoneum during the day), there are a number of options. Some APD machines have

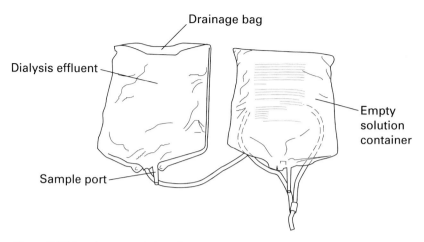

Figure 8.27 Sample port on drainage bag.

a sample bag which can be attached to the drainage tubing. Alternatively, the patient may be taught how to take a sample from the drainage solution containers. If this is not possible, the patient may be asked to detach the drainage solution container from the machine following treatment and take this into the unit. Many APD patients have a supply of CAPD equipment at home for use when travelling if their APD machine is not a portable version; in this case, the patient may be asked to perform a CAPD exchange at home and then attend the clinic with fluid in the peritoneal cavity which can then be drained and sampled in the usual way.

Calculation of peritonitis rates

When evaluating the quality of any treatment it is important to be able to measure its success. Recording the incidence of peritonitis within a group of patients provides us with one way in which we can appraise the standard of patient care. Measuring peritonitis in terms of patient-months giving intervals between episodes of peritonitis is a convenient and reliable way of measuring peritonitis in individual centres on a regular basis. It also allows intercentre comparisons and comparisons at different time points.

Peritonitis rates are expressed as episodes per patient-month and are calculated by dividing the total number of episodes by the total number of patients treated each month. For example, if 100 patients were on PD in January and four had an episode of peritonitis, the rate for January would be 4 in 100 or 1 in 25.

Any patient on PD for 2 weeks is counted as 0.5 of a month. Similarly, a patient on for 1 or 3 weeks is counted as 0.25 and 0.75 respectively. Peritonitis rates have a cumulative value, as demonstrated in Table 8.5. The most accurate peritonitis rate is one which is cumulative for 12 months. Culture-negative or no-growth peritonitis episodes are included in peritonitis rates. Recurrence of the same organism within 14 days of completion of treatment is not included in peritonitis rates.

Table 8.5 Calculation of peritonitis rate. (From Keane et al 1993, with permission.)

Month	Jan	Feb	March	April	May
Episodes	3	1	2	4	1
Patient-month experience	80	86	90	92	94
Monthly peritonitis rate	3/80	1/86	2/90	4/92	1/94
Cumulative	3/80	4/166	6/256	10/348	11/442
Total peritonitis rate	1/26.6	1/41.6	1/42.6	1/34.8	1/40.1
No growth	0	0	1	0	1
Recurrence	0	0	0	1	0

Many peritonitis episodes are mild and can be treated at home. Usually the incubation period from time of contamination for bacterial peritonitis is 24–48 h. Any symptoms should resolve quickly following the initiation of therapy. If the infection shows either a slow response or no response to treatment the choice of antibiotics could be inappropriate.

Those on PD should be taught how to recognise the signs and symptoms of peritonitis during their initial training period and at regular intervals. Ideally the patient, if on CAPD, should complete the bag exchange at home (the presence of PD fluid in the peritoneum may provide some pain relief from inflammation of the peritoneal membrane) and bring the bag of cloudy dialysate effluent into the clinic for sampling. Treatment can then be initiated immediately. The ad hoc advisory committee on peritonitis management (Keane et al 2000) produced a document outlining treatment recommendations for PD-related peritonitis.

There is current debate as to the necessity to perform peritoneal lavage immediately after the diagnosis of peritonitis, as it is thought to reduce the number of phagocytes present in the peritoneum which are available to fight infection. Peritoneal lavage is therefore thought by some to be of benefit only to patients with purulent effluent and abdominal pain as a pain-relieving exercise. There is no evidence to suggest that a transfer set change performed at this time is of any benefit. On admission to the PD clinic the usual fill volume for the patient is medicated with antibiotics.

If the effluent sediment Gram stain suggests Gram-positive bacteria, a Gram-negative organism, or is unavailable, delayed, or negative for any specific organisms, empiric therapy is indicated (Keane et al 2000; Table 8.6).

The patient or carer can be taught how to add the antibiotics to the dialysis fluid to facilitate self-care. Heparin (200–500 units L^{-1}) may also be added to the fluid to prevent the formation of fibrin, which is more likely in the presence of infection.

APD patients may receive antibiotics intraperitoneally by adding the antibiotics to the dialysis solution at the start of the therapy. The i.p. antibiotics may be continued during the long daytime dwell period.

Peritonitis is monitored closely and dialysate effluent should be clear within 48 h of commencing treatment. If the peritonitis resolves, antibiotics are discontinued 7–10 days after the start of therapy.

Table 8.6 Empiric initial therapy, for peritoneal dialysis-related peritonitis, stratified for residual urine volume

Antibiotic	Residual urine output	
	<100 mL day^{-1}	>100 mL day^{-1}
Cefazolin or cephalothin	1 g bag^{-1} q.d.	20 mg kg^{-1} BW bag^{-1} q.d. or 15 mg kg^{-1} BW bag^{-1} q.d.
Ceftazidime	1 g bag^{-1} q.d.	20 mg kg^{-1} BW bag^{-1} q.d.
Gentamicin, tobramycin, netilmicin	0.6 mg kg^{-1} BW bag^{-1} q.d.	Not recommended
Amikacin	2 mg kg^{-1} BW bag^{-1} q.d.	Not recommended

BW, body weight.

Absorption of antibiotics into the serum through the peritoneum from the dialysate is rapid. Therefore, in most cases, administration of intravenous antibiotics is unnecessary.

Permeability changes during peritonitis
The peritoneal membrane permeability tends to increase during episodes of peritonitis, perhaps due to increased blood flow through the peritoneum. Clearances of both large and small molecules increase, as does the absorption of glucose. This can result in marked increases in protein loss through the peritoneum and poor ultrafiltration. Patients need to be educated as to the need to increase dietary protein intake during episodes of peritonitis and to care for their fluid balance ensuring that, if they have no residual renal function, fluid intake is kept to a minimum. Rarely, patients are severely ill with peritonitis and need to be treated in hospital.

There is some evidence to suggest that the administration of amino acid-based solutions during episodes of peritonitis is effective in reducing the amount of protein lost (Dratwa et al 1995).

Culture-negative peritonitis
Occasionally (less than 20%), cultures may be negative for a variety of technical or clinical reasons. If the patient is clinically improving, the first-generation cephalosporin should be continued and the ceftazidime discontinued (Keane et al 2000). Duration of therapy should be 2 weeks. If, on the other hand, no clinical improvement occurs within 96 h, repeat cultures should be taken with consideration of mycobacteria or fungi, and catheter replacement or removal should be considered.

Fungal peritonitis
It is still common practice to remove the PD catheter immediately after fungi are identified by Gram stain or culture. However, recent experience with the newer imidazoles/triazoles and flucytosine (orally or, if available, i.p.) suggests that these drugs may also be effectively administered (Keane et al 2000). However, emergence of resistance to the imidazoles has occurred,

thus raising some concerns. Where available, fungal sensitivities should be obtained and, if successful, therapy should be continued for 4–6 weeks. However, if clinical improvement does not occur after 4–7 days of therapy, the catheter should be removed. Therapy with imidazoles/triazoles and flucytosine should be continued, after catheter removal, orally with flucytosine and fluconazole daily for an additional 10 days.

Relapsing peritonitis

Relapsing peritonitis is diagnosed as a recurrence of the same organism within 4 weeks of completion of the course of antibiotics. These infections should be treated in the same way as the initial peritonitis; however, the reason may be due to abscess formation, colonisation of the catheter or subcutaneous catheter tunnel infection. If there is no response to the antibiotics within 96 h, consideration should be given to catheter removal and replacement at a later date.

Prevention of peritonitis

Factors that can be employed in the prevention of peritonitis are good patient selection, absence of diverticular disease, and excellent education and training for patients and carers along with appropriate system selection. For example, the flush-before-fill procedure has given rise to peritonitis rates as low as one episode in 172 patient-months (Owen & Fair unpublished work) and one episode in 32 patient months (Lewis 1992) and improved peritonitis rates compared to other CAPD systems (Stregmayr 1992, Tielens 1993).

Exit-site infection

An exit-site infection is defined by the presence of purulent drainage with or without erythema of the skin at the catheter–epidermal interface (Keane et al 2000).

A culture of the drainage from around the exit site should be obtained. Antibiotic therapy may be initiated immediately if the infection looks severe, or delayed until the results of the culture are available. Gram-positive organisms are treated with an oral penicillinase-resistant penicillin, cefalexin, or sulfamethoxazole trimethoprim (Flanigan et al 1994). To prevent unnecessary exposure to vancomycin, and thus emergence of resistant organisms, vancomycin should be avoided in the routine treatment of Gram-positive and tunnel infections (Hospital Infection Control Practices Advisory Committee 1995). Gram-negative organisms may be treated with oral quinolones such as ciprofloxacin 500 mg twice daily. Therapy should be continued until the exit site appears completely normal. Prolonged antibiotics may be necessary. If 3–4 weeks of antibiotics fails to resolve the infection, the catheter may be replaced.

Redness and swelling around the catheter exit site without purulent drainage are sometimes an early indication of infection. If infection is suspected, then therapy should be initiated: this may be either intensified local care, a local antibiotic ointment or an oral antibiotic that covers Gram-positive organisms. An alternative approach is careful observation for additional signs of infection.

Tunnel infection

Tunnel infection can present as an extension of the exit-site infection into the catheter tunnel: swelling, pain and redness over the subcutaneous tunnel may be observed. Tunnel infections do not often respond well to antibiotic treatment and it is usual to remove the PD catheter in these cases, reinserting a new one after about 1 month. Antimicrobial therapy should be given to the patient in the interim to resolve the infection, preventing migration of the organisms into the peritoneum, and therefore predisposing to peritonitis.

EDUCATION AND TRAINING FOR THOSE ON PERITONEAL DIALYSIS

It is essential that effective education takes place before patients can be expected to treat themselves at home. Many patients who embark on a dialysis training programme are adults and, as such, their learning needs are seen to be different from those of children (Tarnow 1979). Adults are usually motivated to learn and are often learning from choice. They bring a wealth of life experiences with them that influence their learning and response to teaching. However, there are often many challenges for nurses, including working with patients who have to self-care and assessing possible barriers to learning.

Barriers to learning

People who are just about to start dialysis are often frightened—the prospect of dialysing oneself at home may not appeal. Many new patients are uraemic; symptoms may include nausea, vomiting, sleep disturbances and confusion. Some patients feel so physically unwell by the time they are to commence dialysis that they lack the motivation to learn, feeling that they will never recover.

Teaching this group of patients can be made all the more difficult when other barriers to learning become apparent. A fundamental barrier is language. In the UK, for instance, there is a growing ethnic population, giving rise to a growing proportion of people who speak little English. There are limited resources available for translation and it is frequently the responsibility of a younger member of the family, often a son or daughter, to act as translator during training. It may thus be difficult to assess who is learning, and with no knowledge of the language which is being translated, the trainer finds it difficult to ascertain just who has grasped the concept or answered the question—the patient or the translator? Language may also become a barrier when speaking to patients with no previous medical knowledge. Jargon and clinical terminology can be frightening and confusing.

Many patients who are to learn PD are elderly. Having to learn new concepts and procedures on which their life will depend may seem an overwhelming task. This sometimes makes learners feel vulnerable and inadequate, particularly if they are slow to learn. Short-term memory loss is a problem suffered by many elderly patients and is a source of great frustration to both learner and trainer. These patients frequently have added physical barriers to learning, such as poor vision or lack of manual dexterity. Varying levels of deafness may also be a problem—the learner is trying not only to understand what has been said but is also straining to hear.

A report by the Basic Skills Agency in 2000 found that nearly four out of 10 adults in some parts of England cannot read read or write properly or do simple sums. Across Europe around 10% of the population falls into the low-skills category. In the UK the figure is over 20%: 8 million people are so poor at reading and writing that they cannot cope with the demands of modern life (International Adult Literacy Survey 1998) If we consider this problem in relation to the concepts and procedures which need to be taught to dialysis patients, it becomes apparent that the information given must be clear, unambiguous and readily understood, particularly if the patient's literacy difficulty is paired with a second or even a third barrier to learning.

Social and psychological barriers to learning are discussed in more detail by Thomas (1998).

Training materials

It has been well documented that visual, audio and audiovisual materials are an essential part of any training programme (Frantz 1980, Zappacosta & Lander 1988). It is important, however, that the material used is appropriate to the learner. Patients have many different learning styles and it is important to accommodate these within the training programme.

The learning environment

One of the fundamental needs for effective training to take place is that of a good learning environment. A good training environment is one that is comfortable, non-clinical, free from interruptions and has a welcoming and friendly atmosphere.

Home training

If patients are ultimately to dialyse at home, the clinical environment of a hospital is not an ideal place in which to learn this therapy. Teaching patients in their own home may be the ideal situation, particularly when teaching about CAPD. It will be easier for patients to adapt the therapy to their own lifestyle and if they learn on their own territory some reduction in fear may be achieved. Each patient will almost certainly have uninterrupted one-to-one teaching and the educator will have the opportunity to give practical help and advice about where the dialysis can be performed. Family members may also find it easier to be involved in such education. However, the constraints associated with training patients in their own homes may prevent many renal units from implementing this strategy. One nurse has to be removed from the hospital setting for some days at a time. It may also prove difficult to implement this method of training for patients who were not planned admissions—such as the patient who needs dialysis very shortly after being diagnosed with renal failure. Having a homely setting within the hospital environment or an off-site training centre may bridge the gap between hospital and home (Wild 1992).

Recommendations for training within renal units

- Set aside an area specifically for teaching purposes. The area should preferably be away from the ward, and be non-clinical and quiet. A television and video can be used in this area for teaching.
- Designate a team of nurses for training duties only. Establish some continuity of care by allocating each patient to a designated nurse.
- Invite family members or partners to participate in the teaching programme.
- Use a wide variety of training materials. Five points to good presentation of these materials:
  — Teach the smallest amount possible for the job required
  — Make the point as vividly as possible
  — Review repeatedly
  — Have the learner restate and demonstrate material.
  — The subject matter should be relevant.
- Any material should be presented in a way that is comprehensible to the learner. There are more than 40 different formulae for assessing the degree of difficulty in reading materials (Doak et al, 1985). However, the most common characteristics on which they focus are:
  — difficulty of the vocabulary, particularly the number of syllables in the word
  — average sentence length (Fry 1977, McLaughlin 1969, Seels & Dale 1971).
- Despite the fact that the readability of the material can be measured by the same formula, readers' skills may vary with their interest and background of experience in a particular topic area (Doak et al, 1985).
- Training materials are most effective when presented in an interesting and appropriate manner. Both the language used and the material's degree of complexity need to be taken into account.
- The material should be presented in a memorable fashion. Any visual aids need vivid, simple messages which are easy for patients to remember.
- Finally, but perhaps most importantly; it is essential that the patients want to learn what is being taught.

The training programme should be designed to prepare patients fully for return to the community. The aim of a training programme is to educate patients to a standard whereby they can confidently care for themselves and perform their CAPD in the community. For some learners this may mean that they learn only how to perform CAPD, troubleshoot and manage their renal diet. For others much more detail may be desired, for example, learning how dialysis works.

Group teaching is an excellent way for patients to learn. This not only enables patients to learn from each other, but also helps the teacher, as many patients can be taught the same subject at the same time. The bulk of the training programme should focus on the patients themselves, relating all they are learning to their disease, treatment and, ultimately, their lifestyle. Sessions should be designed to last for no longer than 20 min and visual aids such as flipcharts, acetates and videos are used to make the material interesting and varied.

The internet is becoming an increasingly useful tool in the education of people with kidney failure. It provides many advantages in that the information is available 24 h a day 7 days a week. There are now many websites dedicated solely to the education of patients with kidney failure. The following list proves a useful addition to any training programme:

- www.kidneywise.com
- www.kidneypatientguide.org/uk
- www.kidney.org/uk
- www.nkrf.org/uk.

What to teach patients

It is important that new patients to PD are discharged from the renal unit with enough knowledge to care for themselves safely on dialysis. Broadly speaking, when each patient is taught, priority should first be given to what they must know, then to what they should know, and finally to what they could know. However, all learning objectives should be patient-centred.

The following topics should be included in a PD training programme:

- Medication. The patient's own medication can be used as the central focus for this session. The aim is to ensure that the patient knows how often and why each medicine is taken.

- Normal functions of the kidney. This session can be given in groups using a set of overhead projection acetates to explain in a simple way the basic functions of the kidney, relating these to the symptoms they suffer when kidneys fail.

- CAPD and APD procedures. These are most easily taught on a one-to-one basis. Demonstration techniques can be used to explain the procedure. A PD simulator (plastic torso with a PD catheter) is an excellent tool on which patients can practise their exchanges.

- Catheter and catheter exit-site care. This can be taught to the patient on a one-to-one basis. The PD simulator can be used to practise exit-site dressing technique, as can getting the patient to practise the technique in front of a mirror. Photographs are useful to help explain visually the difference between a healthy and an infected exit site.

- How PD works. Osmosis and diffusion can be explained using simple experiments or diagrams. A video is also available called 'How does CAPD work?' which explains these simple concepts in more detail. (Contact Baxter Healthcare, Wallingford Road, Compton, Newbury, Berkshire RG20 7QW, UK.)

- Diet. Eating is an activity which most people enjoy and which therefore takes up a rather large part of our lives. Maybe it is for this reason that many patients focus on diet and want to know all there is to be taught. Plastic models of food can be used in training sessions to make the learning fun.

- Infections. It has been well documented that peritonitis is a major complication of PD and it is therefore important that peritonitis is explained to patients well, using a purpose-printed flipchart.
- Fluid balance. Fluid overload can be associated with excessive fluid intake and poor education. It is a common experience that one of the most difficult aspects of treatment to adhere to is the reduced fluid allowance. This subject can also be taught in groups using a purpose-printed flipchart. Weighing a jug of fluid can also be useful to demonstrate the difference between fluid weight and flesh weight.
- Fertility and sexuality. It is important to discuss sexuality and body image with PD patients. Having the PD catheter present in the abdomen may inhibit some people (either the patient or partner) and it is essential that any anxieties are discussed. Fertility should also be discussed with patients and partners where appropriate, as it is possible for PD patients to conceive.
- Employment. Having dialysis is not a reason for giving up work. The training period is a good time to discuss work options with patients.
- Ordering and delivery of PD supplies. The practicalities of ordering and delivery of the PD supplies to the patient's home prove a great worry for many patients and their families. This can often be compounded by the problem of where to store this large amount of equipment. A comprehensive video, 'Delivering Dialysis', explains in a simple way the ordering and delivery of the dialysis supplies not only to the patient's home but also to other holiday or travel destinations. (Contact Baxter Healthcare, Wallingford Road, Compton, Newbury, Berkshire RG20 7QW, UK.) Patients can be encouraged to talk amongst themselves to gain ideas from each other as well as utilising the experience of nurses.
- Holidays and travel. It is possible to travel whilst being treated with PD and many patients go on holiday frequently. The practicalities of travel and holidays should be discussed during the training period and on an ongoing basis if appropriate.
- Exercise for PD patients. The nurse's role is to promote a healthy lifestyle for patients. The training period is an ideal opportunity to discuss which type of activities are best suited to that individual patient.

To complement the training programme, reading materials should be made available, along with posters and videos. Many training materials have been translated into other languages for use by those patients whose first language is not English.

Assessment of how much information the patient has retained is difficult to make accurately. Testing can be seen as a threatening procedure, even though it is essential. Games, therefore, make a valuable contribution to the task of assessing learning and can be used in a variety of forms. Simple homemade crosswords, word searches and quizzes can be fun for patients and relatives to do at the end of their training. 'Renal bingo' is an excellent way of assessing groups of patients together (Robinson et al 1988).

SUMMARY

Ongoing education and support are vital to ensure the success of patients on PD. Continuing educational support will help to prevent problems such as peritonitis or fluid overload. As patients gain experience with the therapy, questions may arise which they had not thought of or which were not relevant during the initial training period. It is therefore important to make time available when patients can feel able to ask such questions in an environment where they can be answered fully. Follow-up workshops and home visits by the community nursing team provide an opportunity for patients to discuss the successes and problems they have encountered. Clinical procedure technique can be checked for accuracy by the trainer in a non-threatening environment. Many patients gain an enormous amount from group support sessions (Said 1995); however, other patients may feel threatened in this environment and one-to-one teaching may be more appropriate.

Above all, teaching and learning should be simple and fun, it should be available in an understandable form to all patients all of the time and ultimately it should promote the self-care of the patient.

REFERENCES

Armstrong, A, Cunningham J. The treatment of metabolic bone disease in patients on peritoneal dialysis. Kidney Int 1994; 46 (suppl. 48):S51–S57.

Ash SR, Daugirdas, JT. Peritoneal access devices. In: Daugirdas JJ, Ing TS, eds. Handbook of dialysis. Boston: Little, Brown, 1994:275–300.

Ash, SR, Janle EM. T-fluted peritoneal dialysis catheter. In: Khanna R, Nolph KD, Prowant BF et al, eds. Advances in peritoneal dialysis. Vol. 9. Toronto: Peritoneal Dialysis Publications, 1993:223–226.

Ash SR, Nichols WK. Placement, repair, and removal of chronic peritoneal catheters. In: Gokal R, Nolph KD, eds. Textbook of peritoneal dialysis. Dordrecht: Kluwer Academic, 1994:315–333.

Baxter Healthcare. UK PET Survey. Thetford, Norfolk: Baxter Healthcare, 1992.

Bender K, Swartz MD. The Role Of nephrology nurses and technicians in the implementation of NKF-DOQI. Nephrol News Issues 1999; 13:21–23.

Bergner M, Bobbitt RA, Pollard WE et al. The sickness impact profile: validation of a health status measure. Med Care 1976; 14: 57–67.

Bernardini J, Piraino B, Holley J et al. A randomized trial of *Staphylococcus aureus* prophylaxis in peritoneal dialysis patients: mupirocin calcium ointment 2% applied to the exit site versus cyclic oral rifampin. Am J Kidney Dis 1996; 27:695–700.

Blake PG, Balaskas EV, Izalt, S et al. Is total creatinine clearance a good predictor of clinical outcomes in continuous ambulatory peritoneal dialysis? Peritoneal Dialysis Int 1992; 12: 353–358.

Burkart JM. Adequacy of peritoneal dialysis. Dialysis Transplant 1993; 13:234–243.

Burton HJ, Kline SA, Lindsay RM et al. The relationship of depression to survival in chronic renal failure. Psychosom Med 1986; 48:261–269.

Campbell A. The quality of American life. New York: Russell Sage Foundation, 1976.

CANUSA Peritoneal Dialysis Study Group. Adequacy of dialysis and nutrition in continuous ambulatory peritoneal dialysis: association with clinical outcomes. J Am Soc Nephrol 1996; 7:198–207.

Chen CJ, Moberly JB, Martis L. New developments in peritoneal dialysis solutions Adv Peritoneal Dialysis 1998; 14:116–119.

Churchill DN, Taylor DW, Keshaviah PR and the CANUSA Peritoneal dialysis study group. Adequacy of dialysis and nutrition in continuous peritoneal dialysis: association with clinical outcomes. J Am Soc Nephrol 1996; 7:198–207.

Coles et al. The effect of intra–nasal mupirocin on CAPD exit site infection. Abstract of presentation. American Society of Nephrology Conference, Orlando, 1994.

Consensus Conference on Biocompatibility Review. Nephrol Dialysis Transplant 1994; 9 (suppl. 2):1–186.

Cooper A, Henderson IS, Jones MC. Daytime dwell with 7.5% dextrin in automated peritoneal dialysis (APD). EDTA–ERCA 1995; 21 (suppl. 1):21.

Davies S, Bryan J, Russell GI. Longitudinal changes in peritoneal kinetics: the influence of dialysis and peritonitis. Nephrol Dialysis Transplant 1993; 8: 14–15.

Davies S, Bryan J, Phillips L et al. Longitudinal changes in peritoneal kinetics: the effects of peritoneal dialysis peritonitis. Nephrol Dialysis Transplant 1996; 11:498–506.

Detsky AS, Mclaughlin JR, Baker JP. What is subjective global assessment of nutritional status? J Parenteral Enteral Nutr 1987; 11:458–482.

Diaz-Buxo JA. Intermittent, continuous ambulatory and continuous cycling peritoneal dialysis. In: Nissenson AR et al, eds. Clinical dialysis. Norwalk: Appleton-Century-Crofts, 1984:48.

Di Paolo N, Garosi G, Petrini G et al. Peritoneal dialysis solution biocompatibility testing in animals. Peritoneal Dialysis Int 1995; 15 (suppl.), S61–S70.

Doak CC, Doak LG, Root JH. Teaching patients with low literacy skills. Philadelphia: Lippincott, 1985.

Dobbie J. Monitoring peritoneal hystopathology in peritoneal dialysis. The role of the biopsy registry. Dialysis Transplant 1989; 18:319–335.

Dratwa M. Peritonitis prevention: twin bag better than Y-set. Peritoneal Dialysis Int. XI CAPD abstracts 1992; 72.

Dratwa M, Vladutiu D, Keller N. Nutritional support with nutrineal for CAPD peritonitis. Peritoneal Dialysis Int 1995; 15 (suppl. 4):S32

Dryden MS, Ludlam HA, Wing AT et al. Active intervention dramatically reduces CAPD-associated infections. In: Khanna R, Nolph KD, Prowant BF et al, eds. Advances in peritoneal dialysis. Toronto: Peritoneal Dialysis Bulletin, 1991:125–128.

Dubois D, and Dubois, EF. A formula to estimate the approximate surface area if height and weight is known. Arch Intern Med 1916; 17:863–871.

EDTNA/ERCA Research Board. Post-insertion catheter care project 2001–2002. Available: www.edtna-erca.org 10 Oct 2001.

Enia G, Sicuso C, Alati G, Zoccali C. Subjective global assessment of nutrition in dialysis patients. Nephrol Dialysis Transplant 1993; 8:1094–1098.

Faller B. Amino acid based peritoneal dialysis solutions. Kidney Int 1996; 50 (suppl. 56):S81–S85.

Flanigan MJ, Hochstetler LA, Langholdt D et al. Continuous ambulatory peritoneal dialysis catheter infections: diagnosis and management. Peritoneal Dialysis Int 1994; 14:248–254.

Frantz R. Selecting media for patient education. Topics Clin Nurs/Ed Self Care 1980; 2:77–83.

Fried L, Hutchison A, Stegmayr B et al. Recommendations for the treatment of lipid disorders in patients on peritoneal dialysis. Peritoneal Dialysis Int 1999; 19:7–16.

Fry E. Fry's readability graph: clarifications validity and extensions to level 17. J Reading 1977; 9:242–252.

Fuchs J, Gallagher ME, Jackson-Bey D. A prospective randomised study of peritoneal catheter exit site care. Dialysis Transplant 1990; 19:81–84.

Genestier J, Hedelin G, Schaffer P et al. Prognostic factors in CAPD patients: a retrospective study of a 10-year period. Nephrol Dialysis Transplant 1995; 10:1905–1911.

Gokal R. Peritoneal dialysis, prevention and control of infection. Drugs Aging 2000; 17:269–282.

Gokal R, Jakubowski C, King J et al. Outcome in patients on continuous ambulatory peritoneal dialysis: 4 year analysis of a prospective multicentre study. Lancet 1987; 2:1105–1108.

Gokal R and the Midas Group. A UK multi-centre study of icodextrin in CAPD. Peritoneal Dialysis Int 1994; 14 (suppl. 2): S22–S27.

Gokal R, Ash SR, Holfrich BG et al. Peritoneal catheters and exit site practices. Toward optimum peritoneal access. 1998 Update. Peritoneal Dialysis Int 1998; 18:29–39.

Golper TA, Tranaeus A. Vancomycin revisited. Peritoneal Dialysis Int 1996; 16:116–117.

Gotch FA, Sargent JA. A mechanistic analysis of the National Co-operative Dialysis Study (NCDS). Kidney Int 1985; 28:526–534.

Gotch FA, Sargent JA, Parker TJ et al. National co-operative dialysis study: comparison of the study groups and a description of morbidity, mortality, and patient withdrawal. Kidney Int 1983; 26 (suppl. 23):S42–S49.

Heimbürger O, Waniewski J, Werynski A et al. Peritoneal transport in CAPD patients with permanent loss of ultrafiltration capacity. Kidney Int 1990; 38:495–506.

Hou S. Pregnancy in CAPD patients. Editorial. Peritoneal Dialysis Int 1990; 10:201–204.

Hunt SM, McEwan J. The Nottingham health profile. In: Teeling-Smith G, ed. Measuring health: a practical approach. Chichester: John Wiley 1983:165–169.

Hutchison A. Peritoneal dialysis solutions for the future. Do we have the solution? Dialysis Transplant 1992; 21:57–63.

International Adult Literacy Survey 1998. Online. Available: www.literacytrust.org.uk 18 Oct 2001.

Jacobs C, Issad B, Allouache M et al. The Crucial role of medical and nursing staff in the care of chronic peritoneal dialysis patients. Peritoneal Dialysis Int 1997; 17:23–28.

Jones MR, Gehr T, Burkart JM et al. Replacement of amino acids and proteins losses with 1.1% amino acid peritoneal solution. Peritoneal Dialysis Int 1998; 18:210–216.

Keane WF, Everett ED, Golper TA et al. Peritoneal dialysis related peritonitis treatment recommendations, 1993 update. Peritoneal Dialysis Int 1993; 13:14–28.

Keane WF, Alexander SR, Bailie GR et al. Adult peritoneal dialysis-related peritonitis treatment recommendations: 1996 update. Peritoneal Dialysis Int 1996; 16:557–573.

Keane WF, Bailie GR, Boeschoten R et al. Adult peritoneal dialysis related peritonitis treatment recommendations: 2000 update. Peritoneal Dialysis Int 2000; 20:396–411.

Kelman B. The roles of the peritoneal dialysis nurse. Peritoneal Dialysis Int 1995; 15:114–115.

Kennedy M, Dasgupta M, Chang W et al. Randomized clinical trial of Intraperitoneal amino acids solutions in a North American PD center – preliminary data. Peritoneal Dialysis Int 1999; 19(supp 1): S19.

Keshaviah PR, Nolph KD, van Tone JC. The peak concentration hypothesis: a urea kinetic approach to comparing peritoneal and haemodialysis. Peritoneal Dialysis Int 1989; 9:257–260.

Khanna R, Twardowski ZJ. Peritoneal dialysis access. In: Nolph KD, ed. Peritoneal dialysis. Dordrecht: Kluwer Academic, 1989: 261–288.

Khanna R, Breckenbridge C, Roncari D et al. Lipid abnormalities in patients undergoing CAPD. Peritoneal Dialysis Bull 1983; 3 (suppl.):S13–S15.

Khanna R, Wu G, Prowant B et al. CAPD in diabetics with ESRD: a combined experience of two North American centres. In: Friedman E, l'Esperance F, eds. Diabetic renal retinal syndrome 3. New York: Grune & Stratton, 1986:363–381.

King LK, Kingswood JC, Sharpstone P. Comparison of the efficacy, cost and complication rate of APD and CAPD as long term treatments for renal failure. Adv Peritoneal Dialysis 1992; 8:123–126.

Krediet RT, Pannekeet MM, Zemel D et al. Markers of peritoneal membrane status. Peritoneal Dialysis Int 1996; 16 (suppl. 1):S42–SS49.

Krediet RT, Douma CE, van Olden RW et al. Augmenting solute clearance in peritoneal dialysis. Kidney Int 1998; 54:2218–2235.

Krediet RT, Lindholm B, Rippe B. Pathophysiology of peritoneal membrane failure. Peritoneal Dialysis Int 2000; 20 (suppl. 4): S22–S42.

Lameire M, Dhaene M, Matthys E et al. Experience with CAPD in diabetic patients. In: Keen H, Legrain M, eds. Prevention and treatment of diabetic nephropathy. Lancaster: MTP, 1993; 2:289–297.

Lewis J. CAPD disconnect systems: UK peritonitis experience. Adv Peritoneal Dialysis, 1992; 8:306–312.

Linbald AS, Novak JW, Nolph K et al. (eds) CAPD in the USA. Dordrecht: Kluwer Academic, 1989:63–74.

Lindholm B, Karlander SG, Norbeck HE, Bergstrom J. Hormonal and metabolic adaptation to the glucose load of CAPD in non-diabetic patients. In: Keen H, Legrain M, eds. Prevention and treatment of diabetic nephropathy. Boston: MTP Press, 1983:353–359.

Lye WC, Lee EJ, Tan CC. Prophylactic antibiotics in the insertion of Tenckhoff catheters. Scand J Urol Nephrol 1992; 26:177–180.

McEnzie R Holmes C, Moseley A et al. Bicarbonate/lactate and bicarbonate buffered peritoneal dialysis fluids improve ex vivo peritoneal macrophage TNFα secretion. J Am Soc Nephrol Dialysis Transplant 1998; 9:1499–1506.

McLaughlin GH. SMOG grading—a new readability formula. J Reading 1969; 12:639–646.

Mactier RA. Investigation and management of ultrafiltration failure. Adv Peritoneal Dialysis 1991; 7:57–62.

Mactier RA, Sprosen TS, Gokal R et al. Bicarbonate and bicarbonate/lactate peritoneal dialysis solutions for the treatment of pain on infusion. Kidney Int 1998; 53 1061–1067.

Maki D Improving catheter site care. London: Royal Society of Medicine Services, 1991.

Mistry CD, Mallick NP, Gokal R. Ultrafiltration with iso-osmotic solution during long peritoneal dialysis exchanges. Lancet 1987; ii:178–182.

Moncrief JW, Popovich RP, Seare W et al. New microporous (MP) epidermal cuff at the catheter exit site for access in peritoneal dialysis. Peritoneal Dialysis Int 1996; 16 (suppl. 2):S53.

Mupirocin Study Group. Nasal mupirocin prevents Staph. aureus exit-site infection during peritoneal dialysis. J Am Soc Nephrol 1996; 7:2403–2408.

Norbeck HE, Lindholm B. Long term effects of peritoneal versus haemodialysis on serum lipoproteins. Abstract. Eur J Clin Invest 1982; 12:29.

Park MS, Lee HB, Lim AS et al. Effect of prolonged subcutaneous implantation of peritoneal catheter on peritonitis rate during CAPD: a prospective randomised study. Peritoneal Dialysis Int 1996; 16 (suppl. 2):S54.

Peers E, Gokal R. Icodextrin: overview of clinical experience. Peritoneal Dialysis Int 1997; 17:22–26.

Peers EM, Scrimgeour AC, Haycox AR. Cost containment in CAPD patients with ultrafiltration failure. Clin Drug Invest 1995; 10:53–58.

Piraino B, Bernardini J, Sorkin M. The influence of peritoneal dialysis catheter exit site infections on peritonitis, tunnel infections and catheter loss in patients on CAPD. Am J Kidney Dis 1986; 8:436–440.

Prowant BF, Twardowski ZJ. Recommendations for exit care. Peritoneal Dialysis Int 1996; 16 (suppl. 3):S94–S99.

Prowant BF, Schmidt LM, Twardowski ZJ et al. Peritoneal dialysis catheter exit site care. Am Nephrol Nurses Assoc J 1988; 15:219–222.

Ramos JM, Heaton A, McGurk JG, et al. Sequential changes in serum lipids and their subfractions in patients receiving CAPD. Nephron 1983; 35:20–23.

Randerson DH, Chapman GV, Farrell PC. Amino-acids and dietary status in CAPD patients. In: Atkins RC, Thompson NM, Farrel PC, eds. Peritoneal Dialysis. Edinburgh: Churchill Livingstone, 1989:179–191.

Renal Association. Treatment of adult patients with renal failure. 2nd edn. London: Royal College of Physicians and the Renal Association, 1997.

Robinson JA, Robinson KJ, Lewis DJ. Games: a motivational education strategy. Am Nephrol Nurses Assoc J 1988; 15:277–279.

Routtembourg J. Peritoneal dialysis in diabetics. In: Nolph KD, ed. Peritoneal dialysis. Dordrecht: Kluwer Academic, 1988: 365–379.

Said V. Beyond adventure. Lifeline—CAPD Newslett 1995; 12:2.

Scarpioni L, Ballocchi S, Castelli A et al. Insulin therapy in uremic diabetic patients on continuous ambulatory peritoneal dialysis: comparison of intraperitoneal and subcutaneous administration. Peritoneal Dialysis Int 1994; 14:14–19.

Seels B, Dale E. Readability and reading. An annotated bibliography. Newark: International Reading Association, 1971.

Selgas R, Bajo MA, Paiva A et al. Stability of the peritoneal membrane in long-term peritoneal dialysis patients. Adv Renal Replace Ther 1998; 5:168–178

Starzomski RC. Three techniques for peritoneal catheter exit site dressings. Am Nephrol Nurses Assoc J 1984; 11:9–16.

Stein A, Peers E, Hattersley J et al. Clinical experience with icodextrin in CAPD patients. Peritoneal Dialysis Int 1994; 14 (suppl. 2):S51–S54.

Stregmayr B. Lower incidence of peritonitis in CAPD with integrated disconnect system than with an UV flash system. Peritoneal Dialysis Int 1992; 12:abstract 272.

Tarnow K. Special programmes in continuing education for nursing in working with adult learners. Texas: Texas Woman's University College of Nursing, 1979.

Teehan UP, Schlelfer CR, Brown JM et al. Urea kinetic analysis and clinical outcome in CAPD: a five year longitudinal study. Adv Peritoneal Dialysis 1990; 6:181–185.

Thomas N. Patient education. In: Challinor P, Sedgewick J, eds. Principles and practice of renal nursing. Cheltenham: Stanley Thornes, 1998.

Tielens E. Major reduction in CAPD peritonitis after introduction of the twin bag system. Nephrol Dialysis Transplant 1993; 8:1237–1243.

Tranaeus AP, Mactier RA, Sprosen TS et al. Bicarbonate and bicarbonate/lactate peritoneal dialysis solutions for the treatment of pain on infusion. Kidney Int 1998; 53:1061–1067.

Twardowski ZJ. Clinical value of standardised equilibration test in CAPD patients. Blood Purification 1989; 7:95–108.

Twardowski ZJ. Tidal peritoneal dialysis. EDTNA J 1990; XV: 4–9.

Twardowski ZJ, Nolph KD, Khanna R et al. Peritoneal equilibration test. Peritoneal Dialysis Bull 1987; 7:138–147.

US Renal Data System 2000. Online. Available: www.usrds.org 17 Oct 2001.

Uttley L, Prowant B. Organisation of a CAPD programme—the nurse's role. In: Gokal R, Khanna R, Krediet R et al (eds). Textbook of peritoneal dialysis. Dordrecht: Kluwer, 2000: 363–386.

Vas S. Randomised clinical trial with silver coated PD catheter. Peritoneal Dialysis Int 1996; 16 (suppl. 2):S56.

Verger C, Luzar MA. In vitro study of CAPD Y-line systems. Adv Peritoneal Dialysis, 1986; 2:160–164.

Wang T, Heimbürger O, Waniewski J et al. Increased peritoneal permeability is associated with decreased fluid and small-solute removal and higher mortality in CAPD patients. Nephrol Dialysis Transplant 1998; 13:1242–1249.

Ware JE, Shelbourne CD. The MOS 36 item short-form health survey (SF-36): I. Conceptual framework and item selection. Med Care 1992; 30:473–483.

Welch G. Assessment of quality of life following renal failure. In: McGee H, Bradley C, eds. Quality of life following renal failure. Switzerland: Harwood Academic, 1994:55–98.

Wikdahl AM, Engman U, Stegmayr B et al. One-dose cefuroxime i.v. and i.p. reduces microbial growth in PD patients after catheter insertion. Nephrol Dialysis Transplant 1997; 12:157–160.

Wild JH. Dialysis without tears. Nurs Times 1992; 88:35–36.

Young MA, Nolph K, Dutton S et al. Anti-hypertensive drug requirement in CAPD. Peritoneal Dialysis Bull 1984; 5:85–88.

Young G, Kopple JD, Lindhan B et al. Nutritional assessment of continuous ambulatory peritoneal dialysis patients: an international study. Am J Kidney Dis 1991; 17:462–471.

Zappacosta AR, Lander SM. Components of a successful CAPD education programme. Am Nephrol Nurses Assoc J 1988; 15:243–247.

Zimmerman SW, Ahrens E, Johnson CA et al. Randomized controlled trial of prophylactic rifampin for peritoneal dialysis related infections. Am J Kidney Dis 1991; 18:225–231.

Renal nutrition

Marianne Vennegoor

9

LEARNING OUTCOMES FOR THIS CHAPTER

- To describe the historical background to renal nutrition and dietetics
- To evaluate nutritional management in the predialysis phase
- To identify the dietary principles of haemodialysis (HD) and peritoneal dialysis
- To analyse the role of the nurse in giving dietary advice in the multiprofessional team.

INTRODUCTION

Dietary treatment has always been regarded as an important part of treating patients with end-stage renal failure (ESRF), before and during renal replacement therapy (RRT). During the 1960s many patients were treated by diet alone. The renal diet was adapted to dialysis and transplantation once these modes of RRT became available during the 1970s and early 1980s. Nowadays, chronic fluid overload, hyperphosphataemia and protein-energy malnutrition are amongst the most common problems. These can lead to long term complications if not resolved and adversely affect outcome of treatment and the quality of life of renal patients on decades of chronic treatment. This chapter will address the important issues of dietary management and the role it plays in the overall treatment of ESRF.

Firstly, this chapter would not be complete without an historical introduction to dietary management of each mode of RRT.

HISTORICAL REVIEW OF DIETARY MANAGEMENT

Predialysis treatment (1960–2000)

Dietary treatment has been considered a very important component of the treatment of patients with ESRF for several decades. It was not until the end of the 1960s and the beginning of the 1970s that HD was accepted as a regular form of RRT for selected patients. Prior to this period patients approaching ESRF failure, with gastrointestinal symptoms, were advised to follow a very-low-protein diet (VLPD). The best-known diet was the Giovanetti diet, containing 20 g protein of high biological value to cover essential amino acid requirements. An intake of 50 kcal kg^{-1} body weight (BW) was recommended to prevent loss of muscle tissue and maintain nitrogen balance (Berlyne 1968). This diet was prescribed to selected patients with a serum creatinine clearance of 3 mL min^{-1} or a urea level of 200 mg 100 mL^{-1} (33 mmol L^{-1}) and was the only treatment available to improve the well-being of patients, until regular HD treatment became available.

It became apparent in later years that a badly managed protein-restricted diet contributed to malnutrition before starting HD and that this prolonged the rehabilitation period and also contributed to the outcome of treatment, with an increase in morbidity and mortality.

During the 1980s there was a renewed interest in protein restriction as partially nephrectomised rats showed that protein restriction delayed the progression of renal disease. This was the era of the hyperfiltration/hyper-perfusion hypothesis (Brenner 1983). It was more difficult to prove the same effect in humans. Patients were unable to follow these diets for a long period of time as high-energy diets containing no more than 0.6 g kg^{-1} BW protein were prescribed during the early stages of chronic renal disease to asymptomatic patients.

The National Institute of Health (NIH), USA, initiated the launch of a large multicentre study in 1985. The Modification of Diet in Renal Disease (MDRD) study used four different diets with different levels of protein ranging from usual intake to VLPD supplemented with keto acids and combined with phosphorus restriction. The results of this 2-year study were published in 1994 (Klahr et al 1994).

The NIH stated in 1993 that the nutritional health of a patient prior to dialysis is an important indicator of outcome and that all patients are entitled to receive a nutritional assessment by a trained renal dietitian. In the absence of obvious malnutrition, a moderate low-protein diet of up to 0.7–0.8 g protein kg^{-1} BW day^{-1} should be prescribed. When malnutrition is present, the amount of energy is increased and the amount of protein is raised to 1.0–1.2 g kg^{-1}, to allow for nutritional repletion or to counter the catabolic effects of stress. Dietary prescriptions should include guidelines for energy, fat and carbohydrate, fluid, sodium, phosphate and potassium, as well as other nutrients and micronutrients (NIH 1993).

The MDRD study results showed initially a slower decline in progression of renal disease in the absence of severe proteinuria and hypertension. There appeared to be no further advantage in using a VLPD supplemented with essential amino acids or keto acids (Klahr et al 1994). The report cautioned that, while lowering blood pressure and protein intake appears to be safe, both must be carefully monitored.

CURRENT CONCEPTS OF PREDIALYSIS DIETARY INTERVENTION

As a result of these findings treatment became more focused on prevention of complications due to chronic uraemia. The importance of improving blood pressure control to delay progression is well recognised. Also important is dietary phosphorus restriction to help prevent renal bone disease and secondary tissue calcification, with a modest protein restriction to accommodate phosphorus restriction. Some patients who voluntarily reduce their protein and energy intake to less than recommended need normalisation of their intake. Close supervision to enhance dietary compliance is an important additional component of treatment to prevent malnutrition, which must be detected and treated early. Severe weight loss and a steady decline in serum albumin levels in non-nephrotic patients are obvious clinical signs. The quality of predialysis treatment now includes the principles of healthy eating to help reduce the incidence of cardiovascular disease. This entails the modification of energy sources like carbohydrate and fat.

Starting dialysis early preserves residual renal function for a longer period. It also promotes rehabilitation, and this approach is now accepted as the way forward to reduce complications and unnecessary hospitalisation.

Meanwhile research into the effect of protein restriction on reducing symptoms of uraemia and on the progression of renal failure continues simultaneously and several papers have been published within the last 3 years highlighting some of the known benefits of protein restriction.

Instead of causing protein malnutrition, protein restriction prevents it when protein malnutrition is present and selected patients with advanced renal failure should be given this option of treatment, as a trial if indicated (Walser et al 1999).

Several meta-analyses were conducted including selected previous studies, such as the MDRD study. Fouque et al (1992, 2000), Pedrini et al (1996) and Gin et al (1999) concluded that dietary protein restriction effectively slows the progression of diabetic and non-diabetic renal disease (see also ongoing Cochrane Reviews of abstracts, 2000: www.cochrane-renal.org).

Recently the *Clinical Practice Guidelines for Nutrition in Chronic Renal Failure* were published by the National Kidney Foundation/Dialysis Outcome Quality Initiative (NKF/DOQI: Kopple et al 2000). This publication includes recommendations for protein and energy intake for adults and children. These recommendations are based on evidence and expert opinion. The European Dialysis and Transplant Nurses' Association/European Renal Care Association (EDTNA/ERCA) nutritional guidelines have also been produced (EDTNA/ERCA, 2001). In patients with advanced chronic renal failure, not on dialysis, with a glomerular filtration rate of > 25 mL min^{-1}, a diet with reduced allowance of protein, containing 0.6 g protein and 35 kcal kg^{-1} BW should be initiated. If patients are unable to follow this diet or nutritional status is compromised the protein content can be increased to 0.75 g kg^{-1} BW. The energy intake of less active elderly patients can be decreased to 30–35 kcal kg^{-1}. Refer to page 281 to assess the ideal range of body weight. Any dietary intervention must be implemented by experienced experts and patients must be monitored frequently (Kopple et al 2000).

During the past 3 decades considerable progress was made regarding modes and quality of treatment. Regular HD became available from the mid 1960s onwards.

Patients were initially selected for treatment: they were usually young and free from concomitant disease. HD lasted for 15 or 10 h depending on the number of sessions, twice or three times per week. Dietary management was aimed at controlling the patient's fluid balance and biochemistry. During these early days of dialysis a strict diet by present standards was followed by many patients and consisted of a daily intake of: 50 g protein, 50 mmol sodium, 50 mmol potassium, 3500 kcal and 300 mL fluid.

As the quality of dialysis treatment improved during the 1970s and 1980s, dietary restrictions were relaxed to a daily intake of 60 g protein, 60 mmol sodium, 60 mmol potassium, 2500–3000 kcal and 300–500 mL fluid. Even this type of HD diet was impossible to follow without the help of high-energy, electrolyte-free supplements and several books for patients were published during the following years to promote dietary education (Vennegoor 1982, 1986, 1992).

During the late 1980s and mid 1990s several publications drew attention to the fact that a large percentage of patients on HD and chronic ambulatory peritoneal dialysis (CAPD) showed symptoms of clinical malnutrition. The increase in morbidity and mortality alarmed the renal healthcare professionals to a high degree (Churchill et al 1996, Marckman 1988).

It is not surprising that a multidisciplinary input is required to prevent complications during the predialysis and dialysis phases of treating patients with chronic renal failure and ESRF. Patients with concomitant disease, older patients and those with particular ethnic backgrounds are a challenge to care for. Nutrition guidelines are now in place and continue to be improved as research continues to provide the evidence needed to implement high-quality dietary treatment.

PRACTICAL ASPECTS OF PREDIALYSIS DIETARY MANAGEMENT

The nutritional content of a diet with a reduced protein content should be specifically adapted to each patient's individual needs and personal circumstances. This should result in the reduction of accumulated metabolic waste products, which can be controlled as chronic renal disease progresses.

Regular dietary follow-up should provide maintenance of optimal nutritional status by ensuring that sufficient protein and energy continues to be taken by the patient and that other important nutrients such as vitamins and minerals are prescribed as supplements.

The diet should provide sufficient dietary freedom and enable the patient to lead a near-normal life. This means that dietary flexibility must be incorporated and relatives or friends should be involved while educating the patient to promote maximum dietary compliance.

The following are important in the dietary therapy of conservative management:

- protein
- energy (carbohydrate and fat)
- sodium and fluid
- potassium
- phosphorus
- other minerals, such as calcium, iron and zinc
- vitamins.

Protein

Protein is an important nutrient for the repair and maintenance of tissue and for growth.

Quantity

The level of dietary protein restriction should maintain nitrogen balance and nutritional status, as previously discussed. The calculation should be based on the ideal body weight (IBW), taking the patient's residual renal function into consideration (see Table 9.1). For instance, if a patient consumes a high-protein diet a reduction to 1.0 g kg^{-1} IBW may initially be sufficient which can be reduced to 0.8 g kg^{-1} IBW if renal function deteriorates at a later stage. This is an acceptable degree of protein allowance for long-term use and is well within the limit advised by the World Health Organization of 0.6 g kg^{-1} day^{-1}, assuming the energy content of the consumed diet is sufficient (Table 9.2, World Health Organization 1985).

Quality

It is equally important that the correct type of protein is prescribed for similar reasons, especially when protein restriction is < 0.8 g kg^{-1} IBW. About 50–60%

Table 9.1 Suggested protein and energy requirements versus degree of renal function

GFR (mL min^{-1})[a]	Protein (g kg^{-1} IBW)[a]	Energy (kcal kg^{-1} IBW)
>30	Normalise	30–35
20–30	0.6–1.0[a]	30–35
25	0.6–0.75[a]	30–35
10–5 Dialysis if not yet indicated		

GFR, glomerular filtration rate, IBW, ideal body weight.
[a] at least 50% high biological value (HBV).
35 kcal kg^{-1} IBW for active patients and 30 kcal kg^{-1} IBW for sedentary patients i.e. >60/65 years of age or inactive and disabled.
(Based on K/DOQI recommendations, Kopple (2000) and EDTNA/ERCA nutritional guidelines (2001).)

Table 9.2 Dietary aspects of conservative management of chronic renal failure

Protein	0.6–1.0 g kg^{-1} IBW 50% HBV
Energy	30–35 kcal kg^{-1} IBW Increase with malnutrition Decrease with obesity
Fat	40% of energy Reduce SFA Increase PUFA and MUFA
Carbohydrate	50% of energy Decrease monosaccharides Increase polysaccharides Increase fibre
Phosphorus	600–1000 mg (depending on protein intake) 19–31 mmol L^{-1} Use phosphate binders as needed
Sodium	1800–2500 mg (80–110 mmol day $^{-1}$)
Potassium	Approx. 1.0 mmol kg^{-1} IBW (with hyperkalaemia)
Minerals	Ca (Ca salt) also acts as a phosphate binder Fe with RHuEPO
Vitamins	Water-soluble supplements if needed

IBW, ideal body weight; HBV, high biological value; SFA, saturated fatty acid; PUFA, polyunsaturated fatty acid; MUFA, monounsaturated fatty acid; RHuEPO, recombinant human erythropoietin.
(Protein, phosphorus, potassium and sodium intake are based on EDTNA/ERCA nutritional guidelines (2001).)

of protein should be obtained from high-biological-value sources, such as lean meat, chicken, fish, eggs and some milk. These foods contain a higher percentage of essential amino acids; however, this may not always be achievable as many patients follow a vegetarian diet. Dietary advice must be excellent and this can be achieved by the expertise of an experienced renal dietitian with frequent follow-up sessions either at clinic or by telephone. Well-informed nurses are able to complement the nutritional advice given by the dietitian.

The effect of a reduced-protein diet

An improvement in well-being is first noticed, often with a corresponding decrease in serum urea and creatinine levels. Some patients notice that mild symptoms like 'morning sickness' and a 'metallic taste' in the mouth disappear. The initial fall in creatinine may be due to a reduction in the consumption of muscle protein (i.e. meat or fish).

If urea levels do not show an improvement, the following should be investigated:

- Urinary urea excretion can be measured, indicating the amount of dietary protein intake (Maroni 1994).
- The protein content of the diet may be too high.
- The intake of energy (carbohydrate and fat) is too low and protein is used to supplement energy requirements.

- Other extrarenal catabolic factors can lead to excess breakdown of protein due to lack of energy. This may occur as a result of a serious infection or major surgery.
- Consider steroid therapy, to treat inflammatory disease or to prevent and treat rejection after transplantation. Steroids increase catabolism and this in turn releases nitrogen from tissue, with a corresponding increase of urea. Elevated urea levels then need to be considered as acceptable.

In most cases treatment can continue, after correcting any of the dietary and/or metabolic aspects.

Energy

The amount of energy required for maintenance is just as important as the quantity and quality of the protein itself. Insufficient energy will lead to protein catabolism, a negative nitrogen balance, to protein and protein-energy malnutrition (PEM) and weight loss.

Obesity could be treated safely during the early stages of chronic renal failure, especially with replacement therapy in mind. The formation of a fistula becomes difficult and the possibility of further weight gain with peritoneal dialysis is preventable. A low-energy diet should then be considered and progress closely monitored. The minimum requirement should not be less than 30 kcal (126 kJ) for the 0.8–0.9 g kg^{-1} IBW diet for patients with a normal body mass index (BMI) range.

Example

To calculate energy requirements for a 70-kg person (IBW):

$$70 \times 35 - 30 \text{ kcal } (150 - 126 \text{ kJ}) = 2450 - 2100 \text{ kcal } (14.7 - 8.8 \text{ mJ})$$

Carbohydrate (1 g equals 4 kcal (18 kJ))

Ideally, 50% of dietary energy should be obtained from carbohydrate, the majority from starchy and fibre-containing foods (i.e. wholemeal bread, wholegrain cereals, biscuits, potatoes, brown rice and pasta and small amounts in vegetables and fruit). These foods contain some protein and some are high in potassium and need to be avoided in the case of hyperkalaemia.

Fat (1 g = 9 kcal (38 kJ)

Fat is a concentrated form of energy and makes food palatable, providing a feeling of satiety. The recommended dietary guideline on the intake of fat is about 30–35% of the total energy intake. To achieve a satisfactory energy intake this figure needs to be increased for patients on a reduced-protein diet (1 g protein = 4 kcal (18 kJ); Table 9.2).

Nephrotic syndrome

The nephrotic syndrome is associated with proteinuria. The majority of the protein loss is albumin, but other proteins with an intermediate molecular weight are also secreted. These proteins bind nutrients, such as iron, vitamin D, copper and zinc (Kaysen 1992).

■ BOX 9.1 Management of nephrotic syndrome

Treatment of hypertension

Moderate protein restriction
  0.8–1.0 g kg⁻¹ ideal body weight
  Adequate energy

Treatment of hyperlipidaemia
  Manipulate fat intake
  Lipid-lowering drugs

Hypoalbuminaemia can lead to severe fluid retention, which is difficult to treat by diuretic therapy and dietary sodium and/or fluid restriction alone.

Current practice is to optimise blood pressure control with angiotensin-converting enzyme (ACE) inhibitors and to normalise the dietary protein to 0.8–1.0 g kg⁻¹ IBW. Energy intake should be modified to 35 kcal kg⁻¹ IBW if the patient consumes a high protein diet and/or has a high or low energy intake (Box 9.1). The nephrotic syndrome is associated with hyperlipidaemia due to lipoprotein abnormalities. Hyperlipidaemia and proteinuria disappear when the nephrotic syndrome is successfully controlled. General advice regarding weight loss would be to increase exercise, eliminate smoking and commence a low-animal-fat, low-cholesterol diet which is high in mono- and polyunsaturated fatty acids. This, together with lipid-lowering drugs, may help to reduce the long-term risk of CVD with a morbidity and mortality rate of >50% in patients with CRF (Harris 1994).

Sodium (Na, 1 mmol = 23 mg Na) and fluid

Mild to moderate sodium (Na) and fluid retention occurs in most types of renal disease and contributes to high blood pressure. Diuretic drug treatment controls fluid retention by increasing Na and fluid excretion (urine). A moderate salt-restricted diet (about 80–120 mmol Na) will help to prevent excessive accumulation of Na. In practice, this may not be so simple as many people rely on the purchase of processed foods.

About 80% of our salt intake is hidden in processed foods, including staple food items such as bread and margarine and butter. Some food manufacturers are now replacing salt with salt substitutes which contain potassium, and this may cause problems for those who need a diet that has reduced potassium.

Patients should be advised to:

- Prepare meals using fresh ingredients.
- Use spices and herbs to add flavour to food.
- Use a little salt in meal preparation.
- Avoid adding salt to food after preparation.
- Avoid excessive amounts of salty foods such as cured and processed foods: this includes take-away meals from supermarkets (see Appendix 9.1).

- Avoid using salt substitutes containing potassium salts such as potassium chloride (KCl).
- Avoid meals prepared with monosodium glutamate. Monosodium glutamate is added to enhance the taste of food in restaurants, take-away outlets and ready-to-eat meals sold in supermarkets. Examples are Chinese, Asian and other Far Eastern meals. Monosodium glutamate is an essential ingredient of purchased spice mixes.
- Read food labels and check for additives like monosodium glutamate and salt substitutes.

Patients who are 'salt losers' need to add salt to their meals and/or use salt supplements, such as Slow-Sodium (10 mmol Na).

Potassium (K 1 mmol = 39 mg K)

The total amount of potassium (K) found in a healthy individual is about 50 mmol kg^{-1}. Depending on the dietary intake, approximately 100 mmol K is absorbed from the food and about 90% is excreted by the kidneys. The remainder is excreted via the gastrointestinal route. The intracellular potassium uptake is mediated by insulin.

Progressive renal failure is often complicated by hyperkalaemia, a potassium level of >6.0 mmol L^{-1}, and may occur when renal function has declined to a glomerular filtration rate of 5 mL min^{-1} with normal urine output. Severe hyperkalaemia can also occur at an earlier stage when patients receive ACE inhibitors for blood pressure control combined with a high intake of potassium-rich foods. This is potentially life-threatening, is not associated with physical warning signs and requires immediate treatment. Dietary and non-dietary causes for hyperkalaemia should both be investigated at the same time (Bansal 1992).

A dietary intake of no more than 60–70 mmol day^{-1} (1 mmol kg^{-1} IBW) is sufficient to prevent or treat hyperkalaemia by dietary means in the presence of an adequate urine output or dialysis treatment. However, serum K levels in anuric non-dialysed patients, taking a 50-mmol potassium diet, could rise by 1 mmol day^{-1} despite gastrointestinal adaptation to eliminate dietary K in chronic renal failure (Bansal 1992).

Treatment and prevention of hyperkalaemia

Dietary management

A reduced dietary potassium allowance should be initiated either to prevent or to treat hyperkalaemia alongside correcting other reasons for hyperkalaemia. Most foods contain potassium, but the majority is found in vegetables and fruits; some varieties contain more than others. Staple foods such as potatoes, yam, sweet potatoes, green bananas and plantain are high in potassium, but should be included in a potassium-reduced diet. Potassium-containing salts, such as dipotassium phosphate, are used as food additives but in small quantities.

Patients should receive dietary advice regarding the potassium content of specific foods, avoiding those that are high. A list of fruit and vegetables that are low, medium or high in potassium should be included (see Appendix 9.2). The vegetables should be cut in small pieces and boiled in large amounts of water.

Vegetables prepared in a pressure cooker or microwave or are stir-fried will contain more potassium than if boiled in water.

Potassium and high-fibre foods

Constipation is a common problem for CAPD, older and sedentary patients.

High-fibre cereal products are recommended to help increase the fibre content of a renal diet. A high-fibre diet prevents constipation and has a beneficial effect on hyperlipidaemia. However, some high-fibre foods are high in potassium and some is absorbed, although it is unclear how much (Pagenkemper et al 1994). The overall effect of a high-fibre diet on serum K levels is not significant—about 0.3 mmol (McKenzie & Henderson 1986). It is important to exclude non-dietary causes for hyperkalaemia when exploring the reasons for a patient's difficulty in maintaining normal potassium levels.

Examples of non-dietary causes for hyperkalaemia are:

- metabolic acidosis
- increased catabolism
- endocrine abnormalities
- drugs such as potassium supplements (i.e. Slow-K), potassium-sparing diuretics, ACE inhibitors and non-steroidal anti-inflammatory drugs
- constipation (avoid drugs that contribute to constipation, i.e. phosphate binders)
- excessive exercise, heat stroke and rhabdomyolosis cause hyperkalaemia due to tissue cell destruction (Bansal 1992).

Potassium exchange resins

Potassium binders such as calcium or sodium ion exchange resin (i.e. calcium or sodium resonium) may be used to control hyperkalaemia. Calcium ions are exchanged for potassium ions in the gut and the potassium salt is then eliminated.

Calcium resonium is a gritty textured powder, to be taken in measures of 15 g once, twice or three times daily. The resin is best taken with a sweet soft drink to mask its taste. The long-term use of calcium resonium can lead to severe constipation, unless appropriate laxatives are prescribed (check the potassium content of laxatives and bulking agents). Calcium resonium may be administered rectally in cases of oral intolerance. The dose is doubled to achieve the same effect as oral administration.

Phosphorus (P 1 mmol = 31 mg P)

Renal osteodystrophy

The overall management of renal bone disease is discussed in Chapter 5, but there are some principles of nutritional care that require consideration here. Ca and P are obtained from most foods with a high protein content. Examples are milk and its products: hard types of cheese and cheese spread are especially high in calcium and phosphorus. Phosphorus also appears in high fibre cereal products and fish with edible bones, offal, pulses and nuts. Vitamin D is a fat–soluble vitamin and is obtained from food (i.e. added to margarine and butter) and from exposure to sunlight.

Although hypocalcaemia can be treated by controlling hyperphosphataemia and the maintainance of normal Ca levels with calcitriol administration, great care is needed to avoid hypercalcaemia. Extraskeletal calcification occurs in the presence of an elevated calcium or phosphate product, as previously mentioned. This affects blood vessels, including the coronary arteries and the mitral and aortic valves of the heart. This is now considered one of the major causes of morbidity and mortality in adults (Block et al 1998) and young adults (Goodman et al 2000).

Renal osteodystrophy develops over many years and can be prevented by starting treatment of hyperphosphataemia at an early stage, well before the patient starts dialysis by dietary means and phosphate binders.

Calcium (Ca 1 mmol = 40 mg Ca)

Hypocalcaemia

The recommended daily calcium intake for predialysis patients is 1000–1500 mg. A protein- and/or phosphorus-restricted diet tends to be calcium-deficient as foods with a high phosphorus content are high in calcium. Calcium supplements (i.e. calcium carbonate) may be needed but should be taken between meals, preferably at bedtime to maximise Ca absorption.

Hyperphosphataemia

Hyperphosphataemia is difficult to control by dietary manipulation alone and needs to be combined with phosphate binders. Dialysis helps to eliminate phosphate, but as dietary protein requirements are increased, the intake of phosphorus will also rise proportionally. Likewise, dietary phosphorus restriction reduces the intake of protein when prescribed during the predialysis phase of CRF (see Table 9.2 for the recommended intake of phosphorus).

Foods with a high phosphorus content are to be avoided, in addition to a reduced protein allowance. Foods with a high phosphorus content should either be eliminated or form part of the dietary phosphorus intake (see Appendix 9.3).

Fibre improves bowel habits and the general well-being of patients. Serum phosphate levels may rise slightly, by 0.25 mmol L^{-1} with a high-fibre diet (Pender 1989); however, the benefits of a high-fibre intake outweigh the risk of hyperphosphataemia, which can be treated by increasing phosphate-binding agents.

Phosphate binders

Calcium carbonate is an effective phosphate-binding agent. Phosphate binding occurs in the gut. Phosphate from food forms, with calcium from the binders, an insoluble salt and this product is eliminated via the gastrointestinal route.

Phosphate binders should be taken with food, particularly main meals, and with snacks containing P and with milk-based nutritional supplements.

Aluminium-containing phosphate binders are not routinely prescribed any longer as they may have contributed to aluminium bone disease in the past.

Phosphate binders may be less effective if used with H_2-receptor antagonists to treat gastric and duodenal ulcers by reducing the gastric acid output. Hyperphosphataemia has been reported when ranitidine is used to raise the intragastric pH level in renal patients on phosphate-binding agents (Tan et al 1996).

Sevelamer hydrochloride is a new phosphate binder that does not contain calcium or aluminium and also reduces serum cholesterol levels. It reduces the absorption of phosphorus like the calcium-based binding agents without the risk of hypercalcaemia when calcitriol is prescribed to suppress parathyroid hormone production (Chertow et al 1999).

Magnesium (Mg, I mmol Mg = 24 mg Mg)

Magnesium is retained with impaired kidney function. Magnesium-containing antacids to relieve gastrointestinal problems are potent phosphate binders, but may cause diarrhoea.

Other important nutrients

Iron (Fe I mmol = 56 mg Fe)

The consumption of foods which are high in iron content like red meat, offal, pulses and green vegetables may be reduced in a renal diet. A reduced protein intake may contribute to Fe deficiency. See Chapter 5 for anaemia management.

If oral Fe supplements are used, 200–300 mg Fe day^{-1} is required to restore Fe status when patients are on HD or peritoneal dialysis with a serum ferritin level of < 100 ng mL^{-1} or a relative Fe deficiency with a transferrin saturation of $< 20\%$ (Makoff 1992). Avoid prescribing Fe supplement with phosphate binders to prevent drug interaction; these should be taken between meals (i.e. at bedtime).

It may be necessary to provide a vitamin supplement containing folate, pyridoxine (vitamin B_6), vitamin B_{12} and vitamin C (see Table 9.3). In order to obtain a rapid response to Fe deficiency, intravenous preparations are more often used, whether administered intravenously or subcutaneously (see Ch. 5).

Zinc (Zn)

Meat, fish, pulses and wheat products are rich in zinc and the requirement is 1 mg elemental Zn kg^{-1} day^{-1} for adults. Zinc deficiency is a well-known complication of uraemia and may be due to inadequate dietary protein or excessive losses of protein. Symptoms include impaired taste acuity, metallic taste and impaired wound healing. Renal patients with established Zn deficiency may benefit from supplementation, taken between meals to enhance absorption.

It has been reported that protein catabolic rate improves in patients on HD receiving Zn supplementation (Jern et al 2000).

Vitamins

Vitamins regulate the metabolic pathways of protein, carbohydrate and fat and uraemia alters their serum levels, body stores and function. Vitamin deficiency can occur with a restricted or inadequate diet providing fewer vitamins than recommended for healthy individuals. During HD and peritoneal dialysis the small molecules such as water-soluble vitamins are removed, and losses are higher with high-flux HD. The fat-soluble vitamin A is a larger molecule and vitamin A metabolites are therefore more difficult to remove and could lead to toxicity.

Drug interaction, and the absorption and activity of specific vitamins may also be impaired. Drug interaction more likely affects the activity of vitamins B_6, folic acid and vitamin B_{12}. Vitamin supplements containing these vitamins in appropriate quantities are important as folic acid and vitamins B_6 and B_{12} may improve poor erythropoietic response in those on dialysis. Requirements for these three vitamins may be higher to treat hyperhomocysteinaemia as elevated levels of homocysteine may contribute to cardio-, cerebro- and peripheral vascular disease.

An average of 125 mg vitamin C is lost during each dialysis session and supplementation may be needed, especially in malnourished patients. A high-dose vitamin C supplement should be avoided to prevent hyperoxalosis: 60 mg may be sufficient with a normal dietary vitamin C intake, while a supplement of 200 mg vitamin C may increase serum oxalate levels. Oxalate deposits as crystals in soft tissues like muscle tissue and vital organs and may increase the risk of myocardial infarction, muscle weakness and bone disease.

Vitamin supplements containing the fat-soluble vitamins A, D, E and K are contraindicated in patients with renal failure. Vitamin A metabolites are less well excreted and accumulate over time.

Hypervitaminosis A and toxicity have been reported in patients receiving total parenteral nutrition containing a high dose of vitamin A (Muth 1991). High-dose vitamin E supplementation may be a potential risk factor affecting the clotting mechanism. Considering these risks, routine vitamin A and E supplementation is not recommended.

Vitamin K supplementation is contraindicated unless a patient is on chronic antibiotic treatment (Makoff et al 1996; Rocco & Makoff 1997). Although water-soluble vitamin supplementation is important in dialysis patients, there is no agreement on the amount of each individual vitamin. Renal formula vitamin supplements based on the formula below are available but not as a drug or food supplement in the UK. They should be prescribed according to the specifications of the Medical Control Agency.

Routine supplementation of water soluble vitamins will most likely outweigh the risk of deficiency, especially in patients who are unable to consume an adequate diet as a result of chronic illness, depression or old age. Vitamin supplements should always be taken after an HD session. Table 9.3 lists the suggested daily recommendations (Makoff 1999).

Table 9.3 Suggested daily dosage of vitamins for renal failure patients

Vitamins	Dosage	%RDI (USA)
Vitamin A	0	0
Vitamin E	0	0
Vitamin B_1	1.5 mg	100
Vitamin B_2	1.7 mg	100
Vitamin B_6	10 mg	500
Vitamin B_{12}	6 μg	100
Folic acid	800–1000 μg	200–250
Pantothenic acid	10 mg	100
Niacin	20 mg	100
Biotin	300 μg	100
Vitamin C	60 mg	100

From Makoff (1999) with permission.
RDI, recommended daily intake.

DIETARY MANAGEMENT OF DIALYSIS TREATMENT

Protein and energy requirements

Most patients will receive nutrition information in the predialysis phase. Specific dietary requirements may need adjusting when the mode of therapy (HD, peritoneal dialysis or transplantation) changes.

Current recommendations for dietary requirements are shown in Table 9.4.

Protein

Patients treated by HD or continuous peritoneal dialysis often have PEM and therefore it is very important to maintain an adequate intake of protein

Table 9.4 Dietary recommendations for patients on renal replacement therapy

	HD	PD	TXP
Protein (g kg^{-1} IBW)	1.0–1.2	1.2–1.3	EAR
Energy (kcal kg^{-1} IBW	35	35	EAR
Na (mmol day^{-1})[a]	80–110	80–110	80–110
K (mmol kg^{-1} IBW)	1.0	1.0	Free
P (mmol day^{-1})	31–45	31–45	Free
Vitamins	Yes	Yes	Not required
Phosphate binders	Yes	Yes	Not required

HD, haemodialysis; PD, peritoneal dialysis; TXP, transplantation; IBW, ideal body weight; EAR, estimated average recommendations (national agreement).
Protein intake for HD and PD based on K/DOQI recommendations (Kopple et al 2000).
Energy intake for HD and PD based on K/DOQI recommendations (Kopple et al 2000).
[a] 80–110 mmol equals 1800–2500 mg sodium.
Sodium, potassium and phosphorus intake for HD and PD based on EDTNA/ERCA nutritional guidelines (2001).

and energy. During HD approximately 10–12 g amino acids is lost per treatment. To cover this loss requires a protein intake of 1.2 g kg^{-1} IBW and at least 50% should be of high biological value (HBV).

A daily average of 5–15 protein g albumin is lost during peritoneal dialysis in addition to an average of 3 g amino acids. Protein losses during peritonitis are higher. To cover these losses a protein intake of 1.3 g kg^{-1} IBW is recommended and at least 50% should be of HBV (Kopple et al 2000) .

The protein requirement for a patient with a good functioning transplant returns to normal. However, it must be reduced once again to 1.0 g kg^{-1} IBW in the case of graft failure (Pagenkemper & Foulks 1991).

Energy requirements

An intake of 35 kcal kg^{-1} IBW is recommended to maintain nitrogen (protein) balance and albumin levels in HD and peritoneal dialysis patients. For sedentary and older patients, 30–35 kcal kg^{-1} IBW is sufficient. More information is needed about recommendations for underweight and overweight patients (Kopple et al 2000).

Dextrose (glucose) is used as an osmotic agent for the removal of fluid. Hyperglycaemia with steroid-induced diabetes mellitus, hyperlipidaemia and obesity are common. These problems increase as the osmotic strength of the dialysate increases. When calculating energy requirements for peritoneal dialysis patients, energy from glucose-containing dialysate needs to be included. Glucose absorption may provide between 300 and 700 kcal or more, if strong 3.86% dextrose solutions are used.

Icodextrin

This new solution contains glucose polymers with a larger molecular weight than glucose and it is an effective osmotic agent. The glucose uptake of a dialysate regime including a long dwell time, using 2 L icodextrin instead of 2 L 3.86% dextrose, reduces the energy content attributed to glucose uptake by 50%. See Chapter 8.

Assessment of body weight

In estimating oedema, free body mass weight should be measured after haemodialysis and in peritoneal dialysis after drainage of dialysis fluid, even though patients may still be fluid-overloaded after these procedures.

To estimate IBW, a BMI between 18.5 and 24.9 kg m^{-2} (Garrow 1981) and its corresponding weight in kilograms, is considered within normal range (World Health Organization 1998). These figures should be used to calculate protein and energy requirements for individual patients.

Sodium and fluid

Once a patient becomes oliguric and eventually anuric, the intake of salt and fluid may need to be reduced to control interdialytic weight gain (IDWG) with HD and fluid balance with peritoneal dialysis.

Excessive IDWG in HD patients contributes to hypertension prior to HD treatments, provoking antihypertensive medication. The presence of left ventricular cardiac failure (hypertrophy) is also related to the length of time in ESRF (Ifudu et al 1997).

A reduced fluid allowance is probably the most difficult part of the dialysis diet to cope with. Up to 86% of patients may exceed an IDWG guideline of 1.5 kg and there appears to be no difference between those who have diabetes and those who do not (Halverson et al 1993). Some groups of patients with a different ethnic background appear to have additional problems with IDWG. Indo-Asian patients in particular may often be unable to adhere to their fluid allowances and this is attributed to a higher fluid and salt content of traditional foods and meals (Davidson 2000).

Most renal centres in the UK regard an IDWG ranging from 1.5 to 2.0 kg as acceptable. Considering the differences in size of patients, it may be more appropriate to base IDGW on dry weight using 4% as an acceptable IDWG (EDTNA-ERCA nutrition guidelines 2001). This figure needs to be adapted for obese patients: if BMI is > 25, a weight equal to a BMI of 25 should be substituted for this calculation.

The mechanism of thirst

It is important to remember what causes thirst. Thirst is a direct result of too much sodium as a drink, salty food or just too much added to food. The sodium level in the body is finely tuned in healthy individuals and those with renal failure are no exception. Too much dietary salt will cause the sodium level to rise and the thirst mechanism in the brain to act. It is then necessary to drink sufficient fluid to normalise the sodium level. The most important aspect for maintaining an acceptable IDWG in HD and peritoneal dialysis patients is to reduce the amount of salt, and use herbs and spices to flavour food instead.

Excessive IDWG may not always be due to poor understanding. Solid food contains fluid and patients with a good appetite will have higher IDWGs and this fact can be established with a detailed dietary assessment, indicating a high protein and energy intake (Sherman et al 1995).

Fluid is anything liquid at room temperature and includes jelly, icecream, ice cubes, gravy, soups and sauces, and custard. A daily fluid allowance of 500–750 mL in addition to the previous-day urine output is usually sufficient to prevent excessive IDWG in those on HD. Patients on peritoneal dialysis can increase their intake to at least 750 mL plus their previous-day urine output.

A sodium intake of 80–110 mmol day^{-1} will be sufficient to control thirst and helps the patient to manage the fluid allowance. The use of processed foods (80% of our salt consumption comes from processed and salted food) and adding salt to food after preparation should be avoided. See Appendix 9.1.

Sodium profiling was introduced during the late 1970s to help prevent muscle cramps during dialysis and postdialysis hypotension as a result of shortening dialysis treatment.

Sodium loading during dialysis should and can be prevented by using lower sodium concentrates for HD and automated peritoneal dialysis (Cannata-Andia et al 2000). Patients with a high postdialysis sodium level will have difficulty in maintaining their fluid allowance as the ingestion of salt in between treatment increases serum sodium levels (see above). It is therefore essential to reduce the intake of salt in addition to helping in the-control of excessive IDWG in HD and hypertension (Kooman et al 2000, Krautzig et al 1998).

Hints for patients for keeping to their fluid allowance

- Use little salt in cooking and avoid adding salt afterwards.
- Make use of herbs and spices.
- Avoid or minimise the use of processed food.
- Avoid foods containing monosodium glutamate.
- Measure the fluid allowance in a water jug.
- Divide a fluid allowance evenly through the day.
- Use a small cup or glass instead of a mug or large glass.
- Drink only half a cup each time if possible.
- Ice cubes may be more thirst-quenching, but each cube equals 30 mL fluid (two tablespoons): lemon juice or other flavouring can be added.
- Rinse the mouth with water, gargle, but do not swallow.
- Stimulate saliva production by sucking a slice of lemon or grapefruit, sherbets or chewing gum.
- Take medicines with the main meals unless contraindicated.
- When going out, save the allowance of fluid. This allows for an extra drink when socialising.
- It is important to keep occupied.
- A daily weight check in the morning before breakfast will reveal the rate of fluid accumulation in between HD treatments and the fluid status of peritoneal dialysis.

Potassium

Most patients starting dialysis continue to produce fairly good quantities of urine. This helps with the excretion of sodium, fluid and potassium. At this time, it may be possible to relax the intake of fluid and potassium but urine output must be monitored regularly. Dietary potassium, salt and fluid restrictions should be introduced or adjusted as urine output decreases.

The risk of hyperkalaemia is greater in anuric patients. The dietary intake of potassium should be reduced to 1.0 mmol kg^{-1} IBW day^{-1} for HD treatment. Patients on peritoneal dialysis should be able to relax their potassium intake as potassium is constantly removed.

Hyperkalaemia is a frequent problem, especially with HD, and dietary indiscretion is partly to blame, but the amount of K removed during dialysis can vary as much as 71%. Other reasons for hyperkalaemia should be investigated simultaneously. Some patients on haemodialysis consume foods with a high potassium content during the first or second hour of dialysis. The transit of food and fluid through the gastrointestinal tract may take 9–12 h before any of the nutrients and fluid are absorbed in the blood stream (Gardner 1979). This means that the potassium in food consumed during the early part of dialysis will not be removed during dialysis.

Phosphorus (P)

The recommended intake varies from 1000 to 1400 mg (31–45 mmol day^{-1}) depending on the recommended protein for HD or peritoneal dialysis, to prevent hyperphosphataemia and preserve an adequate and acceptable diet for the patient to follow (EDTNA/ERCA nutritional guidelines 2001).

Dietary P restriction combined with phosphate binders and dialysis helps to prevent severe hyperphosphataemia (see Appendix 9.3).

Table 9.5 shows an example of a patient's dietary phosphorus intake versus HD and peritoneal dialysis. The level of phosphorus retention depends on the amount of dietary protein intake and removal by dialysis. Phosphate clearance by dialysis varies and depends on the efficiency of HD dialysis membranes and the adequacy of both HD and continuous peritoneal dialysis treatment. This table shows that phosphorus intake depends on the recommended protein intake and the resultant amount of phosphorus. Thus a net gain of phosphorus can only be controlled by the appropriate type, dose and use of phosphate binders.

Vitamins

Vitamin supplements are recommended for all dialysis patients with inadequate intake of nutrients as a result of chronic illness, old age and poverty. Table 9.4 lists the recommended intake of vitamins for dialysis patients.

Malnutrition

There have been many papers published since the early 1980s on the consequences of PEM, which is a frequent complication of HD and peritoneal dialysis.

Marckman (1988) concluded that in his cross-sectional study, 47% of HD and 44% of peritoneal dialysis patients suffered from PEM. This related to severe weight loss prior to starting dialysis and during the early 'repletion' stage. Lowrie & Lew (1990) showed that the relative risk of death increases as the serum albumin of the HD patient falls. These authors had already

Table 9.5 Example of dietary phosphorus intake, potential clearance by dialysis and net gain in a patient weighing 70 kg (within normal body mass index range), following a diet based on recommended protein and phosphorus intake

Treatment	Protein (g) (per day)	P intake (mmol) (per day/week)	Clearance (per week)	P gain (mmol) (per week)
HD	82	31–45/217–315	24 mmol[a]	193–291
CPD	91	31–45/217–315	70 mmol[a]	147–245

HD, haemodialysis; CPD, continuous peritoneal dialysis.
[a] Assuming this amount is removed with dialysis.

concluded that longer treatment time and better nutritional status improve the clinical outcome of HD treatment.

In 1991, Young et al concluded that over 40% of CPD patients were mildly to severely malnourished and that there was widespread variation (20–70%) between centres taking part in this international multi-centre study. In 1993, Spiegel et al published their findings about the relationship between serum albumin levels and the risk of morbidity (hospitalisation) in peritoneal dialysis patients. Their results showed that for every 10 g L^{-1} decrease in serum albumin, there was an increase in the odds ratio of 5:2. In diabetic peritoneal dialysis patients the odds ratio increased 10-fold. It was concluded that serum albumin was a marker of increased risk for hospitalisation and that this risk was even greater in diabetics.

However, controversy started to emerge about the reliability of serum albumin used as a marker of nutritional status (Fine & Cox 1992; Heimburger et al 1994).

The Canada–USA Peritoneal Dialysis Study Group published in 1996 the results of a large prospective multicentre study (also referred to as the CANUSA study). This study showed that the relative risk of death increased with age, insulin-dependent diabetes mellitus, cardiovascular disease, low serum albumin and worsening nutritional status. Subjective global assessment and percentage lean body mass were used to assess nutritional status. Malnutrition estimated by subjective global assessment had a strong correlation with an increase in hospitalisation days while a low serum albumin may partly reflect malnutrition as overhydration also results in a decrease in serum albumin. It was concluded that continuous peritoneal dialysis adequacy is an important factor of the clinical outcome of treatment. Dialysis prescriptions need to include any change in renal function (Churchill et al 1996).

Hypoalbuminaemia

Hypoalbuminaemia is an important predictor of morbidity and mortality and there are several reasons for reduced albumin levels in patients with chronic renal failure:

- decreased synthesis due to PEM or the acute-phase C-reactive protein (CRP) response
- redistribution of albumin pools
- albumin losses due to proteinuria and during peritoneal dialysis
- albumin results may be dilutional
- essay methods to measure albumin may differ.

C-reactive protein

The significance of CRP and other acute-phase proteins is a recent topic for research and there are several publications explaining the relationship between raised CRP (normal < 10 mg L^{-1}) and other parameters. CRP levels rise with inflammation, e.g. infection and tissue damage. When serum albumin is corrected for CRP, albumin loses its significance as a nutritional marker (Bergstrom et al 1995).

After correcting dietary treatment and dialysis prescription, serum albumin levels may not always improve and this may be due to other inflammatory processes. Inflammation may prevent the normal anabolic response to adequate nutrition and hence contribute to an increase in the morbidity and mortality rates of dialysis patients (Kaysen 1997).

Raised CRP levels > 50 mg L^{-1} are common in HD patients and less so in peritoneal dialysis. Stimulation of the immune system may be due to the HD treatment itself (biocompatibility of membranes, treatment time, insufficient purification of water used for dialysate, infections of vascular access sites and others (McIntyre et al 1997). Recent studies have suggested the existence of a syndrome consisting of malnutrition, inflammation and atherosclerosis in some patients.

Inflammation is more common in malnutrition and inflammation and there is evidence that both are closely linked to cardiovascular disease in chronic renal failure. It appears that we may have at least two types of malnutrition in those with renal failure: one type without and another type with concomitant inflammatory response with a high morbidity risk. Treatment strategies are different and need further investigations (Stenvinkel et al 2000).

Serum albumin results can vary depending on the assay methods used. There may be a difference of 10 g L^{-1} using bromocresol green or purple or the immunoturdidimetric method. This makes auditing between renal centres also difficult (Carfray et al 2000). Serum albumin levels are usually measured from blood samples prior to HD when a patient may retain additional amounts of fluid. The same applies to a patient on peritoneal dialysis. This should be remembered when a patient presents with unexplained hypoalbuminaemia (Jones 2001).

MANAGEMENT OF PROTEIN-ENERGY MALNUTRITION

Consequences of PEM

- Failure to thrive
- Increased morbidity
  — delayed wound healing
  — decreased resistance to infection
  — electrolyte imbalance
  — prolonged hospitalisation with financial consequences
- Increased mortality.

Prevention and treatment of PEM should start during the predialysis phase of ESRF. Most renal services departments hold multidisciplinary counselling sessions for patients, to provide information on treatment options and other valuable information, and several sessions should be attended by an experienced renal dietitian. All patients should also receive individual dietary advice and frequent monitoring is essential to accommodate any changes in renal function.

There are several reasons for PEM in dialysis patients and these are multifactorial:

1. Reduced dietary intake
   - Reduced appetite (see point 2, below)
   - Existing malnutrition at the start of dialysis due to uraemia and unsupervised predialysis dietary restriction
   - Inadequate dietary nutrient intake. Most patients consume less protein than is recommended. This may not always lead to a negative nitrogen balance in <u>stable</u> HD or peritoneal dialysis patients. Some patients achieve a neutral nitrogen balance on a protein intake of 0.7 g kg^{-1} IBW day^{-1} with a high energy consumption of 35–38 kcal IBW day^{-1} (Bergstrom 1993).
   - Conflicting dietary recommendations: increasing protein and decreasing the intake of phosphorus, and prescription of phosphate binders. Phosphorus restriction may relax once new phosphate binders and vitamin D preparations are prescribed
   - Coexisting gastrointestinal disease (i.e. gastroparesis) and comorbidity such as cardiac failure, cancer or other medical conditions
   - Multipharmacy prescriptions
   - Inadequate provision of nutrients in food provided by hospitals or nursing homes
   - Financial constraints.
2. Reduced appetite
   - Raised serum leptin levels in chronic renal failure. Leptin is a protein/hormone that activates the hypothalamus to reduce appetite and increase energy metabolism. Leptin is excreted by the kidney and levels rise with declining renal function; it is not removed by dialysis. It is thought that hyperleptinaemia may contribute to anorexia and malnutrition in chronic renal failure. Body fat mass, plasma insulin levels and biocompatible dialysis membranes may also contribute to hyperleptinaemia (Stenvinkel 1999, Widjaja et al 2000, Wright et al 2000)
   - Inadequate dialysis, leading to uraemic symptoms
   - Suppression of appetite due to glucose absorption with peritoneal dialysis, intraabdominal compression and constipation
   - Chronic depression and old age.
3. Increase in nutritional losses
   - Water-soluble nutrient losses during dialysis, such as albumin, amino acid and vitamin
   - Persistent proteinuria.
4. Altered metabolism
   - Protein degradation as a result of the dialysis process (HD)
   - Untreated acidosis contributes to protein catabolism
   - Inadequate dialysis
   - Physical activity
   - Intercurrent illness
   - Hyperparathyroidism.

Assessing nutritional status

Prior to implementing nutritional support some documented evidence of PEM will be required.

Body mass index

Height and weight measurements are easy to perform and BMI can easily be calculated by dividing weight in kilograms by height in metres, squared.

Example

A person weighs 65 kg and is 1.70 m tall.

BMI is $\dfrac{65}{1.7 \times 1.7} = 22.49$

Normal range: 18.5–24.9
Underweight: < 18.5
Pre-obese: 25–29.9
Obese class I: 30–34.9
Obese class II: 35–39.9(obese)
Obese class III: 40–60 (very obese).

Methods of dietary assessment

- 24-h recall
- 3-day food diaries, to include one weekend day and one HD day if appropriate
  Both methods depend on patients' recollection of food eaten, a detailed written record and a computer analysis program
- 24-h urine samples in predialysis patients to calculate urea nitrogen appearance and protein losses
- Peritoneal dialysis dialysate collection to estimate protein losses.

Techniques to assess body composition

The best-known techniques are:

- Anthropometry: mid-arm/mid upper arm muscle circumference, skinfold thickness: this is easy to perform and noninvasive, but is influenced by hydration, sensitive to observer error and less sensitive to change over time.
- Bioelectrical impedance: quick and non-invasive, but an indirect method and influenced by hydration and electrode site.
- Dual-energy X-ray absorptiometry (DEXA): direct measurement of bone mineral, lean body mass and other compartments. DEXA is also influenced by hydration, costly and not widely available.

Assessing the nutritional status of dialysis patients using subjective global assessment

It is important to identify malnutrition early to rehabilitate the patient early and to improve the clinical outcome. Subjective global assessment is an assessment of nutritional status and was first performed on surgical patients. It is based on the patient's history and physical examination. The ratings—well nourished, moderately (or suspected of being) malnourished, severely malnourished—are most affected by subcutaneous tissue, muscle wasting and weight loss (Detsky et al 1987).

A simple questionnaire is completed by a trained nurse, dietitian or a member of the medical team.

History
The history includes weight changes, dietary intake, gastrointestinal symptoms, functional status and comorbid disease.

Physical examination
Physical examination takes into account loss of subcutaneous fat, muscle wasting, oedema, ascitis. The overall rating then depends on the score:

- Mild malnutrition to normal: 6 or 7 rating in most categories or significant, continued improvement
- Mild to moderate malnutrition: 3, 4 or 5: no clear indication of normal status or severe malnutrition
- Severely malnourished: 1 or 2 ratings in most categories or significant signs of malnutrition.

The CANUSA study showed that a one-unit increase on the seven-point scale of subjective global assessment rating was associated with a 25% decline in relative risk of death (McCann 1996).

Treatment of protein energy malnutrition
Intervention should start as soon as malnutrition is identified. This consists of dietary review and counselling by an experienced renal dietitian who will:

- increase the existing dietary prescription as required
- modify its consistency if chewing and/or swallowing is a problem
- gradually motivate the patient to improve nutritional intake if active depression is an underlying cause
- introduce nutritional support at an early stage
- monitor progress frequently.

Nutritional support

Methods of nutritional support

- oral or sip feeding for patients who are able to eat and drink normally
- nasogastric or gastrostomy feeding for patients who are unable or unwilling to eat or drink normally. Oral and tube feeding can be combined, for instance tube feeding overnight, while the patient sleeps, and normal eating/drinking during the day
- intraperitoneal amino acids (IPAA) with peritoneal dialysis
- intradialytic parenteral nutrition (IDPN) during HD
- total parenteral nutrition (TPN) for patients who are unable to receive oral/sip or enteral methods of nutritional support.

Nasogastric and sip feeding

Concentrated oral supplements could be used once malnutrition is diagnosed and these should be prescribed as a medicine. The insertion of a percutaneous enteral gastrostomy (PEG) feeding tube enables long-term tube feeding to be carried out without the discomfort of a nasogastric feeding tube. The manufacturers of nutritional support products have improved their range for oral consumption and enteral tube-feeding products. The high protein and energy-dense products are best for the anuric patient who requires additional support, while patients on peritoneal dialysis would benefit from high-protein formulas.

Nutritional peritoneal dialysis

Recent studies indicate that using dialysate with a 1.1% amino acid concentration, providing a net gain of 18 g amino acids in 2 L dialysate, improves the nutritional status of peritoneal dialysis patients. An oral energy supplement must be given during the administration of IPAA (see Ch. 8).

Intradialytic parenteral nutrition

Parenteral formulas containing approximately 65–70 g protein and 1000 kcal (mainly glucose) can be safely delivered during HD treatment. Glucose monitoring during treatment is essential to prevent hyperglycaemia. The fluid balance can be adjusted accordingly. IDPN remains a controversial mode of nutritional support and further research is required to prove its effectiveness. The cost of IDPN is 10-fold compared with enteral nutrition or oral supplementation.

Monitoring nutritional support

It is important to monitor progress after initiating nutritional support. Monitoring patients is an ongoing process and is part of the multidisciplinary auditing process.

Quality standards for dialysis patients

The British Dietetic Association–Renal Nutrition Group published *Standards for Adult Renal Patients: Setting Standards and Achieving Optimal Nutritional Status* (Engel et al 1998). These are being reviewed in 2002.

The EDTNA-ERCA Dietitians' Special Interest Group has published *New European Guidelines for Nutritional Management of Adult Renal Patients* in 2001 (website: www.edtna-erca.org).

The Renal Association and Royal College of Physicians (London) issued standards and audit measures to guarantee adequate treatment in 1997 (Table 9.6). The third edition is being published in 2002.

TRANSPLANTATION

Some nutritional problems occurring after transplantation are specific to immune-suppressive therapy. Side-effects include protein catabolism,

Table 9.6 Nutritional standards for patients on renal replacement therapy

	HD	CAPD
Albumin (g l^{-1})	>35	>35
K (mmol L^{-1a}	3.5–6.5	3.5–5.5
P mmol L^{-1a}	<1.8	<1.8
Ca (mmol L^{-1})	2.2–2.6	2.2–2.6 (within locally agreed normal range, corrected for serum albumin)
Urea kinetic modelling (Kt/V)^a	>1.2 per treatment	>1.7 per week per treatment
Urea reduction rate (URR)^a	>65% per treatment	

HD, haemodialysis; CPD, continuous peritoneal dialysis.
^{a} Reference: Renal Association. Treatment of adult patients with renal failure. 2nd edn. 1997. The third edition is in press.

obesity, hyperlipidaemia and glucose intolerance (steroid-induced diabetes). Dietary guidelines for transplant patients include advice on prevention of obesity and healthy eating.

Nutritional requirements

Protein, energy, vitamin and mineral requirements return to levels as recommended at national level.

Energy

Obesity is common with a successful transplant and is multifactorial:

- The patient's appetite increases due to an increased feeling of wellbeing.
- Steroids stimulate the patient's appetite.
- There may be a lack of exercise.

Obesity contributes to hypertension, hyperlipidaemia and these in turn contribute to cardiovascular disease. Maintenance of IBW for height can be achieved with an energy intake of 28–30 kcal kg^{-1} IBW or less if necessary. The patient should be made aware of the risk of obesity at an early stage.

Hyperlipidaemia post-transplantation

The majority of transplant patients show signs of hyperlipidaemia with elevated serum triglyceride and cholesterol levels. This is due to steroid and ciclosporin drug therapy causing glucose intolerance (insulin resistance) and hyperlipidaemia (Lawrence et al 1995). Changing from saturated to unsaturated fat may not result in a change of serum lipid levels.

Dietary management of hyperlipidaemia

It is obvious that patients with a long history of hypertension, hyperlipidaemia and diabetes are prone to cardiovascular disease. It is important that

Table 9.7 Recommended sources of energy for healthy eating

Carbohydrate	50% of energy intake Increase polysaccharides (i.e. starchy foods) Reduce monosaccharides (i.e. sugar and sugary foods) Increase fibre intake
Fat	30–35% of energy intake Reduce intake of saturated fats (i.e. butter) Increase intake of monosaturates (i.e. olive oil) Increase intake of polysaturated fats (i.e. corn oil) These types of fat can transfer into saturated fat if exposed to high temperatures
Vegetables and fruit	Increase to at least five portions daily
Sodium	Avoid excessive intake of salt. If possible, continue with previous salt restriction to help maintain blood pressure control
Exercise	Include some exercise in general guidelines, but the level depends on physical fitness
Smoking	Patients who smoke should be advised to stop smoking

guidelines for healthy eating and regular exercise are incorporated whenever a renal patient is counselled for dietary advice, in addition to drug (statins) therapy (Table 9.7).

Diabetes mellitus

A major complication of type 1 or type 2 diabetes mellitus is diabetic nephropathy. Studies have shown that a moderate protein restriction (0.8 g kg^{-1} IBW) implemented early (Viberti et al, unpublished work), together with optimal glucose and blood pressure control using ACE inhibitors, will reduce the decline in glomerular filtration rate (Stenvinkel 1993). Hyperlipidaemia is more common in diabetes mellitus and any dietary guidelines will include modification of fat intake. It is also important to reduce energy if the patient is overweight and to provide general advice on healthy eating and living (stop smoking and take exercise). Drugs to control hyperglycaemia will need to be adjusted regularly, as requirements diminish as renal function declines. A renal diet combined with that of diabetes, hyperlipidaemia and possibly energy restriction to treat or prevent obesity is highly complex and needs dedication from the patient, family and carers, especially if started early when the patient feels relatively well.

Dietary management in paediatrics

Chronic renal failure may present shortly after birth or later in life and can proceed to ESRF during childhood (Watson 1991). The profound effects that chronic renal failure can place upon growth (Hokken-Koelega 1995) and development, particularly during infancy, necessitate nutritional management on a long-term basis. Fluctuating clinical and biochemical disturbances with changes in treatment require constant readjustment of the nutritional prescription by an experienced dietitian (Coleman 2001). Infants may present with particular problems such as anorexia and vomiting, and an understanding of the psychosocial effects often proves to be as important as the dietary advice (Norman et al 1995).

Nutritional assessment should include the regular monitoring of growth and dietary analysis by means of food diaries. Biochemical assessment with frequent review of fluid balance and prescribed medication such as phosphate binders is recommended. The maintenance of normal serum calcium and phosphate levels is crucial to achieve normal bone development, and nutritional measures have a large part to play, particularly in controlling phosphate levels (Norman et al 2000).

The dietary aims in managing children with chronic renal failure are dependent upon age, stage of management and nutritional assessment. Oral nutritional supplements, unlike specialist low-protein products, are frequently used and should be encouraged. However, experience has shown that attempting to achieve adequate nutrition this way can be stressful for families.

A proactive approach to maintaining good nutrition and growth without the use of growth hormone has resulted in a programme of early instigation of dialysis in combination with nutritional support (Coleman et al 1998, Lederman et al 1999). Although nasogastric tubes are used successfully, supplementary feeding using a gastrostomy button device may be more suitable in the long term (Watson et al 1998). The button also provides a convenient route for the administration of medication, which has undoubted benefits for the child and family.

Dialysis is seen only as a holding measure before transplantation. Most children do very well and resume normal eating and drinking posttransplant (Coleman et al 1998). However, despite a successful renal transplant with normal renal function there remain concerns that there may be a prolonged transition to exclusive oral nutrition in infants and children who commenced nutritional support via an enteral route early in management (Strologo et al 1997). Such children may continue to require a period of nutritional support. Posttransplantation, energy intake may need to be reduced in some children to prevent rapid weight gain and a healthy, no-added-salt diet should be encouraged with ongoing dietetic advice. Maintaining good nutrition in this group of children requires support from all members of the multidisciplinary team (Collier & Watson 1994). An agreed philosophy of nutritional care and dietetic time to attend ward rounds regularly, outpatient clinics and psychological meetings is essential. Home and school visits with frequent telephone contact are invaluable supportive measures. See Chapter 10 for further reading.

SUMMARY

This chapter has provided the opportunity for the reader to improve current theory and practical knowledge of renal nutrition. However, knowledge is bound to expand over time, with more indepth knowledge and new results from evidence/expert opinion-based research. It is important that as a team, a positive effort is made to review practice continuously, and involve patients in decision making wherever possible. The quality of printed dietary advice, for instance, is one good example where patients can contribute.

Changes in the patient's physical and personal circumstances require dietary adaptation. But so does moving into a different age group and dietary literature for patients should be suitable for the young, middle-aged and the older patient and those from different ethnic groups.

Acknowledgement

With grateful thanks to Janet Coleman who has updated the section on dietary management in paediatrics. Janet Coleman, SRD is Paediatric Renal Dietician, Nottingham City Hospital Trust.

REFERENCES

Bansal VK. Potassium metabolism in renal failure: nondietary rationale for hyperkalemia. J Renal Nutr 1992; 2:8–12.

Bergstrom J. Nutritional requirements of hemodialysis patients. In: Mitch WE, Klahi S, eds. Nutrition and the kidney. Boston: Little, Brown and Co. 1993; 2:263–289.

Bergstrom J, Heimburger O, Lindholm B et al. Elevated serum C-reactive protein is a strong predictor of increased mortality and low serum albumin in haemodialysis (HD) patients. J Am Soc Nephrol 1995; 6:573.

Berlyne GM. A course in renal disease. 2nd edn. Oxford, Blackwell Scientific Publications. 1968.

Block GA, Hulbert-Shearon TE, Levin NW et al. Association of serum phosphorus and calcium phosphate product with mortality risk in chronic hemodialysis patients: a national study. Am J Kidney Dis 1998; 31:607–617.

Brenner B. Hemodynamically mediated glomerular injury and the progressive nature of kidney disease. Kidney Int 1983; 23:647–655.

Cannata-Andia J, Passlick-Deetjen J, Ritz E. Management of the renal patient: experts' recommendations and clinical algorithms on renal osteodystrophy and cardiovascular risk factors. Nephrol Dialysis Transplant 2000; 15 (suppl. 5): 130–131.

Carfray A, Patel K, Whitaker P et al. Albumin as an outcome measure in haemodialysis in-patients: the effect of variation in assay method. Nephrol Dialysis Transplant 2000; 15:1819–1822.

Chertow GM, Burke KS, Dillon MA et al. Long-term effects of sevelamer hydrochloride on the calcium phosphate product and lipid profile of haemodialysis patients. Nephrol Dialysis Transplant 1999; 14:2907–2914.

Churchill DN, Taylor DW, Kesehaviah PR. Adequacy of dialysis and nutrition in continuous peritoneal dialysis: association with clinical outcomes. J Am Soc Nephrol 1996; 7:198–207.

Coleman JE. The kidney in clinical paediatric dietetics. 2nd edn. Shaw V, Lawson M eds. Oxford: Blackwell Scientific Publication, 2001: 158–182.

Coleman JE, Watson AR. Growth post-transplantation in children previously treated with chronic dialysis and gastrostomy feeding. In: Khanna R, ed. Advances in peritoneal dialysis. Toronto: University of Toronto Press, 1998:271–273.

Coleman JE, Watson AR, Rance CH et al. Gastrostomy buttons for nutritional support on chronic dialysis. Nephrol Dialysis Transplant 1998; 13:2041–2046.

Collier J, Watson AR. Renal failure in children: specific consideration in management. In: McGee H, Bradley C, eds. Quality of life following renal failure. Chur: Harwood Academic Publishers, 1994:225–245.

Davidson A. Interdialytic weight gain in Indo-Asians on haemodialysis. Br J Renal Med 2000; 5:23–25.

Detsky AS, McLaughlin JR, Baker JP et al. What is subjective global assessment of nutritional status? J Parenteral Enteral Nutr 1987; 11:8–13.

EDTNA/ERCA nutritional guidelines (2001). Available: www.edtna-erca.org 7 Nov 2001.

Engel B, Vennegoor M, James, G, Singh S. Setting standards and achieving optimal nutritional status. British Dietetic Association renal nutrition group standards for adult renal patients over 18 year olds. 1998.

Fine A, Cox D. Modest reduction of serum albumin in continuous peritoneal dialysis patients is common and of no apparent clinical consequence. Am J Kidney Dis 1992; 20:50–54

Fouque D, Laville M, Boissel JP et al. Controlled low protein diets in chronic renal insufficiency: meta-analysis. Br J Med 1992; 304:216–220.

Fouque D, Wang P, Laville M et al. Low protein diets delay end-stage renal disease in non-diabetic adults with chronic renal failure. Nephrol Dialysis Transplant 2000; 15:1986–1992.

Gardner JL. The GI lag and its significance to the dialysis patient. Dialysis Transplant 1979; 8:132–133.

Gin H, Rigalleau V, Aparicio M. Which diet for diabetic patients with chronic renal failure? Nephrol Dialysis Transplant 1999; 14:2577–2579.

Goodman WG, Goldin J, Kulzon BD et al. Coronary artery calcification in young adults with end-stage renal disease who are undergoing dialysis. N Engl J Med 2000; 342:1478–1482.

Halverson NA, Wilkens KG, Worthington-Roberts B. Interdialytic fluid gains in diabetic patients receiving hemodialysis treatment. J Renal Nutr 1993; 3:23–29.

Harris KPG. Hyperlipidaemia of renal disease: a treatment dilemma? EDTNA-ERCA 1994; XX:26–29.

Heimburger O, Bergstrom J, Lindholm B. Is serum albumin an index of nutritional status in continuous ambulatory peritoneal dialysis patients? Peritoneal Dialysis Int 1994; 14:108–114.

Hokken-Koelega ACS. Growth and growth promotion in children with renal disease. Paediatrics 1995; 8:31–37.

Ifudu O, Dawood M, Homel P et al. Excess interdialytic weight gain provokes antihypertensive drug therapy in patients on maintenance hemodialysis. Dialysis Transplant 1997; 26:541–559.

Jern AN, VanBeber AD, Gorman MA et al. The effects of zinc supplementation on serum zinc concentration and protein catabolic rate in hemodialysis patients. J Renal Nutr 2000; 10:148–153.

Jones CH, Serum albumin—a marker of fluid overload in dialysis patients? J Renal Nutr 2001; 11:59–61.

Kaysen GA. Nutritional management of nephrotic syndrome. J Renal Nutr, 1992; 2:50–58.

Kaysen GA Albumin synthesis, catabolism and distribution in dialysis patients. Mineral. Electrolyte Metab 1997; 23: 218–224.

Klahr S, Levey AS, Beck GJ et al. The effects of dietary protein restriction and blood-pressure control on the progression of chronic renal disease. N Engl J Med 1994; 330:878–884.

Kooman JP, Hendriks EJM, van den Sande FM et al. Dialysate sodium concentration and blood pressure control in haemodialysis patients: letter. Nephrol Dialysis Transplant 2000; 15:554.

Kopple JD, Wolfson M, Chertow GM et al. Clinical practice guidelines for nutrition in chronic renal failure. Am J Kidney Dis/J Renal Nutr 2000; 35:S17–S140.

Krautzig S, Janssen U, Koch KM et al. Dietary salt restriction and reduction of dialysate sodium control hypertension in maintenance haemodialysis patients. Nephrol Dialysis Transplant 1998; 13:552–553.

Lawrence IR, Thomson A, Hartley GH et al. The effect of dietary intervention on the management of hyperlipidaemia in British renal transplant patients. J Renal Nutr 1995; 5:73–77.

Lederman SE, Shaw V, Trompeter RS. Long-term enteral nutrition in infants and young children with chronic renal failure. Paediatr Nephrol 1999; 13:870–875.

Lowrie EG, Lew NL. Death risk in hemodialysis patients: the predictive value of commonly measured variables and an evaluation of death rate differences between dialysis facilities. Am J Kidney Dis 1990; 15:458–482.

McCann L. Subjective global assessment as it pertains to the nutritional status of dialysis patients. Dialysis Transplant 1996; 25:190–202, 225.

McIntyre C, Harper I, Macdougall IC et al. Serum C-reactive protein as a marker of infection and inflammation in regular dialysis patients. Clin Nephrol 1997; 48:371–374.

McKenzie SI, Henderson IS. The effect of increased dietary fibre intake on regular haemodialysis patients. In: Stevens E, Monkhouse P, eds. Aspects of renal care. London: Baillière Tindall, 1986:172–178.

Makoff R. The importance and use of iron supplementation in uremia. Nephrol News Issues 1992; 2:14–19.

Makoff, R. Vitamin replacement therapy in renal failure patients. Mineral Electrolyte Metab 1999; 25:349–351.

Marckman P. Nutritional status of patients on hemodialysis and peritoneal dialysis. Clin Nephrol 1988; 29:75–78.

Maroni BJ. Nutrition in the predialysis patient. Dialysis Transplant 1994; 23:76–94.

Medford S. Medical review criteria—HCFA. J Renal Nutr 1992; 2:77–78.

Muth I. Implications of hypervitaminosis A in chronic renal failure. J Renal Nutr 1991; 1:2–8

National Institute of Health. Morbidity and mortality of dialysis. NIH consensus statement. Bethesda, MD: National Library of Medicine, Office of Medical Applications of Research, National Institutes of Health, 1993:1–33.

Norman LJ, Coleman JE, Watson AR. Nutritional management in a child on chronic peritoneal dialysis; a team approach. J Hum Nutr 1995; 8:209–213.

Norman LJ, Coleman JE, Macdonald IA et al. Nutrition and growth in relation to severity of renal disease in children. Paediatr Nephrol 2000; 15:259–265.

Pagenkemper JJ, Foulks CJ. Nutritional management of the adult renal transplant patient. J Renal Nutr 1991; 1:119–124.

Pagenkemper JJ, Burke KI, Roderick SL et al. Potassium availability in selected bran products: implications for the renal patient. J Renal Nutr 1994; 4:27–31.

Pedrini MT, Levey AS, Lau J et al. The effect of protein restriction on the progression of diabetic and nondiabetic renal disease: a meta-analysis. Ann Intern Med 1996; 124:629–632.

Pender FT. The effect of increasing the dietary fibre content of diets of patients with chronic renal failure treated by haemodialysis at home. J Hum Nutr Dietetics 1989; 2:423–427.

Raine AEG, Margreiter R, Brunner FP et al. Report on management of renal failure in Europe (xii, 1991). Nephro dialysis transplant 1992; 7 (suppl. 2):13–19.

Renal Association and Royal College of Physicians. Treatment of adult patients with renal failure: recommended standards and audit measures. London: Renal Association and Royal College of Physicians of London, Royal College of Physicians Publication Unit. 1997.

Rocco MV, Makoff R. (1997) Appropriate vitamin therapy for dialysis patients. Seminars Dialysis 1997; 10: 272–277.

Sherman RA, Cody RP, Rogers ME et al. Interdialytic weight gain and nutritional parameters in chronic dialysis patients. Am J Kidney Dis 1995; 25:579–583.

Spiegel DM, Anderson M, Campbell U et al. Serum albumin: a marker for morbidity in peritoneal dialysis patients. Am J Kidney Dis 1993; 21:26–30.

Stenvinkel P. Factors influencing the development and progression of diabetic nephropathy. EDTNA-ERCA J 1993; XIX:2–4.

Stenvinkel P. New strategies for management of malnutrition in peritoneal dialysis patients. Peritoneal Dialysis Int 2000; 20:271–275.

Stenvinkel P, Heimburger O, Lindholm B et al. Are there two types of malnutrition in chronic renal failure? Evidence for relationships between malnutrition, inflammation and atherosclerosis. Nephrol Dialysis Transplant 2000; 15:953–960.

Strologo LD, Principato F, Sinibaldi D et al. Feeding dysfunction in infants with severe chronic renal failure after long term nasogastric tube feeding. Paediatr Nephrol 1997; 11:84–86.

Tan CC, Harden PN, Rodger RSC et al. Ranatidine reduces phosphate binding in dialysis patients receiving calcium carbonate. Nephrol Dialysis Transplant 1996; 11:851–853.

Vennegoor M, ed. Enjoying food on a renal diet. London: King Edward's Fund for London, 1982.

Vennegoor M, ed. Nutrition for patients with renal failure. Portsmouth: EDTNA-ERCA, 1986.

Vennegoor M, ed. Enjoying food on a renal diet. London: King Edward's Fund for London, 1992.

Walser M, Mitch WE, Bradley J, et al. Should protein intake be restricted in pre-dialysis patients? Kidney Int 1999; 55:771–777.

Watson AR. Disorders of the urinary tract. In: Levine MI, ed. Jolly's diseases of childhood. 6th edn. Oxford: Blackwell Scientific Publication, 1991:226–268.

Watson AR, Coleman JE, Warady BA. When and how to use nasogastric and gastrostomy feeding for nutritional support. In: Fine RN, Alexander SR, Warady BA, eds. CAPD/CCPD in children. 2nd edn. Boston: Kluwer Academic Publishers, 1998:281–301.

Widjaja A, Kielstein JT, Horn R et al. Free serum leptin but not bound leptin concentrations are elevated in patients with end stage renal failure. Nephrol Dialysis Transplant 2000; 15:846–850.

World Health Organization. Energy and protein requirements. Report of a joint FAO/WHO/UNU meeting. WHO Technical Report Series 724. Geneva: WHO, 1985.

World Health Organization. Obesity. Preventing and managing the global epidemic. Geneva: WHO, 1998.

Wright MJ, Woodrow G, Young G et al. Biocompatible dialysis membranes do not reduce plasma leptin levels. Nephrol Dialysis Transplant 2000; 15:925.

Young GA, Kopple JD, Lindholm B et al. Nutritional assessment of continuous ambulatory peritoneal dialsysis patients: an international study. Am J Kidney Dis 1991; 17:462–471.

FURTHER READING

Canada–USA Peritoneal Dialysis Study Group. Adequacy of dialysis and nutrition in continuous peritoneal dialysis: association with clinical outcomes. J Am Soc Nephrol 1996; 7: 198–207.

USEFUL WEBSITES

K/DOQI National Kidney Foundation: www.kidney.org
EDTNA-ERCA: www.edtna-erca.org
Cochrane Renal Group: www.cochrane-renal.org

Appendix 9.1 Foods with a high and low sodium (salt) content

These foods should be taken in moderation with a salt-restricted diet. It may not be possible to eliminate all the listed foods or meals, unless a low-sodium alternative is available. A compromise may be reached by allowing some salty foods for sandwiches or main meals, but preparing the rest of the meals at home without salt. Adding herbs and spices during meal preparation or thereafter compensates for the loss of salt.

Avoid	Suitable alternative
Dairy products	
Salted butter or margarine	Use unsalted or salt-reduced alternatives
Cheese, cheese spreads	instead
Meat and meat products	
Canned and cured meat products such as:	Fresh-cooked meat
bacon, gammon, salt beef, corned beef,	Fresh-cooked poultry
ham, tongue, all types of sausages, pâtés	Fresh-cooked fish
Meat pies, quiches and sausage rolls	Home-cooked meals
Processed meals	
Fast food-type meals	
Vegetables	
Canned vegetables, sauerkraut, instant	Fresh or frozen vegetables
potato powder, salted potato crisps	
Nuts	
Roasted and salted nuts	
Miscellaneous	
Salt, sea salt, salt substitutes such as	Herbs, spices
Lo Salt, Solo, Selora	Home-made dressings, i.e. French dressing
mayonnaise, salad dressings	Vinegar, lemon, lime juice
Bottled sauces, pickles	
Canned or packet soups or ready-made	Home-made soup
soups	
Pasta sauce, curry paste, soya sauce	Home-made sauces
Meat or yeast extracts and bouillon	Use herbs and spices for curries
cubes, packet gravy, gravy cubes or	Use fresh ingredients for pasta dishes
powders	
Foods containing monosodium	
glutamate	
Salted savoury snacks	
Asian foods	
Poppadums, samosas, other savoury	
snacks, chutneys, pickles, chevra, chana	

Avoid	Suitable alternative
Greek foods	
Taramasalata, canned vine leaves, houmus	
Chinese foods	
Dried fish, salted fish	
Peking duck and similar products	

Appendix 9.2 Foods with high and low potassium content

FOODS WITH A HIGH POTASSIUM CONTENT

Snacks

- Bombay mix, curu snacks, peanuts and raisins, potato crisps, potato hoops, tortilla chips, Twiglets, vegetable samosas.

Sweets

- Chocolate—plain, milk or white—and all sweets containing chocolate or cocoa.
  Liquorice Allsorts, toffees, fudge and other sweets containing nuts, chocolate and dried fruit.

Beverages

- Coffee in excess.
- Milk powder and drinks containing milk powder such as Ovaltine, Horlicks, Complan, Build-up, drinking chocolate, milk shakes, Nutrament, cocoa powder.
- Fruit juices unless exchanged for fruit, tomato juice, carrot juice, vegetable juice, cane sugar juice, pomegranate juice, guava, mango and lychee juice. (This refers to the potassium content of fruit and fruit juice and the amount is equal.)
- Strong ale (e.g. Guinness).

Fruit

- Avocado pear, banana, fresh blackcurrants or redcurrants.
- Dried fruit such as dried apples, dried apricots, dried banana chips, currants, dates, dried figs, prunes, raisins, sultanas and other dried fruits.

Nuts

- All types of nuts, including peanut butter and marzipan.
- All types of seeds such as sesame seeds.
- Chocolate and nut spread.

Vegetables

- Ackee, Jerusalem artichokes, beetroot (only as part of a salad), mushrooms in excess, spinach, celeriac, squash, grilled or fried tomatoes, fried onions in excess, potato waffles.

- Plantain and green bananas.
- Sun-dried tomatoes, tomato purée or sauce in excess.
- Dried pulses such as dried beans, red kidney beans, broad beans, butter beans, black-eyed beans, dried peas, chick peas, lentils.

Vegetables which can be taken instead of potatoes

- Yam, sweet potato, plantain or green banana in small quantities, pulse vegetables and parsnips.

Cereals

- All-Bran, Bran Flakes, oatbran flakes, Fruit and Fibre, oat and wheat bran, Raisin Splitz, Shredded Sultana Bran.

Cakes and biscuits

- Fruit cake, mince pies, Christmas cake, ginger nuts.
- Oat cakes, rye crispbread.
- All biscuits and cakes containing dried fruit, nuts or chocolate.

Pudding and desserts

- Bread pudding and Christmas pudding.
- Desserts containing chocolate.

Meat substitutes

- Fresh soya bean products, vegetarian meat substitutes, bean milk.

Miscellaneous

- Tomato ketchup, tomato chutney, tomato purée, tomato sauce (in small quantities).
- Meat and yeast extracts (dried or paste).
- Salt substitutes containing potassium chloride (i.e. low-salt products).

FOODS WITH A LOW POTASSIUM CONTENT

These can be given as alternatives to high-potassium foods:

Sweets

- Sugar, jam, marmalade, honey, lemon curd, Golden Syrup
- Boiled sweets, barley sugars, peppermints, plain fudge, butterscotch toffee, Turkish delight, fondant sweets, jelly babies, fruit pastilles,

fruit gums, sherbets, marshmallows, lollipops, ice lollies, chewing gum.

Drinks

- Tea—black or with a little milk.
- Soft drinks: tonic, Seven-Up, lemonade, Lucozade (bottled only), soda water, mineral water, dry ginger ale, ginger beer, American ginger ale, bitter lemon, sparkling orange and other soft drinks with a low juice content.
- Fruit squash or barley water with a low natural juice content.
- Whisky, gin, vodka, brandy, rum and liqueurs in small quantities. These can be mixed with water, soda, lemonade, tonic and any of the above soft drinks.

Fruit

- Crystallised or glacé fruit.

Cereal

- Rice, wild rice, noodles, pasta.
- Bread, pitta bread, croissant, puri, chapati.
- Cream crackers, water biscuits.
- Cornflakes, Rice Krispies.
- Plain cake, pastry and biscuits.
- Flour, barley, sago, semolina, tapioca.

Fat (see dietitian's advice on the use of these products)

- Slightly or unsalted margarine, butter, low-fat spreads, oil, olive oil.
- French dressing, mayonnaise, salad cream.
- Double cream, crème fraîche, cream cheese.

Condiments

- Spices such as allspice, cinnamon, ginger powder, mustard powder, nutmeg, pepper.
- Vinegar, Worcester sauce, mustard, chilli sauce.

Dried herbs or spices in moderation

- Basil, bayleaf, caraway seeds, chilli powder, cloves, coriander, curry powder, dill, mint, oregano, paprika, parsley, sage, tarragon, thyme, tumeric, etc.
- Garlic, lemon juice, Tabasco.
- Piccalilli, horseradish, chutney and sweet pickles.

Fresh herbs in moderation

- Basil, bayleaf, coriander, dill, oregano, mint, tarragon, thyme, etc.

POTASSIUM PORTIONS

Potassium portions or exchanges can be used to encourage variety. Most fruits and vegetables contain potassium in varying quantities. Each portion contains approximately 5 mmol (200 mg) potassium. Quantities are based on fresh or boiled vegetables or on fresh, stewed or canned fruit.

Potatoes (one portion contains 10 mmol potassium)

150 g boiled potatoes may be replaced by:

- 150 g new potatoes, peeled
- 75 g baked potato in skin
- 75 g new potatoes, boiled in skin
- 75 g roast potato
- 50 g chips (2 tablespoons) or 6 oven chips
- 25 g = 1 small packet potato crisps (no salt)
- 2 potato croquettes
- 150 g boiled parsnips
- 150 g risotto
- 150 g ravioli or spaghetti in tomato sauce
- 150 g yam, sweet potato, dasheen, eddoes, coco, boiled bread fruit
- 150 g rice and peas (without coconut)
- 75 g boiled green banana or plantain.

Pulses, boiled weight, to be used instead of potatoes (for dialysis patients only)

- 150 g soaked and boiled butter beans, haricot beans, black-eyed beans, baked beans in tomato sauce, dried peas, split peas, chick peas
- 100 g lentils, boiled.
- 75 g red kidney beans, boiled.

VEGETABLES (ONE PORTION IS APPROXIMATELY 5 MMOL (200 MG) POTASSIUM)

Low potassium content

The following vegetables are low in potassium. As a guide, one portion is about 3–4 heaped tablespoons.

Boiled and drained vegetables such as:

- Asparagus (six medium spears)
- Runner beans
- Beansprouts
- Bamboo shoots
- Cauliflower
- Carrots
- Globe artichoke
- Red, white or savoy cabbage
- Chinese leaves
- Marrow

- Pumpkin
- Peas (processed, canned, frozen, mushy peas)
- Onions boiled, pickled or silverskin
- Spring greens.

Medium–high potassium content

The following vegetables have a medium–high potassium content. As a guide, one portion is 2–3 heaped tablespoons of boiled, drained vegetables such as:

- Aubergine
- French beans
- Broccoli
- Celery
- Courgettes
- Curly kale
- Mangetout
- Leeks
- Capsicum (red or green)
- Turnip
- Sweetcorn kernels, on the cob or baby sweetcorn, fresh or canned
- Turnip.

High potassium content

The following vegetables have a fairly high potassium content. As a guide, one unit is 75 g of boiled, drained vegetables such as:

- Brussel sprouts (six)
- Okra (six pods)
- Fennel
- Kohlrabi
- Mushrooms (boiled in water first)
- Tomatoes (canned).

Raw vegetables

A small portion: use a mixture of the following:

- Beetroot
- Red cabbage
- Carrots
- Celery
- Chicory
- Coleslaw
- Corn kernels
- Cucumber
- Lettuce
- Mustard and cress
- Peppers (red, green, yellow or orange)
- Radish
- Spring onions

- Tomato (no more than half a tomato)
- Watercress.

Fruit

Canned, bottled, stewed or baked fruit in water contains less potassium than raw fruit. Drain fruit before measuring a portion, as the juice also contains potassium and should be discarded.

Low potassium content

The following fruits have a low potassium content. As a guide, one unit of fruit is 6 tablespoons of the following:

- Canned apples
- Canned blackberries
- Canned cranberries
- Canned cherries
- Canned fruit cocktail
- Canned gooseberries
- Canned grapefruit
- Canned guava
- Canned loganberries
- Canned lychees
- Canned mandarins
- Canned mango
- Canned paw paw
- Canned peaches (2 halves)
- Canned pears (2 halves)
- Canned pineapple (2–3 rings)
- Canned plums
- Canned raspberries
- Canned strawberries.

or 150 g (or the equivalent) of fresh fruit:

- 1 Apple
- 1 Clementine
- ½ Grapefruit
- Mango
- A thin slice of melon—cantaloupe, galia, honeydew, water
- 1 Small orange
- ½ Ortanique
- 2 Passion fruits
- 1 Medium-sized pear
- 1 Satsuma
- 1 Tangerine.

Medium–high potassium content

The following fruits have a medium–high potassium content. As a guide, one portion is 100 g (canned, 4 tablespoons or fresh):

- Apricots (in syrup or juice only)
- Blackberries (fresh or stewed)
- Blackcurrants (stewed only)
- 12 Cherries
- Gooseberries (fresh or stewed)
- 6–8 Kumquats
- 1 Lemon or lime
- Loganberries (fresh)
- 6 Lychees (fresh)
- 1 Nectarine
- Paw paw (papaya)
- 1 Medium peach (fresh or in natural juice)
- Pineapple (1 medium thick slice)
- 2 Pomegranates
- Plums: depending on size, 1 large or 3–4 small
- Raspberries (fresh)
- Rhubarb (stewed or canned)
- 1 Sharon fruit
- 8 Strawberries.

Fairly high potassium content

The following fruits have a fairly high potassium content. As a guide, one unit is 75 g of canned or fresh:

- Damsons
- 5 Dates (fresh or dried)
- 1 Figs (fresh)
- 4 Greengages (fresh)
- 1 Kiwi fruit
- 6 Prunes.

Appendix 9.3 Foods with high and low phosphorus content

All foods with a high protein content also contain a fair amount of phosphorus. However, some of these foods are an essential part of the diet and cannot be eliminated.

The following foods can be excluded without altering the nutritional quality of the diet.

Foods with a high phosphorus content	Foods with a low phosphorus content
Cereals	
Natural Bran, All-Bran,	All other breakfast cereals
Bran Flakes, Bran Buds,	Porridge
Cereals containing nuts	Wholemeal or white bread, croissant
Rye bread	Yorkshire pudding
Crispbread containing rye	Puri, pitta bread, chapatti, nan
Oatcakes, scones	Flour, barley, sago
Soya flour	Semolina, tapioca, cornflour, custard powder
	Pasta, noodles, rice, wild rice
Dairy products	
Milk, yoghurt (see allowance allocated by renal dietitian)	Cream, crème fraiche
Evaporated and condensed milk	Fromage frais, quark
Milk powder, Horlicks	Cottage cheese and curd cheese
Most types of hard cheese, e.g. Cheddar	Full fat or reduced-fat cream cheese such as Boursin, Philadelphia, roulé,
Stilton, cheese spread	Marscapone, riccota
Eggs (no more than one daily)	Egg white, meringue
However, these quantities may need to be adapted for vegetarian diets	
Meat and meat products	
Liver, kidney, liver pâté and liver sausage, black pudding	Beef, veal, lamb, pork, chicken, turkey, sausages, meat pies (see meal plan suggested by the renal dietitian)
Fish and fish products	
Fish with edible bones such as anchovies, herring, kippers, sprats, whitebait, fish roe, fish paste	Fresh or smoked fish such as cod, haddock, mackerel, salmon, sardines, fish fingers, fish cakes
	Canned fish such as tuna, salmon with all bones removed
	Occasionally use: crab, lobster, mussels, prawns, scampi, squid
Vegetables	
Pulses such as dried peas, dried beans, lentils, baked beans, chick peas	All other vegetables

Foods with a high phosphorus content	Foods with a low phosphorus content
Savoury snacks All types of nuts such as peanuts, peanut butter, Bombay mix, chevra, chana, ganthia, Poppadoms	Popcorn, corn snacks
Sweets Chocolate, cocoa powder Ovaltine, Mars bars, Snickers, Bounty, halva, burfi with nuts	Sweets, barley sugars, butterscotch, mint, fruit pastilles, starburst, sherbets, jelly babies, wine gums, marshmallows Turkish delight, chewing gum, plain toffee and fudge, lollipops, ice lollies
Cakes and pastries Chocolate cake, Battenburg cake Any cakes and pastries containing chocolate or nuts	All other types of cakes, biscuits, pastries Doughnuts, cream cakes, gingerbread
Biscuits Chocolate biscuits, Jaffa cakes All biscuits containing nuts or chocolate	Plain biscuits such as Digestives Cream crackers, Rich Tea, shortbread, sponge fingers, cream-filled biscuits
Puddings Milk pudding, custard, bread pudding, Christmas pudding, fruit pies or crumbles, sponge Chocolate mousse, chocolate icecream, desserts containing nuts and chocolate	Pancakes, pastries, sweet or savoury, fruit jelly, sorbets Plain icecream, cheesecake
Beverages Milk and milk drinks such as milk shakes, Build-up, Complan, Nutrament, drinking chocolate, cocoa, Bournevita, Ovaltine, Jamaican punch	Tea, coffee Soft drinks, Lucozade, fruit squash, lemon barley, blackcurrant drink, lime juice cordial, crusha syrup, rosehip syrup
Condiments and miscellaneous Meat and yeast extracts such as Marmite, Bovril, Vegemite Marzipan, peanut butter Seeds such as sesame, tahini Chocolate and nut spread	Sugar, jam, marmalade, honey Lemon curd, Golden Syrup, gelatine, yeast, pickles, chutney, tomato ketchup, tomato purée, lemon juice, vinegar, mustard, mayonnaise, salad cream, salad dressing, tartare sauce, chilli sauce, soya sauce, herbs and spices, apple sauce, cranberry sauce, redcurrant jelly, horseradish, mint sauce, mint jelly

Renal care in childhood and adolescence

Geraldine Ward

10

■ CONTENTS

■ LEARNING OUTCOMES FOR THIS CHAPTER

- To gain an understanding of the psychological needs of children at different ages
- To analyse the physiological differences between children and adults
- To be able to recognise the main signs and symptoms of childhood renal disorders
- To be able to formulate an appropriate care plan for children on peritoneal dialysis (PD) or haemodialysis (HD).

INTRODUCTION

[Children] are much more susceptible than grown people to all noxious influence. They are affected by the same things, but much more quickly and seriously …
                                                        Florence Nightingale

The purpose of this chapter is to highlight the special healthcare needs of infants, children and adolescents with renal disorders. Kidney disease, especially conditions that lead to renal failure, is relatively rare in childhood. This means that the specialist services comprised of appropriately trained nursing, medical and other staff such as play specialists, hospital teachers, social workers, psychologists and dietitians are to be found in only a limited number of centres in the UK (British Association of Paediatric Nephrology 1995). Many families will thus have to make long journeys to a paediatric renal unit, adding to the stress of caring for a child with a relatively rare medical condition (Hicklin & de Sousa 1997).

Children are emotionally, physically and legally dependent on their parents (or a suitable substitute) for their care and protection and can thus never be treated in isolation from their families or carers. The family is central to the development of any effective treatment plan and provision should be made within the hospital setting to ensure their ease of access to the sick child and their involvement in all aspects of decision making.

Nursing intervention is often best given either directly or indirectly by parents—a factor which must be taken into consideration when planning care (Nicholson 1990). Paediatric healthcare staff must meet the needs of a diverse patient group, comprised of individuals who are constantly changing as they experience the dynamic processes of physical, emotional and intellectual maturation. Chronic health problems in childhood may have long-term negative effects on physical and emotional development, making the passage to independent adulthood a much more difficult experience than normal.

When dealing with children and adolescents the ability to converse with them about their medical condition and treatment in language appropriate to their developmental stage is essential (Douglas 1993). Children, like adults, have a right to be involved in decision making about their medical care and should be aided in this process by receiving information suitable to their level of maturity. Fear and misunderstanding among young patients can result in their unwillingness to cooperate in procedures and therapies; therefore it is vital to take time to win their trust by giving explanations and answering questions as truthfully as possible. Once young people reach the age of 16 years they can legally sign their own consent for procedures. The 1989 Children's Act made it clear that even before this age they have the right to make decisions about their treatment, providing they have 'sufficient understanding and intelligence' (Cretney 1991). There may be scenes of conflict when parents give consent to procedures or treatment which their child refuses—everything from seemingly innocuous blood tests to procedures such as dialysis access surgery can provoke distress and what might be deemed uncooperative behaviour. Encouragement and reassurance must accompany information to help young people to make decisions that are in their best interests. Some young people, however, may consistently refuse to accept treatment which might keep them alive and when they do so, having been fully informed as to the risks and benefits, their wishes must be respected (Doyal & Henning 1994). See Case Study 10.1.

Although great advances have been made in the treatment of renal disorders in childhood, especially in end-stage renal failure (ESRF) management, there are some patients for whom such treatment may be considered inappropriate, such as those with severe multisystem medical problems. The decision not to embark on renal replacement therapy (RRT) in such cases will only be made after detailed discussion with the child's family and the healthcare team (Reiss et al 1996).

DIFFERENCES IN CHILDREN

A newborn child is physiologically very different from an adult, not simply in terms of size, but also in the maturity of its bodily systems. These differences can be summed up as follows:

• A healthy neonate's body is comprised of 80% water; by 1 year of age this has fallen to adult levels of 45–60%. (N.B. An infant has a turnover of body water five times that of an adult so is at greater risk of dehydration: Bradbury & Brocklebank 1995.)

■ **CASE STUDY 10.1**

Joe was 16 years old when his third transplant failed after seven years. His original diagnosis (renal dysplasia) was made soon after birth and his experiences of medical treatment throughout his life had been traumatic. Joe kept up a brave appearance when he was not having any procedures performed but was unable to cope with any treatment which might cause him any pain or discomfort. Family support was limited, particularly because of his mother's religious beliefs, which prevented her from consenting to any of his life-saving treatment (this had been his father's task). His school attendance was very poor and in consequence his achievement record was well below average. The combination of poor school attendance and his mother's religious beliefs restricted Joe's social contacts and his very short stature and obesity added to his low self-esteem. Severe needle phobia prevented his complying with growth hormone therapy (a daily subcutaneous injection). Even when well, Joe repeatedly told hospital staff that he did not want to have another transplant or return to dialysis. Vascular access was a major problem even for routine blood tests and previous abdominal surgery and poor hygiene made either method of dialysis a difficult prospect. Many long conversations went on between Joe, his parents and hospital staff as his renal function deteriorated and he used the fact that he had reached his 16th birthday to insist on his wishes being observed. His parents accepted his decision, as did medical and nursing staff, but Joe was assured he could change his mind at any time. When his transplant stopped functioning, Joe did waiver briefly, venous access was established with some difficulty and he had one session of haemodialysis during which he was completely miserable. When it was over he said he had had enough, he wanted no more treatment and he wanted to go home to die.

- Children grow very rapidly during the first 2 years of life, with another noticeable spurt at puberty.
- By 1 year of age healthy infants have grown approximately 25 cm in length and have achieved around 85% of their ultimate head circumference.
- By 2 years of age they should have achieved half their potential adult height (Betts & Magrath 1974).
- The energy necessary to sustain these rates of growth is greater per kilogram/body weight than that required by adults (Klahr et al 1983).
- Glomerular filtration rate (GFR) does not become proportional to body surface area (BSA) until approximately 3 years of age (Taylor 1994).
- Normal plasma creatinine levels for children are lower than those for adults because of lower muscle mass.
- Children have a higher BSA than adults (for calculation of BSA, see Eq. 10.1.)
- Blood pressure (BP) is much lower in children than in adults; at 1 day of age, a normal term infant has a systolic pressure of around 70 mmHg rising to around 85 mmHg by 1 month of age (Sinaiko 1996). BP continues

to increase with age and gender differences are apparent by the teenage years, with boys having higher readings than girls (Update 1996).

Calculation of body surface area (BSA)

$$BSA = Height\ (cm) \times weight\ (kg) \div 3600 \qquad (Eq.\ 10.1)$$

The following topics will now be discussed: blood pressure, acute renal failure, nephrotic syndromes, chronic renal failure and nutrition in these three conditions; dialysis and transplantation; and psychosocial issues in order to highlight how the paediatric experience may differ from that of adults.

BLOOD PRESSURE

As mentioned above, normal BP in children is lower than that of adults. It can be a challenge when measuring BP accurately in young patients to gain their cooperation. Once this is achieved the following points should be considered:

- To ensure accuracy, the spyhgmomanometer cuff should be of an appropriate size, i.e. the bladder should cover two-thirds of the arm circumference (Dillon 1994).
- Auscultation of BP sounds in children aged less than 5 years is often difficult and Doppler instruments will be needed if conventional sphygmomanometers are used (De Swiet et al 1989).
- Automated BP monitors can be employed but they require frequent calibration and doubts have been expressed about their reliability (National High Blood Pressure Education Programme 1996).
- Several ambulatory BP monitors have been evaluated for use in paediatric practice and are now accepted as a useful tool in determining true hypertension (Portman et al 1991).
- Raised BP, especially in younger children, can rapidly result in seizures or encephalopathy and requires immediate treatment to avoid negative neurological sequelae.

Hypertension in childhood is rare and, though not a cause of renal disease, is almost always due to an underlying renal disorder. Its rarity and the difficulties associated with BP measurement make it impractical to carry out widespread screening of the population; however, any sick child undergoing a general medical examination should have their blood pressure checked (De Swiet et al 1989). Single abnormal BP measurements should never be relied on as an indicator of real hypertension but should prompt further recordings to be made. While some studies suggest that essential hypertension has its origins in early life and that there may be a familial trend to raised BP, the question of whether early treatment of mild hypertension may prevent or delay some of the long-term sequelae is still being considered ((National High Blood Pressure Education Programme 1996).

ACUTE RENAL FAILURE

Acute renal failure (ARF) occurs much less frequently in children than in adults (Arbus et al 1994). Severe disease or late presentation may result in permanent renal or other organ damage. Causes of ARF are similar to those seen in adults (Box 10.1). The neonatal period is a particularly vulnerable time for babies: complications such as prematurity, birth asphyxia or haemorrhage can all cause ARF which may, in some cases, lead to chronic renal failure (CRF). Haemolytic–uraemic syndrome (HUS), which is defined as a triad of microangiopathic haemolytic anaemia, thrombocytopenia and ARF, is predominantly a disease of infants and children. The diarrhoea-associated (D+) type which occurs as a consequence of infection with the *Escherichia coli* 0157 verotoxin is the commonest cause of ARF in otherwise healthy children, accounting for 45% of cases in one series (Moghal et al 1998). It can have serious multisystem effects, resulting in death or neurological deficit as well as permanent renal damage. HUS D+ commonly appears in minor epidemic form, especially in the summer months, sometimes inundating paediatric renal units with patients. ARF may cause, or be part of, multiorgan failure and patients requiring ventilatory support will need to be nursed in paediatric intensive care units.

ARF management requires immediate assessment and stabilisation of the patient with institution of dialysis if necessary. The treatment of choice has traditionally been PD using an automated cycler and a surgically inserted Tenckhoff catheter; however, there is a wide variation in practice (Warady & Bunchman 1996). The choice of initial treatment appears to be dependent on individual centre preferences and experience, so that HD, haemofiltration (HF) and continuous venovenous haemodiafiltration (CVVHD) are as likely to be the treatment of choice as PD (Belsha et al 1995). In some cases PD may be inappropriate or impractical (Box 10.2,) and when plasma exchange is indicated (Box 10.3) HD is the treatment of choice. Dialysis prescription will be determined by assessing each patient's biochemical status, urine output and nutritional needs. Dialysis support may be required for some considerable time and recovery, both physical and psychological, from a prolonged period of hospitalisation may take

---

■ **BOX 10.1 Common causes of acute renal failure in childhood**

Haemolytic–uraemic syndrome

Complications of birth, e.g. asphyxia, prematurity

Poisoning (often iatrogenic, e.g. drug toxicity)

Severe dehydration

Cardiac insufficiency

Meningococcal septicaemia

Severe burns

■ BOX 10.2 Contraindications to peritoneal dialysis

Pleuroperitoneal fistula

Recent intraperitoneal surgery

Severe abdominal burns

Intraabdominal/peritoneal sepsis

Scarring/adhesions from previous major surgery or peritonitis

Severe spina bifida

Prune-belly syndrome (defective abdominal musculature)

Social circumstances, e.g. poor housing, no designated carer

■ BOX 10.3 Conditions which may require plasma exchange

Goodpasture's syndrome

Systemic lupus erythematosus

Henoch–Schönlein purpura

---

many months. Those who have had ARF should be followed up long-term in order to monitor and treat the persistence or development of adverse sequelae such as hypertension.

Nutrition in acute renal failure

Many children presenting with acute renal failure will be too sick to eat and the best way to ensure the high energy intake they require to combat catabolism is to institute nasogastric (NG) feeding immediately. In this way an appropriate mixture of protein, carbohydrate, fat and vitamins can be given to counteract the catabolic effects of uraemia. Some forms of ARF such as HUS or other vasculitic disorders such as systemic lupus erythematosus (SLE) may result in gut involvement and total parenteral nutrition (TPN) is preferred to NG feeding. Fluid restriction may be needed in oliguric or anuric renal failure and the aim should be to balance intake with fluid losses.

NEPHROTIC SYNDROMES

Any disease (Table 10.1) which alters glomerular function, permitting large albumin leakage from the plasma into Bowman's space (Haycock 1994) can cause nephrotic syndrome (NS), which is defined as the presence of heavy proteinuria, hypoproteinaemia and oedema (Clark & Barratt 1994). Patients with NS are often seen in paediatric nephrology wards and depending on their underlying condition will span the entire paediatric age range. Renal biopsy is essential in order to make an accurate diagnosis and to be able to

Table 10.1 Causes of nephrotic syndrome in childhood

Primary	Secondary
Finnish-type congenital nephrotic syndrome (CNS-F)	Systemic lupus erythematosus (SLE)
Diffuse mesangial sclerosis (DMS)	Henoch–Schönlein purpura (HSP)
Minimal-change disease (MCD)	Poststreptococcal nephritis
Focal segmental glomerulonephritis (FSGS)	Immunoglobulin A nephropathy
Mesangiocapillary glomerulonephritis (MCGN)	
Membranous nephropathy	

offer some sort of prognosis to the child and family. This procedure cannot be carried out until the patient is haemodynamically stable. In congenital NS this may have to be delayed until nephrectomy.

Severe NS is a life-threatening condition in which patients may present with gross widespread oedema, respiratory distress, the signs and symptoms of hypovolaemia and thromboembolic complications (Box 10.4). They require immediate assessment and initiation of treatment to prevent serious complications such as stroke or death (Box 10.5). The administration of albumin infusions offers only short-term relief of nephrosis-induced hypovolaemia and may have to be repeated on a daily basis until NS resolves either in response to appropriate therapy or a decline in the underlying disease process occurs.

There are two major categories of NS—primary and secondary (Table 10.1). Amongst primary NS are the congenital nephrotic syndromes (CNS), such as Finnish-type CNS (CNS-F) and diffuse mesangial sclerosis (DMS), which present very early in life and do not respond to steroid or cytotoxic therapy. The young age of patients raises particular management problems and without treatment, death from overwhelming sepsis is the norm in the first few months of life (Holmberg et al 1995). Relatively innocent infections can be fatal because of the loss of large amounts of immunoglobulins (needed to mount immune responses) in the non-selective proteinuria of NS. CNS-F and DMS are autosomally recessive inherited conditions and such diagnoses have important implications for parents considering another pregnancy. Both conditions can be associated with

---

■ BOX 10.4 Indicators of hypovolaemia

Central and peripheral temperature gap >2°C

High/low blood pressure

Abdominal pain

Urinary sodium of less than 10 mmol L^{-1} (in the absence of furosemide (frusemide))

Clotting of major blood vessels

■ **BOX 10.5 Treatment and management of nephrotic syndromes**

Severe cases—rehydrate with 4.5% albumin solution i.v. rapidly to restore circulation

Less severe cases—rehydrate with 20% albumin solution i.v. slowly over 4 h (dose of albumin = 1 g protein kg^{-1} body weight)

Careful fluid balance

Diuretic administration

Core/peripheral temperature monitoring

Initiation of steroid therapy if appropriate

Urine testing for proteinuria (those being treated with steroids/cytotoxic therapy)

Passive/active physiotherapy to prevent pressure sores, deep vein thrombosis and chest infection

Skin care to prevent pressure sores and fungal infections

Prevention/early detection/treatment of infection

Patient/parent education

---

other congenital abnormalities and the early months of these children's lives can be very traumatic for families.

Some important features of treatment for CNS-F and DMS are summarised below (Coulthard 1989, Holmberg et al 1995, Mattoo et al 1992):

- Early unilateral or bilateral nephrectomy minimises or eradicates nephrosis.
- If unilateral nephrectomy is performed, the following treatment will ameliorate the nephrotic state until ESRF occurs:
  — administration of indomethacin to reduce GFR and thus proteinuria and oedema
  — thyroid hormone replacement to make up for urinary losses
  — prophylactic penicillin to prevent sepsis.

After bilateral nephrectomy (possibly staged) there should be a minimum dialysis period of at least 3 months combined with aggressive nutritional therapy to correct protein malnutrition before renal transplantation.

Other primary NS are usually amenable to treatment with steroids in the first instance, though some may relapse frequently and eventually become steroid-resistant, requiring more drastic drug therapy to achieve remission (Clark & Barratt 1994). Such therapy can include treatment with ciclosporin, tacrolimus or even the necessity for alkylating agents (cyclophosphamide, mustine) or vinca alkaloids (vincristine). Having recourse to these latter drugs has implications for future fertility, especially in boys, and this treatment and its potential side-effects should be fully explained before being commenced.

Some patients will respond well to more aggressive therapy while others may continue to suffer a debilitating nephrotic state, eventually progressing to ESRF or undergoing elective bilateral nephrectomy in order to achieve a more acceptable quality of life. Some forms of nephrotic syndrome, such as focal segmental glomerulosclerosis (FSGS), though not CNS-F or DMS, can recur after renal transplantation with recorded recurrence rates of between 20 and 40% (First 1995).

Nutrition and fluid balance in nephrotic syndromes

High-protein diets cannot compensate for urine protein losses but the recommended estimated average protein requirement should be met to ensure that growth is not compromised (Box 10.6). Enteral feeding may be needed when the nephrotic state is severe and the majority of infants with CNS will fail to thrive if left to feed orally. Changes in fluid allowance will only be necessary if oliguria or anuria is present.

CHRONIC RENAL FAILURE

Chronic renal failure (CRF) is an insidious irreversible condition, usually defined as a GFR of below 50 mL min^{-1} 1.73 m^{-2} BSA, (Eq. 10.2), being the level of kidney function at which signs and symptoms start to become evident (Rigden 1994). Even mild renal impairment in childhood can have a significant effect on growth and development (Sedman et al 1996). Although a degree of renal failure may be present from birth, some patients do not come to medical attention until a significant decline in function has already occurred. CRF is rare in childhood, with an annual incidence in the UK of approximately 53 per million child population (pmcp) presenting before ESRF and 9.7 pmcp starting RRT (British Association of Paediatric Nephrology 1995). There are many causes of CRF and the commonest are shown in Box 10.7. Renal failure may be part of a syndrome of problems and other major organs such as the liver or eyes may have noticeable functional deficits requiring specialist attention. For some patients renal failure may be the least of their problems.

$$\text{Calculated GFR} \atop (\text{mL min}^{-1}\ 1.73\ \text{m}^{-2}\ \text{BSA}) = \frac{40 \times \text{height (cm)}}{\text{plasma creatinine (}\mu\text{mol L}^{-1})} \quad \text{(Eq. 10.2)}$$

(Morris et al 1982)

N.B. This is most accurate when GFR is proportional to BSA, i.e. after 2–3 years of age.

■ **BOX 10.6 Recommendations for energy and nutrient requirements in childhood**

Energy and nutrient requirements vary throughout childhood and age-appropriate recommendations can be found in the following publication: Department of Health report on health and social subjects no. 41. Dietary reference values for food energy and nutrients for the United Kingdom. London: HMSO, 1991.

■ BOX 10.7 Commonest causes of chronic renal failure in childhood

Dysplasia/hypoplasia

Obstructive uropathy, e.g. posterior urethral valves

Glomerulopathies

Reflux nephropathy

Juvenile nephronophthisis (medullary cystic disease)

Congenital nephrotic syndromes

Autosomal recessive polycystic kidney disease

Cystinosis

Cortical necrosis

Children with CRF may present in a variety of ways. Renal tract anomalies can be detected on routine antenatal ultrasound screening or early in postnatal life if severe sepsis occurs. However, even congenital defects may not be picked up for many years until renal function has deteriorated to the level at which symptoms become obvious. Presenting symptoms include:

• general malaise, poor concentration and educational difficulties
• nausea, vomiting or anorexia
• failure to thrive—short stature, poor weight gain
• polydipsia or polyuria
• onset of wetting in a previously dry child or inability to attain continence
• headaches
• seizures, encephalopathy or stroke.

All the above are signs and symptoms which may prompt parents to seek medical advice or primary healthcare staff to refer children for further investigation. On presentation some children may require immediate dialysis to treat fluid overload and concomitant biochemical abnormalities. A number will recover sufficient renal function to be treated conservatively. Careful history taking will suggest the relevant investigations to establish the cause of renal failure. It may also be appropriate to check other siblings (even if they have no apparent symptoms) in conditions known to be inherited, such as vesicoureteric reflux (VUR) or juvenile nephronophthisis.

Nutrition in chronic renal failure

A good appetite is considered to be a sign of health and an adequate and well-balanced diet is recognised as vital not only for promoting growth but also providing protection against a whole host of disease processes. Nutritional therapy (Box 10.8) is one of the cornerstones of treatment of CRF in childhood since the negative effect it has on appetite can result not only in significant statural growth retardation but also in brain damage (Rotundo et al 1982). Normal energy requirements are greater per kilo-

---

■ **BOX 10.8 Nutritional therapy for children with chronic renal failure**

The aims of nutritional therapy for children with chronic renal failure, whatever their treatment modalities, are summarised below:

- The provision of an appropriately adequate intake of energy, water, electrolytes, vitamins and minerals
- Protein, carbohydrate and fat intakes balanced to supply body energy requirements
- Sodium supplementation where needed, e.g. in congenital salt-losing conditions such as renal dysplasia or posterior urethral valves
- Fluid intake appropriate to treatment modality/urine output. N.B. Polyuria due to renal concentrating defects is a common feature of some childhood causes of chronic renal failure
- Avoidance of obesity

(Further reading: Haycock 1993, Ridgen & Turner 1997, Ridgen et al 1987)

---

gram/body weight in children compared to adults to meet the demands of growth (Box 10.6). Organs such as the liver and brain, which have a high rate of metabolic activity, comprise a large proportion of body weight, especially in the first 2 years of life (Klahr et al 1983). An energy intake higher than the normal for age will help ameliorate the effects of catabolism caused by renal failure (Rigden et al 1990).

Although some studies have suggested that low-protein diets can delay the progression of renal failure, there is as yet no convincing evidence that this is the case in children and protein restriction may actually be detrimental to growth (Klahr et al 1983, Rigden & Turner 1997).

PD has been shown to increase protein losses in children and the majority will require protein supplementation if growth impairment is to be avoided (Quan & Baum 1996).

Renal failure in childhood is almost universally characterised by a general lack of interest in or positive revulsion towards food. Over 70% of infants and children with CRF have gastro-oesophageal reflux (GOR): the aetiology of this and vomiting and other gastrointestinal motility disorders is ascribed to the effects of uraemia on the polypeptide hormones which regulate gut activity (Ravelli 1995). The knowledge that physical growth is dependent on energy intake makes poor appetite a particularly stressful symptom for parents (Box 10.9). Trying to coax, cajole or otherwise persuade a reluctant child to eat can take many hours a day and may simply result in vomiting, temper tantrums and wholesale refusal to consume anything. Typically, small children with CRF will drink any amount of water, lick salt off crisps but gag and retch if they get anything lumpy in their mouth!

The adequacy of nutritional therapy is assessed by regular measurements of height, weight and head circumference (in infants < 2 years old) which are plotted on growth charts. These measurements demonstrate how

> **■ BOX 10.9 Feeding problems and chronic renal failure**
>
> Some strategies for dealing with the feeding problems encountered in chronic renal failure are listed below:
>
> - Add nasogastric or gastrostomy feeding to ensure adequate calorie and nutrient intake.
> - Appropriate enteral feed can be given either by bolus or overnight (using an automated pump).
> - Encourage breast feeding (with supplemental feeds) and weaning to solids at the usual age (about 4 months).
> - Use low-phosphate formula feeds in babies and toddlers.
> - No cow's milk until at least 2 years of age (should not exceed 250 mL daily).
> - Give daily calorie supplementation (fat emulsions and/or glucose polymers) for all age groups.
> - Encourage oral feeding even if food is refused (touching, tasting and smelling are all part of normal development).
> - Attempt to wean to oral calorie supplements as child approaches school age.
> - Encourage healthy eating in the post transplant phase when steroid therapy and the absence of uraemia often result in an obsession with food and a consequent rapid weight gain.
> - Enteral feeding may need to be continued for younger children who were fed exclusively by this method before transplantation, as it may take some considerable time for them to develop a normal eating pattern.

well or otherwise an individual child is doing in comparison to normal growth standards and facilitate prompt intervention if they are failing to achieve satisfactory progress. A low plasma albumin may indicate an inadequate protein intake, which will need to be increased if growth is suboptimal (Rigden & Turner 1997).

Anaemia

Optimal nutrition and iron supplementation can prevent symptomatic anaemia in patients receiving conservative management (CM). The use of recombinant erythropoeitin (rhEpo) is usually confined to premature infants with conservatively managed CRF and those undergoing dialysis therapy, where it has proved to be a safe and beneficial intervention (Van Damme-Lombaerts & Herman 1999).

Bones

Renal osteodystrophy (ROD) due to phosphate retention and the resulting increase in parathyroid hormone (PTH) levels has serious consequences in childhood, causing rickets and growth failure. To avoid this problem phosphate restriction (reducing the intake of milk, most cheeses and yoghurt) and prescription of phosphate binders, e.g. calcium carbonate, will be needed as renal failure progresses. Aluminium hydroxide is used as a phosphate binder in children only in the short term in the presence of hypercalcaemia since it has been implicated in severe toxicity, causing neurological deficit (Sedman 1992). Giving a hydroxylated vitamin D preparation compensates for impaired vitamin D metabolism. An annual X-ray of the non-dominant hand and wrist will demonstrate the presence of ROD and provide information about growth potential by comparing bone age with chronological age (Rigden & Turner 1997). Obesity in the posttransplant period combined with steroid therapy may cause disease in the weight-bearing joints of the hips and knees and should be avoided.

In the early posttransplant phase significant urinary losses of phosphate and magnesium may occur and supplementation will be needed to prevent unpleasant cramps, possible seizures and bone disease (Meyer et al 1996). Treatment for secondary hyperparathyroidism should be continued post-transplant since it may take some time for parathyroid function to normalise (Nieto et al 1997). Persistent hypercalcaemia combined with raised PTH may indicate tertiary hyperparathyroidism, (a rare occurrence in children) and parathyroidectomy may be needed (Meyer et al 1996).

Growth

Although endogenous growth hormone (GH) levels are high in children with CRF, tissue resistance appears to reduce its effectiveness (Rees & Maxwell 1996). The administration of supraphysiological doses of recombinant human growth hormone (rhGH) has been shown to improve height for some children with CRF (Rees et al 1990), though its use may be limited by its potential to precipitate a decline in renal function, and to cause allograft rejection, and its expense. All conventional means of promoting normal growth by aggressive dietary management and control of biochemical abnormalities such as hyperparathyroidism should be exhausted first (Rees 1997). Alternate-day steroid maintenance regimes are favoured by many paediatric units in order to reduce the potentially growth-retarding effects of prednisolone which are especially noticeable in boys of pubertal age (Guest & Broyer 1991, Rees et al 1988a). Lack of pubertal development by the age of 14 years in boys and 15 years in girls can be a cause of great concern and requires monitoring, investigation and intervention if appropriate (Argente 1999).

Conservative management of chronic renal failure

CM has as its goals the preservation of native kidney function in a well child who is growing and reaching developmental milestones at the appropriate time. Regular and careful monitoring of diet, medication and BP combined with the correction of biochemical abnormalities and the prevention or early treatment of urinary tract infection (UTI) may slow the progression to ESRF and minimise the unpleasant effects of uraemia. Despite these interventions, some renal diseases will proceed more rapidly to end-stage than others. Special clinics for children with conservatively managed CRF can focus on their specific needs and, since the onus of care falls on the family, provide them with the help, advice and support they need to cope.

Preparation for dialysis and transplantation

An important component of CM is the physical and psychological preparation of the child and family for the next phase in treatment. Ongoing discussions about future treatment will lessen the shock when the time for change arrives. Pre-emptive transplantation (PET), where possible, is the goal of many paediatric renal units and obviates the need for dialysis access surgery or the disruption to family life which dialysis itself entails. It is vital, however, that patients being offered this option demonstrate the ability to adhere to the treatment regime since non-compliance with drug therapy, in particular, is likely to result in graft failure (Flom et al 1992). Preparing for PET requires early evaluation of the patient so that any potential problems such as bladder abnormalities can be dealt with (Matas et al 1996). The optimal condition for transplantation is one in which the patient is fully immunised, has a 'safe' bladder, i.e. one which will not compromise transplant function (30–40% of potential paediatric transplant recipients do not satisfy this criteria: Churchill et al 1996). Conditions which may necessitate bladder surgery and/or the initiation of self-catheterisation are shown in Box 10.10. Since a high proportion of paediatric allografts fail as a result of vascular thrombosis, any underlying defects in clotting need to be identified (Andrew & Brooker 1996) so that anticoagulant or other therapy can be initiated posttransplant. Ultrasound examination of relevant abdominal vasculature is necessary to check for abnormalities so that the surgeons can plan the placement of the graft (Box 10.11).

Dialysis must be discussed and tentative plans made, even if PET is the goal, since renal function may deteriorate more rapidly than anticipated or the wait for a donor organ may be longer than expected.

A prospective live donor, if there is one, will need to be referred to the adult nephrology service for assessment and work-up. Since most live donors in paediatrics are parents who are by definition almost always the patient's prime carers, consideration must be given to the psychosocial and financial implications of parental donation as well as the potential morbidity risks. Live donation offers the benefits of being able to plan a transplant date to suit the family but the work-up procedure may reveal some previously unknown health problem, adding further worries to an already anxious situation.

■ **BOX 10.10 Patients needing bladder assessment**

Obstructive uropathy, e.g. posterior urethral valves

Neuropathic bladder

Spina bifida

Prune-belly syndrome

Reflux nephropathy

Dysplasia (if there is a history of wetting or urinary tract infection)

■ BOX 10.11 Transplant preparation checklist

Blood group, tissue type, human leukocyte antigen antibodies

Routine immunisations completed, including bacillus Calmette Guérin (BCG) and varicella vaccine (if antibody-negative)

Hepatitis B and C status

Bladder assessment—possibly augmentation surgery and/or institution of catheterisation if required

Thrombophilia screening

Imaging of major blood vessels—inferior vena cava and iliac vessels

Dental check

Information, education and orientation

Pre-emptive transplantation

The goal for all children in ESRF is a successful renal transplant as this provides the best chance of enjoying a normal life. Transplantation without prior dialysis is practised in many paediatric renal units but the feasibility of this approach is dependent on the availability of donor organs, degree of renal failure at presentation, underlying renal disease, and the patient's suitability for transplantation (Box 10.12). Although malignant disease in childhood is rare it is usual to delay transplantation and the introduction of immunosuppression until at least 1 year posttreatment (in the case of Wilm's tumour: Ettenger 1996) or longer (2–5 years) in non-renal malignancies (Wilkinson 1996). The optimum time for PET is when GFR falls to 10 mL min^{-1} 1.73 m^{-2} BSA, i.e. before dialysis therapy becomes necessary.

Currently in the UK the number of patients waiting for kidney transplants greatly exceeds the number of cadaveric organs being offered. In 1999 paediatric patients (i.e. those less than 18 years) accounted for 2% of the total waiting list for kidneys in the UK and they received 6% of the grafts. Sixty per cent of these 115 children received grafts from paediatric donors (data from the United Kingdom Transplant Special Support Authority (UKTSSA) 1999). The number of live donor grafts performed in the UK has also increased in the last few years in both paediatric and adult centres. In the author's centre, 40% of the total paediatric transplants

---

■ BOX 10.12 Contraindications to pre-emptive transplantation

Active disease, e.g. antiglomerular basement membrane disease

Congenital nephrotic syndromes

Recent malignant disease

Difficulty in accepting healthcare advice

performed in 1999 were from living donors. Human Leukocyte antigen (HLA) type, HLA antibodies, blood group and matching criteria may all unfavourably influence waiting time.

DIALYSIS

Although the ideal treatment for ESRF is a successful transplant, this cannot be achieved without preparation if its chances of success are to be enhanced. Some patients will present to tertiary centres in established ESRF and discussions about renal transplantation cannot take place until they are stable. Others, as mentioned above, require a period of time on dialysis to improve nutritional status or to allow a disease process to 'burn out' before transplantation can be safely considered.

Dialysis, whilst an excellent holding treatment, is fraught with risks and with decreasing patient size, care becomes more complex (Knight et al 1993). Gaining access to the blood stream, whether for PD or HD, is technically difficult in very young children whose increased susceptibility to infection and small-calibre blood vessels may compromise that access. Although in paediatric practice, PD is usually the treatment of choice, between 25 and 50% of patients will undergo HD at some stage (Warady & Bunchman 1996).

Peritoneal dialysis

The popularity of PD is due to its relative simplicity (compared with HD) and the fact that it is less disruptive to normal functioning than HD. In very small children in particular, inserting a peritoneal catheter is generally easier than trying to establish vascular access, although there will be patients in whom PD is impossible or impractical (Box 10.2). Most paediatric units favour automated PD (APD) over continuous ambulatory PD (CAPD) as it appears to provide more efficient dialysis (Lewis 1999, Warady & Bunchman 1996). APD machines can be programmed to deliver small fill volumes, making it possible to dialyse successfully very young children at home overnight, leaving the family free during the day to attend school and work. APD, by reducing the number of times that access to the peritoneal catheter is made, lessens the potential for infection entering the system.

The choice of peritoneal catheter will depend on local preference and patient size but those with double cuffs appear to be associated with lower infection rates (Warady & Bunchman 1996). Reported peritonitis rates among paediatric patients on PD vary from 1 every 8.2 to 1 every 13.3 patient-months (Warady & Bunchman 1996). Causative organisms are most commonly Gram-positive (around 42%), with *Staphylococcus aureus* accounting for the majority of cases of peritonitis (Kuizon et al 1995). Repeated or severe infection can result in sclerosis of the peritoneum, rendering it unusable for dialysis. Infants often become systemically ill quite quickly, as they seem unable to contain bacterial infections within the peritoneum, so even vague symptoms should be responded to quickly (Keane 1996). Exit-site infection is also commonly due to *S. aureus* which, if persistent, may result in PD catheter removal and the need for a respite period on HD until the infection has completely cleared (Levy et al 1990). Infection, whether of the peritoneum, tunnel or exit site, must be taken seriously since it can compromise dialysis delivery. A revision of hygiene and connection techniques is vital after any such episode. Dialysis efficiency can be measured using peritoneal equilibration tests adapted for paediatrics (Hanna et al 1993).

The surface area of the peritoneum is related to BSA and the amount of fluid that can be tolerated in the peritoneal space is proportional to the size of the patient. Children therefore will have a reduced capacity for accommodating PD fluid and their fill volumes (FV) are calculated according to their BSA (Eq. 10.3).

$$FV = 1.1 \text{ L m}^{-2} \qquad \text{(Eq. 10.3)}$$

Haemodialysis

Paediatric HD should only be undertaken by staff with the relevant expertise in an environment with adequate medical and technical back-up should complications occur. Such preconditions may thus limit the availability of this treatment option. Safe HD in children requires consideration of several factors, including venous access, extracorporeal blood volume (ECBV) and appropriate dialyser size.

Venous access

For HD to be effective, safe access to the blood stream has to be established and maintained. This can be difficult to achieve, especially in the very young where the small calibre of blood vessels makes access surgery technically demanding, and is best performed by those with appropriate experience. Factors to be considered when planning venous access are summarised below:

- Central venous catheters (CVCs) can be used in the short or long term for acute/chronic dialysis for children of all ages.
- Uncuffed catheters are usually only viable for periods of less than 2 months.
- One or more internal cuffs are more durable and allow CVCs to function for up to a year or longer (Goldstein et al 1997).
- Arteriovenous fistulae (AVF) can be created in children; they may only be possible in the older patient with adequately sized radial or brachial blood vessels, though microsurgery techniques can achieve functional AVF even in children who weigh less than 10 kg (Bourquelet et al 1990).
- Heterologous grafts using expanded polytetrafluoroethylene (PTFE) have been successfully created, even in quite young children (Brittinger et al 1997) where other methods have failed and long-term permanent access is required.
- There may be considerable resistance from children and parents to AVF or graft formation with concerns about the potential disfigurement and pain from needling.

- CVCs and PTFE grafts are particularly prone to infection and thrombosis.
- CVC infection, usually due to *S. aureus*, may occur at the exit site or within the catheter lumen; if persistent, or if bacteraemia develops, removal of the CVC may be the only solution (Goldstein et al 1997).
- Needling of AVF and PTFE grafts should be done by experienced staff using appropriately sized needles to minimise trauma that might cause scarring or thrombosis.

Practicalities of paediatric haemodialysis

Most paediatric HD in the UK is carried out in hospital since it is intended to be a short-term holding measure until successful transplantation can be carried out. Despite this intention, some patients may be on HD for considerable periods of time, especially those in whom previous transplantation has failed. Attending for dialysis sessions two or three times a week is disruptive for family life and schooling and there is evidence that psychosocial dysfunction among this group is more common than with other treatment modalities (Reynolds et al 1988).

For safe HD the following points must be observed:

- Dialysers and dialysis lines must be of an appropriate size for the child being treated (such equipment is available commercially).
- The safe ECBV is no more than 80 mL blood (Box 10.13).
- Bicarbonate is the buffer of choice in paediatric centres since it corrects acidosis and reduces dialysis-associated symptoms.
- Dialysis efficiency should be measured with urea kinetic models adapted to paediatrics, as children's urea generation and protein catabolic rates are more prone to fluctuation than those of adults (Buur et al 1994).

TRANSPLANTATION

The ideal treatment for ESRF is a successful transplant, not least for the benefits to cognitive function which it achieves (Fennell et al 1996), but attainment of this goal is dependent on a number of factors. The most important of these is the patient's suitability as a recipient and the availability of donor organs. To enhance the chances of success thorough prepar-

---

■ **BOX 10.13 Extracorporeal blood volume (ECBV)**

Children's circulating blood volume (CBV) is lower than that of adults but increases with age (Table 10.2).

ECBV must be calculated accurately before initiating haemodialysis if the dangers of hypovolaemia are to be avoided. A safe ECBV is approximately 8–10% of total CBV.

Table 10.2 Calculation of circulating blood volume

Age	Blood volume (mL kg^{-1})
Neonates	85–90
Infants	75–80
Children	70–75
Adults	65–70

ation is necessary (see above). This requirement means that the minimum age at transplantation is likely to be no less than 6 months and most centres would not consider patients until they have reached at least 6 kg in weight. However, the larger and older the child, the easier the surgery and the lower the risks of morbidity and mortality. Size-matching of organs is not necessary; however, placing a large adult kidney into a small child (< 20 kg) may be difficult for the surgeon. A large kidney on being connected to its blood supply can sequester between 150 and 250 mL blood immediately, thus making careful intraoperative fluid management crucial (Ettenger 1996). Very small children may require elective ventilation posttransplant since respiratory function can be temporarily compromised by the resulting increased intraabdominal pressure created by the placement of a large adult kidney within a small space (Najarian et al 1990). Intensive nursing care is vital in the immediate postoperative period (Box 10.14).

Children are susceptible to many of the same complications as adults, e.g. bacterial and viral infections, urine leaks, renal artery stenosis and malignancy. Reports of the incidence of posttransplant malignancy vary from 1.4% (Kohaut & Tejani 1996) to 7.1% (Srivasta et al 1999). B-cell lymphoma associated with Epstein–Barr virus (EBV) infection is the commonest lesion seen.

Young children have more active immune systems than older children and adults and this factor enhances their tendency to rejection. When combined

---

■ BOX 10.14 Care immediately posttransplantation

Monitor fluid balance—using central venous pressure, core–periphery temperature gap, urine output, fluid intake, blood pressure

Maintain central venous pressure at 5–10 cm water

Maintain central–peripheral temperature gap of less than 2°C (using space blanket)

Dopamine infusion as needed to increase renal perfusion

Analgesia infusion

Monitor all vital signs

Nil by mouth until bowel sounds return

Nurse patient in sitting position to aid respiratory function with their higher metabolic rates, achieving optimum immunosuppression can be problematic (Kohaut & Tejani 1996). Paediatric immunosuppression is prescribed according to BSA and total load is heavier than in adult patients to counteract increased immunoreactivity and metabolic rates (Ferraresso & Kahan 1993; Box 10.15).

In children, especially those receiving adult kidneys, the signs of rejection can be much subtler than an obvious rise in creatinine (Box 10.16). Other indicators include a BP that may be raised for up to a week before creatinine becomes elevated (Bunchman et al 1990). This may be accounted for by the disproportionate size of the graft relative to the recipient's body mass, where such a difference exists. Renal transplant biopsy is an invaluable tool in confirming rejection in the presence of ambiguous signs and symptoms. However, the majority of paediatric patients will require either heavy sedation or even general anaesthesia for this procedure—a factor that complicates its performance.

Close monitoring is vital at all stages of the transplant process if morbidity and mortality are to be minimised and the ultimate goal of a fit, healthy child is to be achieved. The frequency of this monitoring process will decrease with time, but throughout the childhood period and even in the presence of a well-functioning graft, care must be taken to ensure that

---

■ **BOX 10.15 Immunosuppression**

Pharmacokinetic studies are more difficult to perform in children because of ethical constraints and the comparatively small numbers of patients. Immunosuppression drug combinations may be similar to those used in adults but the use of new agents will often be delayed until adequate clinical trials have taken place.

Current protocols rely on prednisolone, ciclosporin/tacrolimus and azathioprine/mycophenalate mofetil with the use of T-cell antibodies or interleukin receptor blockers at induction (Smith & McDonald 2000).

■ **BOX 10.16 Signs and symptoms of transplant rejection in children**

Creatinine raised by >10%/falling creatinine becoming static

Tender painful graft

Fever

Hypertension

Sudden weight gain

Decreased urine output

Diarrhoea (more common in younger children)

Flu-like aches and pains

Irritability, particularly in small children

the side-effects of treatment are kept to a minimum and that normal growth and development occur. If this is not the case then intervention may be needed.

PSYCHOSOCIAL CARE

Renal disorders in childhood and adolescence, particularly those requiring intensive treatment and/or leading to chronic renal failure, have a significant impact on the psychosocial functioning not just of the affected individual but also of the whole family. The child's illness and the resulting need for medical and nursing interventions undermine the parent's role as protector and carer and may cause financial difficulties which affect the whole family's quality of life. Paediatric nephrology nurses can enhance the family's ability to care for their child by offering teaching and support to help increase parental self-esteem and restore their sense of control (Frauman & Gilman 1990).

Cultural and religious beliefs concerning illness may be an additional factor complicating the acceptance and implementation of medical treatment. Being sensitive to such beliefs should help to avoid misunderstanding and conflict. Ill health increases the vulnerability of children, particularly in situations where appropriate care is not possible within the family setting. This may result in the need to invoke official child protection procedures to guarantee that the relevant care and treatment are delivered. Nurses, always the patient's advocate, may thus have to play leading roles in interactions with agencies such as social and legal services and the police.

The pressures of ERSF vary according to treatment modality, with the families of children on hospital haemodialysis finding it most stressful (Reynolds et al 1988) and those with successful transplants reporting fewer problems (Brownbridge & Fielding 1991). Normal family functioning is severely disrupted by the need for frequent hospital attendances, inpatient stays, administration of medication, ensuring adequate nutrition, carrying out dialysis and general monitoring of their child's condition. A successful transplant can reduce the intensity of care although many parents and older patients still report high levels of anxiety when attending for routine outpatient clinics.

Poor statural growth and delayed puberty as well as the alterations to body image that occur as the result of immunosuppressive therapy are stress factors for teenagers with renal problems. While administration of rHGH can help some patients achieve an acceptable height it may not work in every case and its administration may not be well tolerated. Medication side-effects are a potent cause of non—compliance; a problem that is well recognised among renal patients of all ages (Wolff et al 1996). Early studies of adult survivors who had started RRT therapy in childhood demonstrated their inability to integrate fully into society and establish meaningful relationships (Henning et al 1988). It is to be hoped that improved treatment regimes will significantly reduce this negative outcome of otherwise successful treatment.

Emotional distress resulting from healthcare experiences is common among children and adolescents and may have long-term negative sequelae (Hart et al 1992). Therapeutic play under the auspices of qualified hospital play specialists is integral to any treatment programme, providing an opportunity for children and adolescents to express their fears and anxieties and enabling them to develop coping strategies. The use of distraction techniques by play specialists can be invaluable in helping patients through unpleasant procedures with minimal fuss. Hospital teachers can maintain educational continuity and the classroom as well as the playroom are important centres of escape and enjoyment where at least a temporary respite from treatment can be obtained.

The British Association of Paediatric Nephrology defines 15–18-year-olds as adolescents and believes they are most appropriately cared for in paediatric units (British Association of Paediatric Nephrology 1995). However, some in this age group, presenting with renal problems for the first time, may be referred directly to adult nephrology services. Staff in these areas may find themselves challenged as they encounter emotionally labile teenagers whose attempts to be mature are shaken by illness. As children grow older it is appropriate to encourage them to take increasing responsibility for their own care. They have to learn not just about their condition and its treatment but to take the initiative in reporting problems, organising appointments and ordering medication. Paediatric nephrology staff can aid them in this process, supporting them and their parents who may be finding it difficult to allow them such independence. The most logical time for transfer to adult renal services is at the end of secondary education but some young people with long-standing renal problems (especially renal failure) may still be too emotionally and physically immature for this transition (British Association of Paediatric Nephrology 1995). Those who have spent their entire childhood attending one hospital where all is familiar and reassuring may find moving on a momentous and frightening event. These young people may benefit from a transition clinic held jointly with adult and paediatric staff where they can be introduced to their new healthcare team in the presence of familiar faces (Watson et al 1996).

SUMMARY

Ill health in early life can have a profound impact on children's growth and development. To minimise the negative effects associated with renal disease and its treatment, paediatric nephrology staff must form a therapeutic partnership with child and family to try to ensure that the young people for whom they care have the opportunity to grow into healthy intact individuals capable of taking their place in adult society.

This chapter has attempted to highlight some significant aspects of paediatric nephrology nursing but it has only skimmed the surface. For those who are interested in learning more, a closer examination of the reference material will provide further information.

REFERENCES

Andrew MA, Brooker LA. Hemostatic complications in renal disorders of the young. Pediatr Nephrol 1996; 10:88–99.

Arbus GS, Farine M, Guignard JP. Acute renal failure. In: Postlethwaite, RJ ed. Clinical paediatric nephrology 2nd edn. Oxford: Buttterworth Heinemann, 1994: 248–265.

Argente J. Diagnosis of late puberty. Hormone Res 1999; 51 (suppl. 3):95–100.

Belsha OW, Kohaut EC, Warady BA. Dialytic management of childhood acute renal failure: a survey of North American pediatric nephrologists. Pediatr Nephrol 1995; 9:61–73.

Betts PR, Magrath G. Growth patterns and dietary intake of children with chronic renal insufficiency. Br Med J 1974; 2:189–193.

Bourquelet P, Cussenot O, Corbi P et al. Microsurgical creation and follow-up of arteriovenous fistulae for chronic haemodialysis in children. Pediatr Nephrol 1990; 4:156–159.

Bradbury MG, Brocklebank JT. A simple guide to understanding fluid balance. Curr Paediatr 1995; 5:94–97.

British Association of Paediatric Nephrology. Report of a working party. London: BAPN, 1995.

Brittinger WD, Walker G, Twittenhof WD et al. Vascular access for hemodialysis in children. Pediatr Nephrol 1997; 11:87–95.

Brownbridge G, Fielding DM. Psychosocial adjustment to end stage renal failure: comparing haemodialysis, continuous ambulatory peritoneal dialysis and transplantation. Pediatr Nephrol 1991; 5:612–616.

Bunchman TE, Fryd DS, Sibley RK et al. Manifestations of renal allograft rejection in small children receiving adult kidneys. Pediatr Nephrol 1990; 4:255–258.

Buur T, Bradbury MG, Smye SW et al. Reliability of urea kinetic modelling in children. Pediatr Nephrol 1994; 8:574–578.

Churchill BM, Jayanthi RV, McLorie GA et al. Pediatric renal transplantation into the abnormal urinary tract. Pediatr Nephrol 1996; 10:113–120.

Clark G, Barratt TM. Minimal change nephrotic syndrome and focal segmental sclerosis. In: Holliday MA, Barratt TM, Avner ED, eds. Pediatric nephrology. 3rd edn. Baltimore: Williams & Wilkins, 1994: 767–787.

Coulthard MG. Management of Finnish congenital nephrotic syndrome by unilateral nephrectomy. Pediatr Nephrol 1989; 3:451–453.

Cretney SM. Implications of the Children Act 1989. Arch Dis Child 1991; 66: 536–541.

De Swiet M, Dillon MJ, Littler W et al. Measurement of blood pressure in children: recommendations of a working party of the British Hypertension Society. Br Med J 1989; 299:497.

Dillon M. Hypertension. In: Postlethwaite RJ, ed. Clinical paediatric nephrology. 2nd edn. Oxford: Butterworth Heinemann, 1994: 175–195.

Douglas J. Psychology and nursing children. Basingstoke: PS Macmillan, 1993.

Doyal L, Henning P. Stopping treatment for end-stage renal failure: the rights of children and adolescents. Pediatr Nephrol 1994; 8:763–771.

Ettenger RB. Kidney transplantation in children. In: Danovitch GM, ed. Handbook of renal transplantation. 2nd edn. Boston: Little, Brown, 1996: 271–296.

Fennell RS, Edwards JR, Vehaskari M. Psychosocial aspects of the care of the child with moderate renal failure. J Pediatr 1996; 129:S8–S12.

Ferraresso M, Kahan BD. New immunosuppressive agents for pediatric transplantation. Pediatr Nephrol 1993; 7:567–573.

First MR. Living-related donor transplants should be performed with caution in patients with focal segmental glomerulosclerosis. Pediatr Nephrol 1995; 9:S40–S42.

Flom LS, Reisman EM, Donovan JM et al. Favourable experience with pre-emptive renal transplantation in children. Pediatr Nephrol 1992; 6:258–261.

Frauman AC, Gilman CM. Care of the family of the child with end stage renal disease. ANNA J 1990; 17:383–387.

Goldstein SL, Maceriowski CT, Jabs K. Hemodialysis catheter survival and complications in children and adolescents. Pediatr Nephrol 1997; 11:74–77.

Guest G, Broyer M. Growth after renal transplantation: correlation with immunosuppressive therapy. Pediatr Nephrol 1991; 5:143–146.

Hanna JD, Foreman JW, Todd WBG et al. The peritoneal equilibration test in children. Pediatr Nephrol 1993; 7:731–734.

Hart R, Mather PL, Slack JF et al. Therapeutic play activities for hospitalised children. St Louis: Mosby, 1992.

Haycock GB. The influence of sodium on growth in infancy. Pediatr Nephrol 1993; 7:871–875.

Haycock GB. Steroid responsive nephrotic syndrome. In: Postlethwaite RJ, ed. Clinical paediatric nephrology. 2nd edn. Oxford: Butterworth Heinemann, 1994:210–225.

Henning P, Tomlinson L, Rigden SPA et al. Long term outcome of treatment of end stage renal failure. Arch Dis Child 1988; 63:35–40.

Hicklin M, de Sousa M. Children with renal problems. In: Smith T, ed. Renal nursing. London: Baillière Tindall, 1997: 363–382.

Holmberg C, Antikainen M, Rönnholm K et al. Management of congenital nephrotic syndrome of the Finnish type. Pediatr Nephrol 1995; 9:87–93.

Keane WF. Peritoneal dialysis related peritonitis treatment recommendations. Update. Advisory committee on peritonitis management of the International Society of Peritoneal Dialysis. Peritoneal Dialysis Int 1996; 16:557–573.

Klahr S, Buerkert J, Purkerson ML. Role of dietary factors in the progression of chronic renal disease. Kidney Int 1983; 24:579–587.

Knight F, Gorynski L, Bentson M et al. Hemodialysis of the infant or small child with chronic renal failure. ANNA J 1993; 20:315–323.

Kohaut EC, Tejani A. The 1994 annual report of the North American Pediatric Renal Transplant Cooperative Study. Pediatr Nephrol 1996; 10:422–434.

Kuizon B, Melocoton TL, Holloway M et al. Infectious and catheter related complications in pediatric patients treated with peritoneal dialysis at a single institution. Pediatr Nephrol 1995; 9:S12–S17.

Levy M, Balfe JW, Geary D et al. Exit site infection during continuous and cycling peritoneal dialysis in children. Peritoneal Dialysis Int 1990; 10:31–35.

Lewis M. Report of the Paediatric Renal Registry. In: UK Renal Registry. 2nd Annual Report. Bristol: Renal Association, 1999.

Matas AJ, Chavers BM, Nevins TE et al. Recipient evaluation, preparation and care in pediatric transplantation. The University of Minnesota protocols. Kidney Int 1996; 49:S99–S102.

Mattoo TK, Al-Sowailen AM, Al-Harbi MS et al. Nephrotic syndrome in the 1st year of life. Pediatr Nephrol 1992; 6:16–18.

Meyer MM, Norman DJ, Danovitch GM. Long-term post-transplant management and complications. In: Danovitch GM, ed. Handbook of kidney transplantation. 2nd edn. Boston: Little, Brown, 1996:154–186.

Moghal NE, Brocklebank JT, Meadow SR. A review of acute renal failure in children: incidence, aetiology and outcome. Clin Nephrol 1998; 49:91–95.

Morris MC, Allanby CW, Toseland P et al. Evaluation of a height/plasma creatinine formula in the measurement of glomerular filtration rate. Arch Dis Child 1982; 57:611–615.

Najarian JS, Frey MD, Matas AJ et al. Renal transplantation in infants. Ann Surg 1990; 212:353–365.

National High Blood Pressure Education Programme. Update on the 1987 task force report on high blood pressure in children and adolescents: a working group report from the National High Blood Pressure Education Program. Pediatrics 1996; 98:649–658.

Nicholson A. Childhood cancer, an overview: nursing care. In: Thompson J, ed. The child with cancer. London: Scutari Press, 1990:1–16.

Nieto J, Ruiz-Cuevas P, Escuder A et al. Tertiary hyperparathyroidism after renal transplantation. Pediatr Nephrol 1997; 11:65–68.

Nightingale F. Notes on nursing. Skretkowicz V, ed. London: Scutari, 1992:160.

Quan A, Baum M. Protein losses in children on continuous cycler peritoneal dialysis. Pediatr Nephrol 1996; 10:728–731.

Portman RJ, Yetman RJ, West MS. Efficacy of 24-hour ambulatory blood pressure monitoring in children. J Pediatr 1991; 118:842–849.

Ravelli AM. Gastrointestinal function in chronic renal failure. Pediatr Nephrol 1995; 9:756–762.

Rees L. Human growth hormone in renal disease. Br J Renal Med 1997; 2:9–12.

Rees L, Maxwell H. The hypothalamo-pituitary growth hormone insulin-like growth factor 1 axis in children with chronic renal failure. Kidney Int 1996; 49 (suppl. 53):S109–S114.

Rees L, Green S, Adlard P et al. Growth and endocrine function in steroid sensitive nephrotic syndrome. Arch Dis Child 1988a; 63:484–490.

Rees L, Green S, Adlard P et al. Growth and endocrine function following renal transplantation. Arch Dis Child 1988b; 63:1326–1332.

Rees L, Rigden SPA, Ward G et al. Treatment of short stature in renal disease with recombinant human growth hormone. Arch Dis Child 1990; 65:856–860.

Reiss U, Wingen AM, Schärer K. Mortality trends in pediatric patients with chronic renal failure. Pediatr Nephrol 1996; 10:41–45.

Reynolds JM, Garralda ME, Jameson RA et al. How parents and families cope with chronic renal disease. Arch Dis Child 1988; 63:821–826.

Rigden SPA. Chronic renal failure. In: Postlethwaite RJ, ed. Clinical paediatric nephrology. Oxford: Butterworth Heinemann, 1994: 266–281.

Ridgen SPA, Turner A. Chronic renal failure. In: Ryan SW, ed. Nutritional Support. London: Baillière, 1997:233–248.

Rigden SPA, Start KM, Rees L. Nutritional management of infants and toddlers with chronic renal failure. In: Nutrition and health. Great Britain: AB Academic Publishers, 1987; 5: 163–174.

Rigden SPA, Rees L, Chantler C. Growth and endocrine function in children with chronic renal failure. Acta Paediatr Scand 1990; 370 (suppl):20–26.

Rotundo A, Nevins TE, Lipton M et al. Progressive encephalopathy in children with chronic renal insufficiency in infancy. Kidney Int 1982; 21:486–489.

Sedman A. Aluminium toxicity in childhood. Pediatr Nephrol 1992; 6:383–393.

Sedman A, Friedman A, Bolneau F et al. Nutritional management of the child with mild to moderate chronic renal failure. Pediatrics 1996; 129:S13–S18.

Sinaiko AR. Hypertension in children. N Engl J Med 1996; 335:1968–1973.

Smith JM, McDonald RA. Progress in renal transplantation for children. Adv Renal Replace Ther 2000; 7:158–171.

Srivasta T, Zwick DL, Rothberg PG et al. Post transplant lymphoproliferative disorder in pediatric renal transplantation. Pediatr Nephrol 1999; 13:748–754.

Taylor CM. Assessment of glomerular filtration rate. In: Postlethwaite RJ, ed. Clinical paediatric nephrology. 2nd edn. Oxford: Heinemann, 1994: 87–100.

UKTSSA. Transplant activity 1999. Bristol: United Kingdom Transplant Special Support Authority, 1999.

Van Damme-Lombaerts R, Herman J. Erythropoietin treatment in children with renal failure. Pediatr Nephrol 1999; 13:148–152.

Warady AB, Bunchman TE. Update on peritoneal dialysis and hemodialysis in the pediatric population. Curr Opin Pediatr 1996; 8:135–140.

Watson A, Philips D, Argles J. Transferring adolescents from paediatric to adult renal units. Br J Renal Med 1996; 1: 24–26.

Wilkinson AH. Evaluation of the transplant recipient. In: Danovitch GM, ed. Handbook of kidney transplantation. 2nd edn. Boston: Little, Brown, 1996: 109–122.

Wolff G, Strecker K, Vester U et al. Non-compliance after transplantation (abstract S21). Pediatr Nephrol 1996; 10:C43.

Renal transplantation

Patricia M Franklin

11

■ CONTENTS

■ LEARNING OUTCOMES FOR THIS CHAPTER

- To analyse the risks and benefits of renal transplantation
- To identify the contraindications to transplantation
- To understand the importance of pretransplant assessment and the nursing role in the pretransplant clinical care pathway
- To explore donor and recipient matching and its importance to graft survival
- To understand cadaveric and living-related donation
- To evaluate critically the possible options to increase cadaveric donor supply
- To outline the nursing care for the renal transplant recipient in the pre-, peri- and postrenal transplant phase
- To explain the use of immunosuppressive regimens in individual recipient situations.

INTRODUCTION

Renal transplantation is now widely acknowledged as the treatment of choice for those with end-stage renal failure (ESRF). Since the time of the first transplants in the 1950s, advances in antirejection therapies, surgical techniques and tissue matching have enabled kidney transplantation to evolve from an experimental procedure to the treatment that can offer the best quality of life and the most cost-effective care for kidney patients.

Many patients view a kidney transplant as the gateway to 'personal liberation' and as the opportunity to restore 'control over one's life' (Galpin 1992). A successful transplant offers freedom from the practical and psychological difficulties and restrictions of long-term dialysis; freedom from dependence upon a machine, fluid bag or partner; freedom from fluid and dietary restrictions; a return of sexual functioning and fertility with the possibility of parenthood; and a return to an almost normal lifestyle.

A small study in Oxford in 1990 demonstrated fewer changes in life satisfaction score after transplantation in an older age group (> 60 years, $n = 30$), but major changes in life satisfaction for the two younger groups, namely 18–35 years and 35–60 years. A study from the University of Maryland reported similar findings, noting that 'Older age was associated with smaller, but still significant, improvement in quality of life' (Connerney & Bartlett 2001). Thus, older patients may wish to spend more time evaluating the risks and benefits associated with transplantation before joining the transplant waiting list.

Most research studies clearly show that for the majority, kidney transplantation has the greater rehabilitation potential and that the quality of life for patients with functioning grafts is superior to that which is usually achieved on dialysis (Evans et al 1985, Jofre et al 1998, Morris & Jones 1988). However, research into quality of life has received much criticism, and individual perception and assessment of quality of life is known to be affected by a wide range of independent and personal variables. But, for many of those with renal failure, transplantation offers an improved quality of life, and may be the most significant factor for patients when considering transplantation.

Cost-effective care

Transplantation is the most cost-effective treatment option for end-stage renal disease. The cost of 1 year of haemodialysis or peritoneal dialysis is similar to that of a renal transplant in the first year. However, thereafter the cost of continuing care for the transplant patient is one-fifth of the cost of dialysis per year.

National waiting-list figures for kidney transplant

The improvement in quality of life and cost-effectiveness of this treatment support the suggestion that renal transplantation is the treatment of choice for the majority of patients. Unfortunately, such a goal is not possible at present because of the limited supply of cadaveric organs. The current UK waiting list for kidney transplantation stands at more than 5000 patients (Fig. 11.1). On average, 1700 renal transplants are performed in the UK each year.

We therefore need to explore ways of increasing donor numbers in order to offer all suitable patients the chance of a transplant.

CONTRAINDICATIONS TO RENAL TRANSPLANTATION

Although the majority of patients may request a transplant, transplantation may not be suitable for all those with ESRF because of possible medical complications.

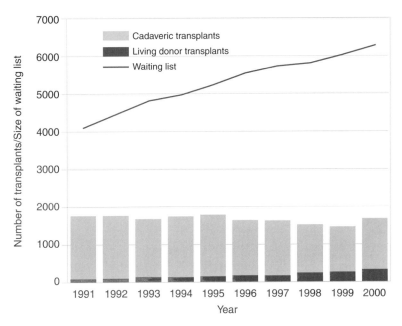

Figure 11.1 Kidney transplants and waiting list at year-end 1991–2000. Statistics prepared by UK Transplant from the National Transplant Database maintained on behalf of Transplant Services in the UK and Republic of Ireland.

Malignancy

Malignant disease must be excluded prior to transplantation as the immunosuppressive regime may cause accelerated growth of the tumour and may encourage secondary spread. If the patient is known to have had a tumour removed in the past, it is important to ascertain the type of tumour, the stage of tumour development and the treatment received. In selected cases transplantation may still be possible provided that curative treatment has been given and sufficiently long follow-up has occurred to exclude recurrence.

Recurrent disease

It is also important to consider the patient's primary renal disease as in some cases the disease may recur and destroy the new kidney (Table 11.1). Renal disorders with a very high recurrence rate include focal segmental glomerulosclerosis (FSGS) (causing massive proteinuria and scarring of the glomeruli) and mesangiocapillary glomerulonephritis (an immunological disorder of the glomeruli). However, transplantation may still be considered but only after counselling and explanation of the risks to the patient. Most centres would advise against living related donation in this situation.

Other conditions, such as Goodpasture's syndrome and the other vasculitic illnesses, need to have been fully treated before going ahead with transplantation because of the risk of damage in the new kidney in the presence of active disease. Twelve months is normally considered the earliest that transplantation would be considered, to allow antibody levels to

Table 11.1 Recurrence of glomerulonephritis in renal transplants

Type of glomerulonephritis	Recurrence (%)
Focal segmental glomerulosclerosis	30
Membranous nephropathy	10
Mesangiocapillary type I	20–30
Mesangiocapillary type II	95
Immunoglobulin A nephropathy	50
Henoch–Schönlein purpura	80
Antiglomerular basement membrane nephritis	5
Idiopathic crescentic glomerulonephritis	?

Data from Mathew (1991) with permission.

fall. Several other diseases, such as diabetes, can cause microscopic changes in the kidney after many years but rarely lead to graft loss.

Hepatitis virus and human immunodeficiency virus

Patients who are hepatitis B or hepatitis C positive may be at risk of progressive liver disease after transplantation due to the impact of the immunosuppressive therapy. Similarly, the immunosuppression would have an adverse effect in the presence of human immunodeficiency virus (HIV), reducing life expectancy. In most centres, infection with HIV is classed as an absolute contraindication to transplantation. Opinions differ with regard to transplantation in the presence of hepatitis B and hepatitis C. Decisions are taken on an individual basis with regard to level, type of infection and the extent of liver damage. However, many patients with hepatitis B and C have no or quiescent disease.

Diabetes mellitus and cardiovascular disease

Many people with diabetes can receive a renal transplant, but they are at risk from other complications of their diabetes. Cardiovascular disease is seen primarily in those with type 2 diabetes, and may contribute to higher levels of morbidity and death. Also, it is important to assess vessel patency prior to transplantation, as severe atherosclerosis of the iliac vessels may at worst preclude transplantation and at best complicate the transplant surgery.

EVALUATION FOR TRANSPLANTATION

Age

Morbidity and mortality after kidney transplantation tend to increase with age and therefore the age of the recipient must be classed as a risk factor. Age must also be considered within the context of other risk factors, such as advanced cardiovascular disease. Most centres do not have age barriers for transplantation. Health is assessed on an individual basis, and physiological rather than chronological age and the existence of other risk factors

> ### ■ BOX 11.1 Ethical discussion point on shortage of donor organs
>
> * Renal transplants: demand far exceeds supply
> * Younger patients are shown to gain greater life satisfaction after a transplant
> * Older patients are at greater risk of complications
>
> Discussion
> * Should younger patients be given priority over the older group?

are seen as the important assessment issues. Many units have patients of 70 years and over who have progressed well following a kidney transplant. With demand far exceeding supply and studies reporting smaller changes in improvements in quality of life for the older age groups, some may question the use of such a precious and scarce resource in older people. This debate continues, with some centres now attempting to match kidneys from older cadaveric donors with the older recipients, although tissue match is always the major deciding factor (Box 11.1).

Polycystic kidney disease

This inherited kidney disease can result in several members of a family receiving ESRF treatments. The native cystic kidneys may be very large, thus leaving little space for the transplant, and there may also be an increased risk of bleeding and infection. Occasionally, it may be necessary to perform a unilateral, or in severe cases a bilateral, nephrectomy prior to transplantation.

Urinary tract

It is important to assess that there are no problems with the bladder and urethra and that there will be no difficulties following transplantation; if it is felt that the bladder capacity is unacceptably low, surgical enlargement may be possible. In the presence of a history of repeated urinary tract infections with bilateral reflux, it may be necessary to undertake a bilateral nephrectomy prior to transplantation to reduce the risk of posttransplant infection.

Cardiac disease

Routine investigations such as an electrocardiogram (ECG) and cardiac history are essential for all patients. Those patients who are in the high-risk groups for cardiovascular disease (e.g. older patients, those with diabetes or ischaemic heart disease) should be reviewed by a cardiologist and undergo further investigation. Patients who have a history of myocardial infarction should be symptom-free for 1 year prior to transplant.

Gastric ulceration

A history of indigestion and/or gastric ulceration must be noted and endoscopy undertaken if active ulceration is a possibility, as those with active ulceration risk bleeding after transplantation due to the action of the steroid therapy. Treatment with H_2 receptor blocking agents (such as ranitidine) should be given prior to transplantation if active disease is present. Many centres also use ranitidine prophylaxis in all recipients during the first 6 postoperative months.

Respiratory disease

Routine chest X-ray is essential for all patients, and any infection must be treated. Pulmonary tuberculosis will require treatment before transplantation. Patients with a history of tuberculosis and those who have visited or lived in high-risk areas will require prophylactic treatment with isoniazid and pyridoxine for at least 1 year following transplantation.

Patients should also be strongly advised to stop smoking and should be offered information regarding smoking cessation strategies and support systems.

Obesity

Obesity may make the transplant surgery difficult and increase the risk of postoperative complications. Nutritional advice should be given pre- and posttransplantation (Chapter 9).

Oral hygiene

Dental hygiene and assessment of dental state are essential. Any gum infection or dental problems should be dealt with prior to transplantation. Ciclosporin can cause gum hypertrophy, which is made much worse in the presence of poor hygiene.

PRETRANSPLANTATION PREPARATION

Patients may be referred for transplantation during different phases of the disease process; some may be in the predialysis stage, others may already be established on dialysis therapy. Early transplantation before the need for dialysis therapy is often welcomed from a clinical perspective but may prove difficult psychologically if emotional adjustments have not been successfully negotiated and the patient and family are still reeling from the impact of the disease. An overview of the psychological support required for those pretransplantation is outlined in Chapter 3.

An important part of this support is the pretransplantation information group for patients and families, and details are provided in Chapter 3. Tables 11.2–11.5 show useful checklists for the pretransplant stage.

SPECIFIC PRETRANSPLANT ANXIETIES AND FEARS

Specific issues concerning body image are discussed in Chapter 3: other anxieties include acceptance of the transplant as part of the 'self' and guilt over benefiting from traumatic death. There are also very specific challenges

Table 11.2 Pretransplant information and assessment proforma: checklist used by the transplant nurse specialist in stage 1: information and discussion

1. Desire to receive a transplant

2. Benefits of a renal transplant
   - Improved quality of life
   - Freedom from dialysis
   - Normal healthy diet
   - Freedom from fluid restrictions
   - Travel freely (may require special vaccinations)
   - Employment
   - Improved fertility (majority)—contraception

3. Risks/disadvantages of a renal transplant
   - Immunosuppression
   - Adherence with medication and healthcare advice
   - Drug side-effects
     — Ciclosporin
        Hirsutism (electrolysis available)
        Gum hyperplasia (dental care)
        Tremor
        Nephrotoxic/hepatoxic
     — Steroids
        Body image changes
        Weight gain/hunger
        Mood swings
        Bone problems
        Changes in control of diabetes
     — Azathioprine
        Some hair loss
        Susceptible to infections
     — Tacrolimus
        Increased blood glucose levels
     — Mycophenolate mofetil
        Diarrhoea
        Nausea
        Leukopenia
   - Susceptible to infections and viruses
   - Lymphoma and cytomegalovirus infection—risks and treatment
   - Risk of rejection/biopsies
   - May lose financial benefits—annual prescription

4. Clinical
   - Blood pressure
   - Pulse
   - Dental check: date of last check
   - Last cervical smear: date of last smear
   - Breast self-examination
   - Weight
   - Height
   - Body mass index >25 <35

relating to patients' education and understanding of their immunosuppressive therapy.

It is vital that patients understand the need to continue with their anti-rejection therapy for as long as they have their transplant. Many patients

Table 11.3 Pretransplant information and assessment proforma: checklist used by the physician to evaluate clinical assessment and information

Clinical assessment: discussion

Clinical history
1. Renal disease and disease progression: dialysis status
2. Previous medical history, noting previous blood transfusions, pregnancies and previous transplants
3. Previous surgery
4. Current clinical status
5. Social history, family status
6. Smoking, alcohol, recreational drugs
7. Current medications, allergies
8. Immunological status, blood group

Clinical assessment
1. Cardiac assessment
2. Respiratory assessment, tuberculosis risks/contacts
3. Urological assessment
4. Gastrointestinal assessment—previous gastric ulceration, treatment and outcome
5. Abdominal assessment—previous surgery, Tenckhoff site
6. Vascular assessment—assess pulses
7. Dentition
8. Gynaecological status

Information: discussion
1. Risks
   • Surgical, anaesthetic, death rates, patient survival rates
   • Graft survival rates–cadaveric and living donor
   • Lymphoma
   • Cytomegalovirus
   • Cardiovascular
   • Skin cancer
2. Further investigations required
3. Live donor possibility or cadaveric list
4. Immunosuppression regimen required
5. Decision
   • On cadaveric transplant waiting list
   • For live donor programme
   • Await further investigations
   • Patient undecided—does not want a transplant
   • Unsuitable for transplant due to ....

believe that it will only be necessary to take the drugs until the kidney settles into the body. There are great challenges for the transplant team to ensure that patients are well informed about their medication.

An American study involving 531 kidney transplant recipients with ciclosporin regimens was conducted by Didlake et al in 1988. Results reported graft loss in 2.8% of the sample and rejection episodes in 1.99% of the sample, possibly due to reluctance to take the prescribed medication. Of 295 transplant recipients who responded to the questionnaire, 13% reported missing more than three doses per month of their medication.

Table 11.4 Pretransplant assessment proforma used by the transplant nurse specialist in stage 3: routine investigations

1. Blood group
2. Tissue typing
3. Biochemistry
4. Haematology
5. Liver function tests
6. Lipid levels
7. Virology
   - Hepatitis B and C
   - Cytomegalovirus
   - Human immunodeficiency virus
   - Epstein–Barr virus
   - Varicella zoster virus
8. Chest X-ray
9. Electrocardiogram—cardiac referral if required
10. Midstream urine
11. Further specific investigations required:
    -
    -
    -

Table 11.5 Pretransplant assessment proforma used by the transplant nurse specialist in stage 4

1. Orientation	Tour of the unit
2. Waiting list	How it works, how to manage waiting time
3. Planning for the transplant call	Arrange child/pet/others care
4. Transplant call	What to expect, transport
5. Contact numbers	Holiday arrangements
6. Inpatient care	Ward environment and policies—information booklet
7. Final cross-match	
8. Pre- and postoperative care	
9. Transplant nurse specialist	Contact card—further contact

Further evidence suggests that there are difficulties in taking medication across different transplant groups (Rovelli et al 1989).

A variety of explanations have been given for these difficulties. These include the effects of immunosuppression on physical appearance, inability to accept the lifestyle limitations, misinformation given by one patient to another, poor education given by staff and fear of long-term side-effects. Sometimes, those who have had difficulty in accepting dialysis are exemplary transplant recipients because the posttransplant lifestyle is especially precious.

It is inappropriate to refuse transplantation to patients who are perceived as high risk for noncompliance (Case Study 11.1). It is important to offer extensive pretransplant counselling to explore the reasons for not taking healthcare advice and, if necessary, offer additional posttransplant support in order to help facilitate adherence to medication therapies.

■ CASE STUDY 11.1

Claire, a 16-year-old, received a cadaveric transplant and her initial recovery was excellent. But, at 3 months posttransplant, she missed several appointments and refused to discuss her feelings with her parents or staff. At this time, Claire moved in with a friend and did not attend clinic for 3 weeks. Frequent contact by family and transplant personnel was ignored. Finally, she was admitted with acute rejection which resulted in graft loss. She returned to dialysis.

One year later, she asked to go back on the transplant list for a second graft. Some medical and nursing staff were reluctant to offer a second chance due to the shortage of kidneys, and difficulties with taking medication. Discussions with Claire highlighted the difficult issues for her with the previous graft which included changes in body image and a desire to be a 'normal teenager' experiencing life without parental control.

If she received a second transplant, Claire agreed to work closely with the transplant nurse specialist in the posttransplant phase to explore future difficulties. The medical staff agreed to plan a specific immunosuppressive regimen that would minimise the particular side-effects that she had found distressing.

Claire received a second transplant and made an excellent recovery.

TRANSPLANT WAITING LIST

Once the pretransplant assessment has been completed satisfactorily and the tissue- typing and blood-grouping details are finalised, the name of the patient will be added to both the local and national waiting lists. Waiting time is impossible to predict.

It is important to explain to patients that the transplant waiting list is very different from other hospital waiting lists in that they do not simply have to wait until their name reaches the top of the list to receive a graft. The transplant list is essentially a pool of recipients, and each transplant is allocated on the basis of the closest match, irrespective of time waiting. Therefore, their name will join the recipient pool and they must wait for the best match for them. This is a difficult concept to understand and some patients become distressed if another patient, who has waited less time, is transplanted before them.

It is also important that patients do not sit by the phone all day waiting for 'the call', thus greatly restricting their lifestyle. Patients are encouraged to keep as active and as healthy as possible whilst waiting and to continue as normal a lifestyle as possible. Some patients may still feel ambivalent about a transplant at this time. Specific fears and anxieties may need to be explored and support given within the context that patients must be allowed the time to decide the best treatment for themselves. Ongoing contact with the transplant nurse specialist is vital during the waiting time and it is recommended that those who are waiting are contacted every 12 months and offered support and reassurance. Support is especially important at times of additional stress such as when a fellow dialysis patient receives or rejects a kidney.

DONOR AND RECIPIENT MATCHING

Immune system: overview

The human body has a complex system of defences that can provide protection against infection and disease. This system has the ability to target, isolate and destroy potentially harmful invaders. This destruction is achieved in three stages—first by the recognition of structures on the invader (antigens) which are not present in the host. Antibodies and T cells that can recognise the antigens as 'foreign' are then produced. These antibodies and T cells then attach to the invader and destroy it both directly and by recruiting other mechanisms of destruction. Exactly the same happens to a transplant unless it is from an identical twin. The 'foreign' antigens on the transplant induce antibodies and T cells. These target the transplanted organ and do their very best to destroy it. The term 'transplant antigens' is used to describe those antigens which are most important in this regard. Only two are really important: the human leukocyte antigen (HLA) system and the ABO system (see below). In order to prevent rejection it is necessary to circumvent the immune system (matching and cross-matching) and to suppress the immunological response.

Components of the immune system

Leukocytes (white blood cells)

These comprise the cells which produce the antibody (B lymphocytes), recognise the foreign antigens (T lymphocytes), directly destroy invaders (activated T lymphocytes), or can be called in to help with the destruction process (monocytes, polymorphs and eosinophils). Thus, it can be seen that the lymphocytes play several roles and therefore have the major influence on graft acceptance.

Lymphocytes

These comprise 20% of the total white blood cell count (WBC) and are made up of several groups of cells with specialised functions. The term 'orchestra' is often used to describe the mode of operation. Each section of the orchestra is made up of individuals with similar but not identical characteristics. The overall result of the orchestra playing is a result of each section performing in concert with the others.

Lymphocyte types

- T cells: these have antigen recognition structures fixed to their surface.
- B cells: these have antigen recognition structures that can be secreted (antibodies).

T cells and B cells can be naive or activated. T cells can be activated to various functions, namely helper, killer or tolerant status. B cells can be activated to produce antibody or memory.

Each naive lymphocyte has an antigen recognition structure that is unique, for example different from other members of its section and thus capable of seeing a different antigen. In this way literally millions of 'foreign' antigens can be recognised. Each time a recognition event occurs, a naive cell becomes activated and divides. Thus, even if a single cell recognises an antigen as foreign it keeps dividing until it forms a significant number of identical cells (a clone), all capable of recognising the antigen.

Depending on influences from other sections, T cells can help B cells produce antibody (helper T cells), kill targets bearing the antigen directly (killer T cells), or become tolerant (i.e. capable of recognising the antigen but not producing a damaging response to it). B cells can produce antibody in around 8–10 days if they see it for the first time (naive B cells) or within 24 h if they have seen it before (memory B cells). B cells produce much more antibody if they get help from the T cells which can themselves see the same antigen.

One point about antibody production which is relevant to transplantation is that the process which produces it is long-lived. This is very positive for vaccination programmes, where having antibody around for years and years is very beneficial, although negative of course for transplantation.

ABO blood groups

The ABO system of human blood groups was described by Landsteiner in 1902. Blood group is determined by A and B antigens on the surface of the red blood cells. Each individual has one of the four basic blood group types—O, A, B or AB.

Each individual has antibodies to the blood group antigens that they do not express (Table 11.6). Antibodies against the blood group antigens can cause hyperacute rejection and therefore matching of blood group between donor and recipient is vital. Blood group O organs can be transplanted into all groups; O is classified as the universal donor. Blood group AB recipients can receive organs from all groups; AB is classified as the universal recipient.

Table 11.6 The ABO blood group system

Blood group	Percentage of population	Antigens expressed	Antibodies expressed	Acceptable donor blood group
O	47%	None	Anti-A, Anti-B	O
A	42%	A	Anti-B	O, A
B	8%	B	Anti-A	O, B
AB	3%	AB	None	O, A, B, AB

Histocompatibility antigens

A further set of proteins that can trigger the B and T cell response are the transplantation antigens or the histocompatibility antigens. The histocompatibility antigens can be divided into two groups—major and minor.

Major histocompatibility complex (MHC)

This system, first discovered in the mouse by Peter Gorer at Guy's Hospital in the late 1930s is, as the name suggests, the most important system in transplantation and indeed in immunity to infection. The human system is termed HLA (for human leukocyte antigen) and was identified by Dausset, van Rood and Payne in the 1960s (Klein 1986). The sera from pregnant women were found to have antibodies that recognised lymphocytes from their partners and from some random blood donors. The reason for this is that pregnancy is in some ways like a transplant. Passage of blood from partner or child to mother results in T cells and antibody being produced to the foreign antigens on the blood cells. Since the most potent foreign antigens are those of the HLA system, most of the mother's response is directed against them and the long-lived antibody-producing cells remain in her blood. These antibodies can persist for over 40 years.

The HLA system is complex. There are four main series important for transplantation—A, B, C and DR. There are over 30 antigens in each series. Each person can have two from each series (one from each parent). The permutation on 2/30 from A, 2/30 from B, 2/30 from C and 2/30 from DR means that, outside of a family, it is very rare for individuals to have identical HLA types. Luckily for matching in renal transplantation, DR is dominant. However, most of the antibody and T-cell response is produced to A, B and C.

The rules for HLA and matching are not nearly so clear-cut as the rules for ABO, but there are several strong guidelines:

• Transplantation of a kidney into someone who has antibodies directed to a foreign (mismatched) HLA antigen on that kidney will result in hyperacute rejection.

• Transplantation of a kidney into someone who has strong memory to a foreign (mismatched) HLA antigen on that kidney will result in very rapid rejection.

• Transplantation of a kidney with two mismatches at DR will have more rejection than one with one mismatch at DR, and both will have more rejection than a kidney with no DR mismatches. However, rejection episodes can be treated or mismatched patients given additional immunosuppression (Fig. 11.2).

Donor and recipient matching

The majority of organs for transplant come from cadaveric donors. It is essential to match for blood group and to achieve the best DR match possible. Since antibodies can be induced to pregnancies or transfusions or previous transplants and can be boosted by infection, regular screening of patients on the waiting list is necessary to maintain knowledge of their

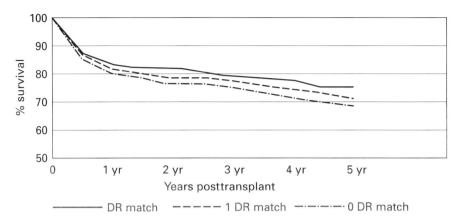

Figure 11.2 Influence of human leukocyte antigen DR matching on renal allograft survival. Data from Oxford Transplant Centre (2001).

current antibody status. Donors are avoided if they contain any mismatch to which the recipient is responding to or has responded to.

Donor and recipient cross-matching

As a final check for current antibody and for the accuracy of past screening, a recent sample and selected past samples from the recipient are always checked against donor cells before transplantation.

UK matching system

Within the UK, each transplant centre has a local list of recipients awaiting transplant. There is also a national list held at UK Transplant in Bristol. Each cadaveric donor is tissue-typed at the local transplant centre and the details sent to Bristol, where the closest tissue match is found from the central computer. The kidneys are then sent to the recipient centre for transplant.

A new scheme for the national allocation of kidneys was adopted in the UK in July 1998, replacing the previous Beneficial Matching Scheme (Gilks et al 1987). The new scheme was the result of work by Task Forces of the UK Transplant Kidney and Pancreas Advisory Group and is based on rigorous analyses of the National Transplant Databases to determine factors that influence renal transplant outcome in the age of modern immunosuppression (Morris et al 1999). The scheme is based on HLA matching, gives priority to paediatric patients, some priority for highly sensitised patients (i.e. patients with high levels of HLA antibodies) and uses a point score to differentiate between equally matched patients. Local patients have priority over national patients. The scheme has three tiers. Tier 1 kidneys are offered to patients with no mismatched HLA antigens at HLA-A, -B and -DR (termed a 000 mismatched transplant). If there are no such patients in tier 1, then kidneys are offered in tier 2 to favourably matched patients (i.e. no mismatch at HLA-DR and a maximum of one mismatched antigen at both the HLA-A and HLA-B locus; 100, 010, 110 mismatch grades). If there are no patients in either tier 1 or 2 and the kidneys cannot be used locally, then the kidneys are offered in tier 3 to the transplant unit with the highest balance of exchange. Monitoring the scheme has shown an increase in the proportion of well-matched transplants and of the number of highly sensitised patients transplanted in the UK (Fuggle et al 1998).

Pretransplant cross-match

Prior to transplant, a cross-match test is performed in the tissue-typing laboratory. A blood sample from the recipient is mixed with lymphocytes from the donor. If the donor cells react (die), the result is termed a positive cross-match; the recipient is adversely reacting to the donor antigens. In the presence of a positive cross-match, transplantation cannot proceed, as the transplant would be rejected.

Sensitisation

When there is a positive cross-match, the recipient is sensitised to that donor. The higher the level of sensitisation, the greater will be the difficulty in finding a transplant that will not reject.

Sensitisation can occur during pregnancy (to partner's antigens), during blood transfusion and after transplantation. In order to reduce the risk of sensitisation it is important to minimise the giving of blood transfusions.

Some recipients may have a high level of sensitisation (highly sensitised). Many cross-matches are performed for each recipient. If recipients do not react with the various donors tested then they are classified as unsensitised. If the blood reacts with 50% of donors they are 50% sensitised, and if blood reacts with 100% of donors they are highly sensitised. Unfortunately, some highly sensitised candidates wait many years for a compatible transplant.

CADAVERIC (HEART-BEATING) DONATION

The majority of renal transplants result from cadaveric donation. Cadaveric donors are patients who have suffered irreversible brain stem damage (brain stem death) and are maintained on a ventilator within a critical care unit.

Causes of brain stem death

The most common causes of brain stem death are listed in Box 11.2.

Cerebral swelling resultant from trauma or anoxia and intracerebral bleeding can cause raised intracranial pressure which forces the cerebral hemispheres through the tentorial hiatus thus compressing the brain stem and interrupting its blood supply. Such herniation of the cerebral tissue is usually described as 'coning' and results in irreversible damage to the brain stem.

Brain stem functions

The brain stem is responsible for the capacity to breathe spontaneously and the capacity for consciousness. If the brain stem is irreversibly damaged

---

■ **BOX 11.2 Common causes of brain stem death**

Intracerebral bleed or infarction
Head trauma
Cerebral hypoxia due to:
- Respiratory arrest
- Cardiac arrest
- Smoke inhalation/carbon monoxide poisoning
Cerebral tumour
Drug overdose
Intracranial infection

---

then there is loss of function and it is argued that the 'irreversible loss of the capacity for consciousness and the irreversible loss of the capacity to breathe' constitutes brain stem death, which constitutes death of the person (Pallis 1994).

Brain stem death diagnosed by signs of irreversible damage to the brain stem is an accepted concept in most countries of the world.

Brain stem death diagnosis

Tests to diagnose brain stem death originated from the Harvard Medical School criteria (Harvard Medical School 1968) which were published in the USA in 1968. A UK Code of Practice for the diagnosis of brain stem death was agreed by the Conference of Medical Royal Colleges in 1976, 1979,1991 and 1998 (UK Code of Practice 1998).

The clinical diagnosis of brain stem death involves three steps. The first step is to ascertain that the following preconditions have been met:

- The patient is deeply comatosed and on a ventilator.
- The patient has been maintained on the ventilator for sufficient time to ascertain that the brain damage is irreversible.
- There is a positive diagnosis of the cause of the coma.

The second step is to exclude other possible causes of coma which are:

- primary hypothermia ($< 35°C$)
- drug intoxication or alcohol intoxication
- metabolic and endocrine disturbances.

The third step is to perform testing to ascertain:

- absent brain stem reflexes
- apnoea (loss of capacity for spontaneous breathing).

Tests for brain stem death: absent brain stem reflexes:

- The pupils are fixed and dilated: there is no response to light.
- The corneal reflex is absent; the patient does not blink when the cornea is stimulated.

- Vestibulo-ocular reflexes are absent; there are no eye movements during or after slow injection of 20 mL of ice-cold water into each external auditory meatus.
- Cranial nerve response to pain is absent: there is no response to stimulation of any somatic area.
- Gag reflex is absent: there is no response to tracheal and bronchial stimulation by a suction catheter.
- No respiratory movements occur when the respiratory centre is stimulated (apnoea testing).

Declaration of brain stem death

The UK Code of Practice recommends that brain stem death testing should be carried out by two medical practitioners 'who have expertise in this field'. One should be a consultant and the other a consultant or senior registrar. Neither of the doctors should be a member of the transplant team or associated with potential transplant recipients.

Repetition of testing

The Code of Practice also recommends that testing should be performed twice to ensure that there has been no observer error. The interval between the tests is normally at the discretion of the critical care staff who will also consider the needs and circumstances of the family.

Time of death

The time of completion of the first set of tests is legally the time of death, and this should be recorded as such on the death certificate.

Criteria for multiple organ donation

- The patient is aged 0–80 years.
- The patient has suffered severe and irreversible brain damage resulting in brain stem death.
- The patient is maintained on a ventilator.
- The patient has no major untreated sepsis (discuss with transplant team).
- The patient has no malignancy—except primary brain tumour (discuss with transplant team).
- The patient is HIV- and hepatitis B- and C-negative (discuss with transplant team).

Patients with some degree of sepsis that have been treated may be considered, as may hepatitis B- or C-positive cases, in certain instances. Conversely, other diseases may preclude donation of specific organs. Therefore it is recommended that critical care staff consider organ donation in all those with brain stem death and refer to the local transplant coordinator for a decision regarding medical suitability.

Patients from high-risk groups (as defined by the Department of Health 2000) should also be excluded. In order to keep transplants safe, the Department of Health guidelines state that 'certain medical and social information' must be given. Therefore, donor families are given an information sheet (Table 11.7) and asked to read these questions and answer 'to the best of their knowledge'.

Table 11.7 Keeping transplants safe: information sheet given to proposed kidney donor families

In order to proceed with organ and tissue donation, the Department of Health[a] guidelines state that we need to ask for certain medical and social information.

Therefore to the best of your knowledge:
Is there a history of behaviour that might increase the risk of HIV, syphilis, hepatitis A, hepatitis B and hepatitis C?

Has your relative ever:
• had any acupuncture, tattoos, ear and/or body piercing within the last 6 months?
• been tested for or known to have HIV, hepatitis B and/or hepatitis C?
• had sex with another man (if a man)?
• received money or drugs as payment for sex?
• injected or snorted drugs?
• been sexually active in Africa (excluding Morocco, Algeria, Tunisia, Libya and Egypt)?
• had sex with anyone in the above list during the last 12 months?

Does your relative have a risk of having an infection of unknown origin? Has he or she ever had:
• a past medical history of jaundice?
• a family history of CJD or confusion?
• an occular tissue transplant (cornea, sclera or occular stem cells)?
• human pituitary-derived growth hormone or gonadotrophin before 1989?
• neurosurgery or operations on tumours or cysts on the spine or implantation of dura mater before August 1992?

Has your relative:
• had a history of neurodegenerative disease of unknown aetiology?
• had a history of disease of unknown aetiology (i.e. multiple sclerosis, Alzheimer's disease, Parkinson's disease or Crohn's disease)?
• had a history of encephalitis?
• had a history of animal bites received overseas in the last 6–12 months?
• had a history of rabies, herpes simplex or unknown virus?
• travelled outside western Europe and had an infection whilst abroad?
• travelled overseas in the last few months? Has he or she contracted malaria or lived for more than 3 months in a malaria risk area (Africa, Asia, south and central America, Mexico, Mississippi Valley, West Indies, California, Texas, Japan and the Caribbean)?
• had Lyme disease, tuberculosis or brucellosis?
• been tested for toxoplasmosis?
• been tested for cytomegalovirus?
• had a recent viral infection or rash, such as chickenpox, shingles, measles or Epstein–Barr virus?

Thank you for taking the time to read this sheet. If it would be more appropriate, please feel free to discuss the above with the transplant coordinator in private before the donation. All information is treated with the strictest of confidence.

[a] *DOH Committee on Microbiological Safety of Blood and Tissue Transplantation (2000, revised). Crown copyright material is reproduced with the permission of the Controller of HMSO and the Queen's Printer for Scotland.*
HIV, human immunodeficiency virus; CJD, Creutzfeldt–Jakob disease

Requesting donation

In the UK, the legal requirements for organ donation are contained in the Human Tissue Act 1961. The Act states that:

The person lawfully in possession of the body of a deceased person may authorise the removal of any part from the body for use for the said purposes, if having made such reasonable enquiry as may be practicable, he has no reason to believe:

(a) *that the deceased had expressed an objection to his body being so dealt with after death ... or*
(b) *that the surviving spouse or any surviving relative of the deceased object to the body being so dealt with.*

Therefore, in practice, it is the next of kin or the patient's executor who is usually approached to give permission for donation. If the patient has signed a donor card there is no statutory requirement to approach the family, but in practice the views of the family are always sought and if objections are raised donation does not occur.

If the next of kin cannot be notified, the body remains in the possession of the hospital. In such cases the hospital manager can give permission for donation as long as reasonable enquiries have been made and that there is no reason to believe that the deceased had expressed objections.

Religious beliefs

As far as it is known, no major religious groups in the UK object to the principles of organ donation and transplantation. Some groups feel that it is only permissible if donors themselves had requested donation. These groups include, in particular, Orthodox Jews, Christian Scientists and some Hindu groups. Jehovah's Witnesses have religious objections to blood transfusions, but feel that donating or receiving organs is a matter for all Jehovah's Witnesses to decide for themselves.

It is often thought that the Muslim faith does not support donation and anecdotal evidence suggests that British Muslims are, in general, reluctant to donate organs. However, recent legislation has approved donation and transplantation in Muslim countries such as Saudi Arabia. Also, a recent fatwa issued by the Muslim Law Council has stated that Muslims may donate organs. They may carry donor cards and their next of kin may give permission for donating (Carlisle 1995). Previous reluctance to donate may have been cultural rather than religious and therefore information and liaison with Muslims will be vital in order to encourage donation.

Birmingham is one centre within the UK that has appointed a renal recipient transplant coordinator for the Asian community. The aim of this role is to provide 'continuous direct rapport and liaison with this community by developing specific educational material relevant and appropriate to the patient population' (Jain 1999).

Jain (1999) states that there is a documented two- to fourfold increased prevalence of ESRF in the Asian patient group. The major causes are the higher incidence of hypertension and diabetes combined with other reasons which are, as yet, unknown. In Birmingham, although the Asian population, comprising a variety of groups, forms 14% of the general population, they represented 30% of the transplant waiting list in 1997. There are fewer cadaver organ donations from this community and after enquiry the author suggests that the 'reasons for this are complex and multi-factorial'. She states that there appear to be religious misconceptions. Although the three major Asian religions, Hinduism, Sikhism and Islam, encourage organ donation, there is a fear and mistrust coupled with a lack of awareness about brain stem death, the scope and value of organ donation and transplantation. Language and cultural barriers seem to have inhibited the uptake of public health messages pertinent to organ donation and transplantation.

Awareness campaigns have been initiated and living donation has been seen as a possible interim solution as dialogue develops. Culturally sensitive education and support have been introduced coupled with a significant drive to increase public awareness in the Asian community in the UK. It is too early to assess the impact of these initiatives but a more positive perception of organ donation and transplantation is now reported from within this community.

Other issues inherent to the UK may also be adversely affecting the cadaveric donor rate from within all groups, particularly aspects relating to gaining consent from the bereaved.

Fear of increasing the distress of the family

Critical care staff have expressed fears that offering donation may increase the distress of the bereaved (Wakeford & Stepney 1989); however, experience suggests that offering the choice to donate, if performed with empathy, does not increase distress. Indeed, donor families report that the act of donation brings comfort and something positive in an otherwise negative situation (Buckley 1989). American and UK studies have noted that a fundamental need for relatives during a 'crisis time' is 'to feel there is hope' (Coulter 1989, Molter 1979, Wilkinson 1995). In the presence of a diagnosis of brain stem death there can be no hope for the patient but donation can be an option of hope with life for others.

Acceptance that death has occurred

It is crucial that the bereaved family have accepted the fact that death has occurred before donation is requested. In the case of brain stem death the acceptance of death is more difficult for the family as they are asked to accept a 'new concept of death'. The accepted concept and image of death involves a cold, lifeless body without a heartbeat; however, in the case of brain stem death the family are presented with an image of a warm patient with a heart beat who appears (due to the ventilator) to be breathing. Therefore, the visual message is one of life but the verbal message is one of death. In such cases denial is often enhanced and relatives must struggle to understand and accept the situation. Denial may be particularly acute in the case of an intracerebral bleed where there is no outward sign of injury or trauma.

Clear communications must ensue, the core message being that there is no hope of recovery. Irreparable damage has occurred and the brain has died—death of the brain stem is death of the person.

When to offer donation

It is damaging to approach the family too early, as trust may be lost. A recent study to examine the reasons for relatives' refusal (Mori/UKTCA/BACCN 1995) notes that a refusal may have been because the family were 'approached too early by inexperienced staff'. This study also reports that 'Consent for donation rates are higher in cases where the request is made after the second set of brain stem tests'. Furthermore, a study from the USA noted that relatives were more likely to agree to donation if the explanation of brain stem death and the request for organ donation were clearly separated in time (Garrison et al 1991). Thus it is important for the family to have accepted that death has occurred before donation is offered, also to inform the family of the death and to request donation at separate meetings.

Who should offer donation?

All studies report that the person who has established a trusting relationship with the family is the most appropriate person to offer donation. It is important that the requestee has a positive view of donation and can offer it in a positive way.

How to offer donation

There are no 'right' words; each situation is unique and families will have their own individual responses. The family should be asked if they have any objection to donation rather than for permission to proceed. Some families will require time to consider their decision. Many relatives will have additional questions concerning the process of donation and its implications at this time. It may be helpful for the family to meet with the transplant coordinator, who can answer specific questions. The family may require reassurance on the following issues:

- The donor will feel no pain.
- There will be dignity and respect throughout the donor surgery.
- The body will not be grossly mutilated or disfigured.
- The surgical wound will be sutured.
- They can view the body after surgery and the funeral will not be delayed.

The transplant coordinator will work closely with other healthcare professionals to answer further questions and to facilitate the wishes of the family. The coordinator can also reassure the family that he or she will be present throughout the surgery and at the end to oversee and continue care. The coordinator will ensure that the bereaved can see the deceased after surgery in the chapel of rest if this is their wish.

Unconditional gift

It is important to stress that organ donation is a voluntary 'unconditional gift.' A recent case, much publicised, reported that the bereaved had stated that the organs 'must only be given to white recipients'. Such a condition is totally unacceptable and there is now legislation which prohibits the placing of any conditions when agreeing to organ donations.

■ CASE STUDY 11.2

A 58-year-old female who had been investigated as a living donor for her son suddenly collapses from a subarachnoid haemorrhage 1 month before the planned transplant and is declared brain stem dead.

The family agree to cadaveric donation but stipulate that one kidney *must* be given to her son.

It is illegal to place this condition upon the donation.

Discussion question:
• Should the son receive one of the kidneys donated?

Continuing care after donation

Letters of thanks containing brief anonymous information concerning the transplant recipients are given or sent to the donor family after the donation. Further help and support are also offered. Many families state that the news of the successful transplants is a source of comfort. More recently, transplant coordinators have arranged meetings between donor families and recipients. Such meetings have been requested by both parties and have followed careful counselling and preparation to ensure the willingness of all individuals involved.

Refusal to donate

A study by Gore et al (1989) reported that approximately 30% of relatives of potential donors within intensive care units refused consent. The Mori/UKTCA/BACCN (1995) study also reports a 38% refusal rate. The five most common reasons given for refusal were:

• The relatives did not want surgery to the body (24%).
• The patient had stated in the past that donation was not to take place (21%).
• The relatives felt that the patient had suffered enough (21%).
• The relatives were divided over the decision (19%).
• The relatives were not sure whether the patient would have agreed to organ donation (18%).

Refusal rates of 30% represent a desperate lost potential. Therefore, it is vital that information programmes to allay fears and to present the successes of transplantation continue. It is also helpful to implement education for healthcare staff to examine the issue of requesting donation so that personnel will feel comfortable when offering this option of hope to the family.

Transplant coordinator groups have introduced workshops on breaking bad news and the approach for donation for nursing and medical colleagues working in intensive care and emergency departments. Such workshops utilise informed actors and provide a forum and a safe environment for staff to examine sudden traumatic death, the reactions of relatives and responses that will facilitate the approach for donation.

If the family agree to donation, the ventilation continues and the preparations for the donor surgery are made, but if the family refuse donation then ventilation will cease.

It is always helpful for the family if the deceased carried a donor card, was registered as a donor on the National Register or had discussed the issue with them. Most families want to fulfil the wishes of their loved one and if they know the thoughts of the deceased with regard to donation, then the question and decision are no longer difficult for them.

Clinical care of a potential organ donor

Brain stem death results in changes to normal homeostatic mechanisms; such changes will ultimately result in cardiac arrest. Once permission has been given for donation it is important to stabilise the condition of the donor to ensure optimal condition of the organs for transplantation. The care can be very complex and is outside the scope of this book; but further reading can be found in Novitzky (1998).

The role of the transplant coordinator

All renal transplant centres within the UK employ transplant coordinators. The transplant coordinators are senior practitioners (usually with a nursing background) who offer a 24-h service to intensive care units with regard to organ donation. The role of the transplant coordinator at the time of donation is to offer:

- advice regarding suitability of a potential organ donor
- advice regarding donor clinical care
- advice and/or help with the approach to relatives
- organisation of the organ donation procedure and surgery
- support of the family and staff.

Organisation of the organ donation procedure and surgery

The transplant coordinator will usually attend at the donor hospital to offer advice and support to the donor family and critical care staff. Organisation of the organ donation is complex and the transplant coordinator will attempt to make all arrangements with a minimum of distress to the donor family and the critical care staff. The majority of organ donations today are multiple donations and it is the transplant coordinator who organises the necessary blood and clinical tests, liaises with the heart, liver, renal and ophthalmic teams and arranges the donor surgery (Table 11.8).

Permission from the coroner

If the case comes under the jurisdiction of the coroner (or procurator fiscal in Scotland), then permission must be obtained to proceed to organ donation. Cases usually requiring the coroner's permission include:

- road traffic accident
- suspicious deaths/suicide
- deaths less than 12 h after surgery
- traumatic deaths.

Table 11.8 Organ donation: role of the transplant coordinator

Arrival at donor hospital
Meet with critical care staff
Assess potential donor suitability
Advice regarding donor clinical care (if requested)
Meet with donor family; offer advice and support (if requested)
Permission from the coroner or coroner's officer
Organise clinical tests and blood tests:

Clinical tests	Blood tests
12-lead ECG	ABO blood group
Chest X-ray	Biochemistry
Approx. size and weight of donor	• Urea and electrolytes
Arterial blood gases	• Liver function tests
	• Full blood count
	Virology screen
	• HIV
	• Hepatitis B and C
	• Cytomegalovirus
	• Toxoplasmosis
	• Syphilis

Contact UK Transplant re super-urgent cases
Liaise with heart, liver, renal and ophthalmic teams
Liaise with theatre staff and obtain theatre time:
  • Accompany donor to theatre
  • Assist surgical teams
  • Support theatre personnel
Final care of donor
Contact with donor family offering information and/or support
Information and thanks to donor hospital personnel

ECG, electrocardiogram; HIV, human immunodeficiency virus.

It is unusual for permission to be withheld except in the case of suspected murder.

Removal of kidneys from a multiorgan donor

It is most common now for kidneys to be taken out as part of an operation from a multiorgan donor. This requires careful coordination between the liver, renal and thoracic teams involved to make sure that there is no compromise to viability in any of the transplanted organs (Plates 2–4).

The exact details of the operation vary from centre to centre, but the principles include a generous incision giving good exposure to the organs of interest with the heart still beating, and placement of cannulae for in situ perfusion and cooling.

• A bilateral subcostal incision with a midline sternotomy is a common approach to the chest. The heart and lungs are inspected and mobilised first to allow rapid removal at a later stage.

• A careful laparotomy is carried out before dissection of the major blood supply to the liver. The common bile duct is transected and the gallbladder incised and flushed to prevent biliary autolysis.

- Cannulae are placed into the aorta and portal vein via the mesenteric vein for perfusion. The distal inferior vena cava is cannulated and used for vascular drainage. Ventilation ceases when the aorta is cross-clamped. Perfusion starts simultaneously to minimise warm ischaemia.
- The organs are removed; first, heart and lungs, followed by the liver and then the kidneys. Careful cooperation between teams is required to minimise damage to the various organs. The pancreas is used for transplantation with increasing success; concurrent retrieval with the above organs has not been associated with adverse outcome.

Before closure of the abdominal incisions, specimens of donor lymph nodes and spleen are removed for histocompatibility and tissue typing.

Surgical technique for cadaveric donor nephrectomy

If the kidneys are to be removed alone, bilateral nephrectomy is accomplished through a long midline incision or a bilateral subcostal incision. The kidneys are either taken out en bloc or individually on patches of inferior vena cava and aorta. The technique preferred in this centre entails the removal of an individual kidney on a patch of aorta and inferior vena cava. The technique is as follows:

- Abdominal incision and laparotomy are performed as for multiorgan retrieval.
- The aorta is dissected up to the superior mesenteric artery and the inferior vena cava dissected above the renal veins.
- Slings are placed around the aorta and the inferior vena cava above the bifurcation ready for tying at a later stage.
- A catheter is passed into the aorta through an incision just above the bifurcation. The balloon of the catheter is distended with fluid and ties placed around the aorta distal to the balloon to hold it in place. Care must be taken not to overdistend catheter balloons as this can obstruct the lumen of the catheter.
- A similar procedure is carried out with the inferior vena cava just above the confluence of the right and left common iliac veins, and the aorta and inferior vena cava below the catheters are tied off.
- The aorta is tied off in the upper abdomen and perfusion is started through the Foley catheter (Fig. 11.3). As perfusion starts, ventilation is discontinued.
- The kidneys begin to get cold at this stage and, while the perfusion fluid is running through into the kidneys and out through the renal veins, the kidneys should be surrounded by ice to assist cooling and prevent rewarming from the adjacent tissues.
- The inferior vena cava above the renal veins is ligated and the blood from the kidneys drains out through the catheter in the inferior vena cava.
- After 2 L of perfusion fluid has flushed through the kidneys and the kidneys are cold, they can be mobilised and the cannulae removed.

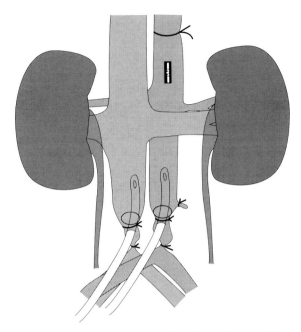

Figure 11.3 Perfusion catheters in situ for cadaveric donor nephrectomy.

• The inferior vena cava is split up the middle and along the back, taking care not to divide the right renal artery. The aorta is also divided anteriorly and posteriorly, taking care to avoid damaging the left renal vein which crosses in front of the aorta. Having done this, each kidney is taken out with a section of aorta, inferior vena cava and long length of ureter and placed in iced saline, where it is reflushed with preservation fluid.

• Normally, no further dissection is done at this stage, but the kidney is placed in sterile bags and sent at 4°C to the receiving centre. Further dissection of the kidney is performed immediately before subsequent transplantation into the recipient.

Following removal, each kidney is examined for any surgical injury and unusual anatomy and is placed in a sterile bag with a small amount of perfusion fluid. This bag is then placed inside two further polythene bags to ensure sterility. The kidney is finally packed into a transport container with ice.

Organ preservation

The aim of preservation is to maintain the organ in an optimal condition until transplantation can occur. All living cells require oxygen to survive. Once the blood supply to the organ ceases, the lack of oxygen will result in cellular ischaemia. Cooling the organ will reduce the cellular metabolism and thus help to minimise subsequent damage. Ischaemia that occurs before the organ is cooled is termed warm ischaemia.

Warm ischaemia

If the blood supply to the kidneys is interrupted without cooling, the tubular cells suffer warm ischaemia resulting in acute tubular necrosis (ATN). ATN may be reversible if the warm ischaemia time is limited (approx. 45 min). However, should the warm ischaemia extend longer than 1 h the glomeruli are likely to suffer irreversible damage and the kidney may not regain function. During cadaveric donation (heart-beating donation) the ventilation and blood supply continue until the perfusion system is in place. As perfusion with cooled fluid commences, the ventilation ceases. Thus, the kidney is immediately cooled and the warm ischaemia is limited to approximately 1–2 min only.

Cold ischaemia

The ice should maintain the kidney at approximately 4°C, thus minimising ischaemic damage and enabling transport to the transplant centre. The time from the beginning of cooling to reperfusion and rewarming at the time of transplantation is termed the cold ischaemia time. Most kidneys can be stored for 24–48 h if necessary. However, recent studies suggest that prolonged cold ischaemia does reduce the function of the transplant, particularly if the kidney is from an elderly donor. Therefore, most transplant centres transplant kidneys within 24 h of removal when possible.

LIVING RELATED DONATION

In the early days of transplantation, live related transplants were the only possible option but, with the advent of cadaveric donation from brain-dead donors and improved immunosuppression regimes, most centres concentrated, in the main, on cadaveric donation with fewer live donor transplants. This was due, in part, to the fact that some clinicians struggled with the ethical issue of subjecting a healthy and fit person to the risks of major surgery that had no personal benefit for them, albeit there would be benefit to their family member.

Ethical issues

The core factors of the living donation debate involve the critical issue of a balance between 'doing good without doing harm' and the concept of altruism.

Physical well-being—doing good without doing harm

The donation will most certainly 'do good' in benefiting the recipient but may also 'do harm' to the donor, as the surgical procedure exposes the living donor to major clinical risks. Mortality from living donor surgery is difficult to assess because the statistics are not confirmed; however, donor deaths have been reported. A figure of 1 in 2000 may be correct. Early postoperative complications may also occur and may include chest infection, deep vein thrombosis, wound infection and postsurgical depression amongst others. Long-term complications have not been demonstrated, with follow-up studies of living related donors, for as long as 20 years, finding no functional abnormalities. A major study undertaken by Najarian et al (1992) at the University of Minnesota followed living kidney donors for 20 years after donation by comparing renal function, blood pressure and proteinuria in donors with siblings ($n = 57$). The study conclusions found that the donor group had had no progressive rise in serum creatinine; the frequency of hypertension was not higher than in the general population or in sibling controls; and finally, that although 23% of these donors had proteinuria, so did 22% of their siblings. Such proteinuria was mild in most and not associated with hypertension or renal dysfunction. The study postulated that renal transplant donors were not at an increased risk of developing renal failure.

Psychological well-being—doing good without doing harm

Undoubtedly, many living donors gain psychologically from the act of giving. Studies suggest that donors describe the act 'as one of the most meaningful experiences in their lives' (Fellner & Marshall 1968) and 'view themselves as more worthwhile because of donation' (Simmons et al 1971). The satisfaction of helping a 'loved one' return to a normal lifestyle is very rewarding for many. Indeed, it has been suggested that there may be psychological harm if a donor is prevented from giving (Simmons et al 1977). Thus, living donation presents physical risks but psychological gain for the donor.

Altruism

Altruism—the act of unselfishness—means giving freely without thought of reward. Much debate has surrounded this concept, with writers in the 1960s and 70s questioning the fundamental reasons for giving. Kemph (1966) reported that although donors were 'consciously altruistic' there was 'considerable unconscious resentment' towards the recipient and towards hospital personnel who requested or encouraged the donation. Other studies suggested the presence of a degree of coercion or subtle familial pressure. There were also reports of financial incentives or other 'material rewards' offered by recipients to donors to encourage donation. Although many of these early studies involved small numbers of donors and recipients, the negative findings led many centres to pursue cadaveric options.

Later studies in the 1970s and the 1980s reported more positive psychological findings. Smith et al (1986) found that 97% of donors reaffirmed their decisions and fewer than 15% said that they felt pressurised to donate.

Such positive reports encouraged some centres to increase live donor programmes but many continued with a strong stance against it, mainly because of the physical risks to the donor. However, a study by Levey et al (1986) noted that the physical risks to the donor were 'minimal' and that the benefits to the donor were 'considerable' with regard to self-esteem and self-worth. Surman (1989) stated that 'kidney donation has a favourable outcome for both donor and recipient and that the participation of living related donors in kidney transplantation was now widely accepted'.

Studies in the 1990s have been supportive of live donation but have also noted psychological issues that may need to be addressed. Russel & Jacob (1994) reported that 'psychological side effects, namely donor depression and family conflict were noted but these risks were generally under-emphasised'. More recent studies have also reported positive findings. Jacobs et al (1998) investigated follow-up of 529 living donors who had donated between 1985 and 1996. Study conclusions noted that 'donors scored higher than the general population with regard to quality of life issues'. If given the opportunity only 4% of the donors said that they would not donate again and 9% were unsure.

Benefits for the transplant recipient

Although the ethical issues have been recognised and much debated, the decision to continue with living related donation has usually been based upon the very real benefits that ensue for the recipient. Living related donation has always demonstrated higher graft survival rates than cadaveric donation. Although recent advances in immunosuppression have narrowed the gap between the two groups (Fig. 11.4), in most cases the living related grafts still have a 10% better survival rate at 1 year and a significantly higher probability of function in the long term. The closer tissue match achieved with related donation usually results in fewer rejection episodes and a reduced amount of immunosuppression.

The living donation can be planned to take place at the most suitable time (medically and socially) for the recipient. As renal function deteriorates, transplantation can be planned for the predialysis phase, thus avoiding the physical and psychological stress of dialysis adjustments. Similarly, planning can minimise disruption to family and working patterns.

Such benefits have encouraged units to continue with living related donation. Indeed, with the increasing shortage of cadaveric organs, many centres are seeking to increase the numbers of living related grafts and are also considering living unrelated programmes.

Transplant rates

Living related donation programmes vary throughout the world. Norway has the highest rate, with 40% of the total transplant programme resulting

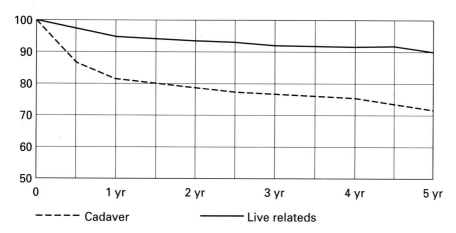

Figure 11.4 Cadaver allograft compared to live related allografts. Data from Oxford Transplant Centre 1984 to the present time.

from living donation. Sweden, the USA, Denmark and Greece also have relatively high rates. Until recently, the UK had a low rate with only 5% of the total transplant programme resulting from living related donation (Fig. 11.5).

However, with the positive results reported from both Norway and the USA in live related and live unrelated programmes, many UK centres have increased live donation. Indeed, transplant clinicians and the Department of Health are now actively promoting live donation (see Fig. 11.6).

Living unrelated donation (genetically unrelated—emotionally related)

In Norway, parents, siblings, adult children, uncles, aunts, grandparents and spouses are accepted as donors. Spouses are, of course, genetically unrelated but are recognised as 'emotionally related'. The Norwegian experience suggests that transplantation between spouses (partners) can achieve graft survival rates equal to the best achieved with cadaveric organs. Similar results for transplantation between partners have been reported in the USA (Terasaki et al 1995). Most UK centres are now utilising spousal/partner donors and also other donors, who have a demonstrable long-term relationship with the recipient, such as close friends. However, all centres stress that the donor must be well motivated and well informed and that the offer must be 'altruistic' and come from within a 'stable relationship'.

Buying and selling of organs

Living related and living unrelated transplantation in the UK is controlled by strict laws to prevent the possibility of illegal practices such as financial payments and coercion. The unrelated group are monitored by a government committee entitled ULTRA (Unrelated Live Transplant Regulatory

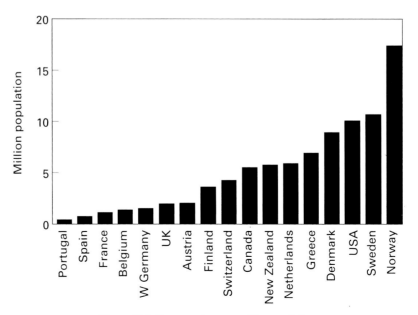

Figure 11.5 Live transplants per million population.

Kidney transplants and number of patients waiting for kidney transplant at year end 1991 – 2000 UK			
Year	Cadaveric transplants	Living donor transplants	Kidney waiting list
1991	1776	89	4113
1992	1772	100	4482
1993	1685	142	4830
1994	1749	135	4968
1995	1793	156	5241
1996	1643	183	5559
1997	1632	178	5734
1998	1524	250	5811
1999	1468	269	6045
2000	1487	336	6284

Figure 11.6 Live and cadaveric kidney transplants and number of patients waiting for kidney transplants. Statistics prepared by UK Transplant from the National Transplant Database maintained on behalf of Transplant Services in the UK and Republic of Ireland.

Authority). The aim of this body is to ensure that there is no reward or coercion and that a 'long-standing relationship' is evident between donor and recipient. At present, legislation precludes the use of altruistic donors who wish to give anonymously to the donor pool. Such donors are being utilised in the USA and New Zealand and at present discussions are taking place with regard to the possibility of such altruistic donations occurring in the UK.

The buying and selling of organs does occur in some of the developing countries and is an accepted practice. Indeed, some clinicians have suggested that a similar system, strictly controlled by legislation, could be introduced in the UK to increase transplant rates. The ethical and moral ramifications would be immense and at present such a concept is illegal and totally unacceptable to most.

Donor and recipient matching

Individual tissue type is inherited as half from each parent. Therefore, matching within a nuclear family unit will result in a potential donor who is HLA-identical, a one-haplotype match or a mismatch.

Immunological aspects (example as for donor-related (DR) matching)

Matching for the MHC will take place, however. Figure 11.7 demonstrates tissue-type inheritance using the DR locus.

Therefore, potential donors may be:

- HLA-identical, as with DR1:3 (siblings)
- a one-haplotype match, as with DR1:3 and DR1:8 (siblings)
- DR1:4 and DR1:3 (parent–child)
- unmatched, as with DR1:3 and DR4:8 (siblings).

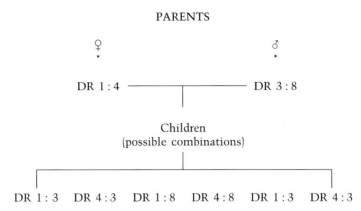

Figure 11.7 An example of tissue-type inheritance.

The results of HLA-identical and one-haplotype matches demonstrate higher graft survival rates than cadaveric transplants. Therefore, parents and siblings are usually the most suitable living donors from a tissue-matching perspective. Donor and recipient must also be matched from an ABO blood group perspective.

Parents are usually very willing to donate but siblings may be ambivalent and experience a crisis of loyalties between the family of birth and the family of marriage.

Psychological issues

The question of the possibility of living related donation may bring unity to a family group but it may also bring conflict. Parents will often offer early in the disease process and are extremely well motivated, but problems can arise if one parent is 'more suitable' due to tissue matching or physical constraints. The 'less suitable' parent may feel rejected and excluded from the donation and transplant process.

Siblings may be willing or ambivalent and it may be difficult to express ambivalent feelings because of societal concepts of family loyalty and love. A sibling of a patient has expressed the wish that 'the request had never been made, as once verbalised it was impossible to refuse without feeling enormous guilt'. Married siblings may wish to donate but may encounter hostility from their partner who feels that the risks are too great and that responsibilities to the family of marriage are more important than loyalty to the family of birth.

Ongoing psychological support is a necessary part of a living donor programme. Donor and recipient must be well informed concerning the risks and benefits and also the psychological difficulties that may develop. Separate meetings, both for the donor and the recipient, with medical staff and nurse/counsellor should be planned so that feelings, fears and anxieties can be discussed with honesty. The motivation to donate should be explored and, if appropriate, the donor offered the opportunity to withdraw without guilt or family conflict.

Similarly, the decision to receive should be explored and the recipient offered the opportunity to refuse. Several patients at this centre have refused living donation, preferring to wait for cadaveric grafts so as not to 'inflict my disease on my family'. The dynamics of the donor and recipient relationship must be well understood so that help and advice may be offered if difficulties arise.

Assessment and preparation of donors

The living donor must be:

- well motivated
- in excellent health with two normal kidneys and normal renal function
- compatible for blood group and tissue match with the recipient.

The assessment and preparation for living donation are extensive and normally carried out in stages over several weeks or months. Different centres will conduct tests at different stages but most units complete the same catalogue of tests in order to ensure that the criteria are fulfilled. Usually the assessment involves three stages. At each stage the donor meets with medical staff and the nurse counsellor. Various tests are grouped together for each visit, thus minimising the disruption to the donor's working and personal life. Prior to stage 1, the donor will have received written information regarding the risks and benefits and the pre- and postoperative experiences. Preliminary blood grouping and tissue typing may have occurred before the stage 1 visit (if not, they will be completed during this visit).

Stage 1

The donor and recipient and other family members are invited to the transplant centre to meet with the transplant surgeon and the nurse counsellor. At this meeting the risks and benefits are explored, as are the forthcoming tests and the pre-, peri- and postsurgery experiences.

The donor and recipient have the opportunity to meet separately with the nurse counsellor alone, so that individual thoughts and anxieties can be explored in privacy. This is also an opportunity to explore the donor–recipient relationship. Such meetings help to initiate a trusting relationship with the nurse counsellor so that support can be available throughout the experience.

Assessment at stage 1

- Age: the donor must be above the age of consent and below the age of 70–75 years (age limits may vary in specific circumstances). The assessment criteria is for physical health rather than chronological age.
- Informed consent: the donor must be able to understand the risks that may ensue.
- Preliminary medical history: hypertension, if severe or of long-standing, untreated diabetes and other problems that would suggest anaesthetic risk to the donor may prevent donation.
- Renal disease: familial renal disease may exclude from donation.
- Smoking: smokers in our centre are asked to stop prior to donation because of increased anaesthetic risks. They are also referred for lung function tests if smoking has been heavy over a prolonged period of time.

- Drug or alcohol abuse: this is investigated fully and may preclude from donation.
- Obesity: donors who have an unacceptable body mass index (BMI) will be asked to reduce weight prior to surgery.
- Blood and clinical tests: taken at visit 1 stage 1 (Box 11.3).

If the initial assessments are satisfactory and the donor still wishes to donate, further tests are completed prior to a medical assessment which should be performed by a nephrologist who is not responsible for the recipient (Boxes 11.4 and 11.5).

If the results of the tests and the medical evaluation are satisfactory, the donor assessment will proceed to stage 4. Stage 4 includes glomerular filtration rate (GFR) estimation, renal angiography and dimercaptosuccinie acid (DMSA).

Throughout the assessment programme the donor is assured that it is possible to retract the offer to donate at any time. Such a decision will be strictly confidential and support and advice will be available. If the donor wishes, a medical reason not to donate can be provided. This medical reason is seen within the context of a 'benevolent decision' to enable the donor to retract without family conflict or distress, thus promoting full

---

■ **BOX 11.3 Stage 1 donor blood and clinical tests**

- Blood group
- Tissue typing: T- and B-cell cross -match
- Urea, electrolytes, creatinine
- Liver function tests: fasting glucose
- Haemoglobin and clotting screen
- Viral screen
- Urine tests (midstream urine and urinalysis)
- Blood pressure, pulse, weight and height

■ **BOX 11.4 Investigations at stage 2 prior to medical assessment**

Blood tests
- Repeat tissue typing
- Urea and electrolytes ⎫ two readings of these tests are preferable at
- Liver function test ⎬ stages 1 and 2
- Haematology ⎭

Clinical tests
- Chest X-ray
- Electrocardiogram
- Ultrasound scan of renal system

Urine tests
- Midstream urine, urinalysis, 24-h urine (× 2) for creatinine clearance

---

■ **BOX 11.5 Stage 3: medical assessment**

The nephrologist in this centre will meet with the donor and ascertain that the donor is well informed, able to consent, really motivated and altruistic. He/she will tell the donor that he/she is 'their doctor and their advocate'. He/she will then proceed to anwer three critical questions:

1. Is the donation safe for the recipient?
2. Is the donor fit for a nephrectomy?
3. Can the donor afford the gift?

Is the donation safe for the recipient?
Assessment of:

• Donor infection
• Donor age, blood pressure
• Donor—exclude history of cancer
• Donor kidney function

Is the donor fit for a nephrectomy?
To establish donor health, an in-depth medical history will be taken and a physical examination completed, paying specific attention to the following issues:

• General health and past medical history, especially cardiac and respiratory
• Anaesthetic and bleeding history
• Thrombosis history/oral contraceptive (the donor will be asked to stop contraceptive 3 months before surgery)
• Drugs, alcohol and smoking
• Allergies
• Specific evaluation for undeclared cancer, hypertension, cardiac disease, respiratory disease, risk of deep vein thrombosis
• Anatomically safe: how many arteries?

Can the donor afford the gift?
• Is the blood pressure acceptable? (Any hypertensive damage should exclude the donor)
• Is renal function normal for age and gender?
• Is the 24-h urine protein < 300 mg?
• Is the fasting glucose normal?
• Is there a risk of renal disease in later life?

---

altruism. Other centres have reported using such a technique successfully within their programmes (Hilton & Starzomski 1994).

Once the tests are completed the donor and partner will meet with the nurse counsellor and the surgical team that will be performing the nephrectomy. The nurse counsellor can further explore any fears and anxieties and can fully outline the pre- and postoperative procedures. The surgeon can give details of the kidney to be removed and size and placing of surgical scar.

Two separate surgical teams are usually involved with a living related donation. The donor team assume responsibility for donor care and the transplant team take responsibility for recipient care. In this centre, the donor and recipient are both nursed within the transplant centre in separate rooms. However, they may be nursed together if they so wish, if there are language or other difficulties.

The recipient will also be offered the opportunity to meet the nurse counsellor and the transplant surgeon to discuss pre- and postoperative care and any specific fears and anxieties. The recipient clinical preparation will be completed as outlined above. Providing all the assessment tests are satisfactory, the preoperative assessment for both donor and recipient will occur in the week before surgery (Box 11.6).

The donor and recipient are usually admitted on the day before transplant and at this stage a further medical history and physical examination will be performed, along with an anaesthetic and physiotherapist assessment.

Preoperative care for the donor

The immediate preoperative care for the living donor will be similar to that given to patients undergoing conventional nephrectomy. However, particular attention is paid to informed consent, preoperative hygienic care and premedication.

Surgical technique of nephrectomy

Living related donor nephrectomy is always emotionally taxing surgery and can be technically difficult. The estimated mortality from living related donor nephrectomy is 1 in 2000. Thus, while very rare, the risks are certainly not negligible and major morbidity or death is very traumatic not only for the relatives but for the members of the surgical team themselves.

The two approaches for removing a kidney from a live donor are either transabdominal, intraperitoneal, or via the loin over the 11th or 12th rib, either spreading or removing the 11th or 12th rib. The intraabdominal approach is usually through a transverse incision in the right or left upper quadrant.

■ **BOX 11.6 Stage 4: preoperative assessment of donor and recipient**

Blood tests
• Final cross match and tissue typing
• Methicillin-resistant swabs (throat, nose, axilla, groin) *Staphylococcus aureus*
• Midstream urine, urinalysis
• Biochemistry
• Liver function tests
• Haematology and clotting screen
• Electrocardiogram, blood pressure, pulse, temperature
• Chest X-ray

Preoperative dialysis plan for the recipient will be agreed, if required

The kidney may be approached via the abdominal cavity (transperitoneal) or from the loin (extraperitoneal). The kidney is carefully exposed and meticulous dissection is carried out with careful handling of the kidney and careful exposure of the renal vein and artery. The gonadal and adrenal tributaries of the renal vein are ligated and divided and often a posterior lumbar vein needs ligating and dividing as well.

The renal artery is cleaned and exposed at its junction with the aorta and the ureter is identified and dissected down to the pelvic brim or just below, where it is ligated and divided. It is very important to avoid too much dissection in the hilum of the kidney and it is also essential to avoid stripping the ureter of its adventitia. The blood supply to the ureter normally comes from the renal artery, branches from the gonadal vessels and the external iliac artery and branches of the superior vesicle artery. In a transplant kidney the blood supply to the ureter is entirely dependent on the renal artery and it is essential to keep a good amount of adventitia around the ureter to allow the blood to reach the distal ureter. One of the major complications after transplantation is ischaemia of the lower end of the ureter and this is normally due to stripping of the ureter at the time of the donor surgery.

When the kidney is free and attached just by the artery and the vein, the artery is ligated and divided first, followed by the vein. The kidney is removed and placed in iced saline where perfusion is started immediately and, after careful inspection, any further dissection is carried out and a renal biopsy is taken.

Postoperative management: living donor
The postoperative care for the living donor is similar to the care given for a conventional nephrectomy. Nephrectomy is recognised as painful surgery requiring frequent analgesia in the early postoperative phase. In most centres, patient-controlled analgesia using an opiate is utilised.

Hydration: fluid and electrolyte balance
Paralytic ileus may occur as a result of the retroperitoneal dissection and the handling of the bowel. Therefore, the intake of oral fluids must commence slowly and only increase as ileus resolves and bowel sounds are evident. In practice, hydration is maintained by intravenous infusion for the first 24–48 h until oral intake is sufficient. Close monitoring of fluid and electrolyte balance is necessary until dietary intake is adequate.

The passing of urine may prove difficult due to the pain of movement and anxiety, so often a urinary catheter is inserted under anaesthetic so that urinary output can be closely monitored and pain minimised. The catheter is usually removed on the second postoperative day. Regular midstream urine specimens should be obtained for microscopy, culture and sensitivity during hospitalisation. Monitoring of urine output is important to determine the function of the remaining kidney.

Wound management
Wound management should include regular inspection to exclude complications of bleeding and infection.

Emotional support

During the early postoperative period, emotional support should be offered, as should frequent information regarding the progress of the recipient. Donor and recipient should be reunited at the earliest opportunity and encouraged to spend time together. The donor may experience a feeling of anticlimax after the surgery due to a release of the preoperative tension and anticipation. Such anticlimax may combine with postanaesthetic 'blues' to form a mild depression with emotional lability. Staff should recognise the altruism of the act and offer understanding and reassurance.

Discharge

The majority of living donors will be discharged between the fourth and fifth postoperative day. It is recommended that they continue their postoperative recovery at home for approximately 6 weeks to 2 months. Return to work will be variable depending on type of employment and its physical and psychological demands. Physical monitoring may include two further assessments by the surgical team.

Most centres now monitor donors at 1 year postdonation and then long-term care is referred to the general practitioner who may assess renal function and physical health annually. Emotional support should continue as appropriate, with help available if difficulties arise (UK Guidelines for Living Donor Kidney Transplantations 2000 prepared by the working party of the British Transpant Society and Renal Association: obtainable from British Transplantation Society Secretariat, Triangle House, Broomhill Road, London SW18 4HX).

Laparoscopic donor nephrectomy

The advent of laparoscopic surgery has introduced the possibility of laparoscopic donor nephrectomy. Transplant centres in the USA started this type of donor surgery in 1995 and are now reporting the results of their experience. Several centres in the UK have also commenced laparoscopic donor nephrectomy: at this time Leicester has the greatest experience.

Donor mortality and morbidity rates

Montgomery & Ratner (2001), from the Johns Hopkins University Hospital, Maryland, USA, report 200 laparoscopic donor procedures without a mortality. They also state that they 'are not aware of any donor mortalities associated with the procedure although it is alleged that they have occurred'. Furthermore, they state that the laparoscopic donor complication rate was significantly less when compared with the open donor surgery group (9% versus 22.2%).

Further reports from another centre compared their first 70 laparoscopic donors with a historic open nephrectomy group and found comparable morbidity rates (Flowers et al 1997). These two groups conclude that 'in centres with a large experience and expertise in advanced laparoscopic techniques, the donor operation can be performed safely and without excess morbidity'. However, most UK surgeons remain ambivalent and believe that the transperitoneal approach for the open operation has less morbidity than has been previously reported. Further larger studies are necessary before true comparisons can be drawn between the two techniques.

Advantages to the donor

The laparoscopic donor studies suggest that the advantages to the donor include 'reduction in the operative blood loss, reduction in postoperative pain, reduction in length of hospitalisation and a speedier recovery in relation to normal activities and return to work'.

Risks to the kidney transplant

There have been some reported problems with the kidneys retrieved via laparoscopic techniques. However, after several refinements to the surgical technique, the Montgomery & Ratner study (2001) reports that 'the kidney that is produced by the laparoscopic donor nephrectomy can be transplanted using standard techniques without excess recipient morbidity and has equivalent short-term and long-term function as that achieved by open nephrectomy'.

For further reading and explicit diagrams showing the laparoscopic surgical technique, refer to Morris (2001).

INCREASING DONOR ORGAN SUPPLY

As stated earlier, cadaveric organ donor rates and kidney transplant rates in the UK have remained fairly constant during the last 10 years. Such rates are insufficient to meet demand and the renal transplant waiting list has risen to 5750 and continues to rise. If the renal transplant rate continues at approximately 1700 per year, many hopeful dialysis patients will be denied their 'treatment of choice' (Fig. 11.1). Extending the living related and unrelated programmes will increase the supply of kidneys, livers and in some cases lungs for transplantation but it is crucial that the UK explores and introduces alternative initiatives to increase the cadaveric organ supply.

A document released in June 2000 by the British Medical Association highlights the inability of the current system of organ donation to meet the increasing demand and outlines various ways of overcoming the difficulties by increasing the availability of organs for transplantation. This report believes that a multifaceted approach is needed. One way is to have more direct appeals for people to register as potential donors by:

- addressing common concerns and misconceptions
- facilitating registration on the National Health Service organ donor register.

Also, the British Medical Association suggests improvements to the UK transplant coordination system and infrastructure by:

- placing 'key donation' personnel in every hospital. These personnel will work with the regional coordinators
- adoption of required referral, whereby all staff routinely refer any suitable patient who has died to the transplant coordination service
- developing a national transplant coordination service, with an increase in the number of transplant coordinators

- the establishment of additional critical care beds
- making the list of criteria for exclusion of patients as potential organ donors less restrictive.

These suggested changes are, in part, based upon the very successful Spanish organ donation system (Table 11.9).

As can be seen from Table 11.9, Spain has 31.5 cadaveric donors per million population, compared to only 13.5 cadaveric donors per million in the UK and Ireland.

In 1989 the official agency for transplantation in Spain, the National Transplant Organisation, created a national network of specially trained, dedicated and strongly motivated hospital physicians to take charge of the whole process of organ donation in 139 hospitals. The aim of these appointments was to improve:

- detection of potential organ donors
- management of the donors
- approach to the family
- the support of the mass media and to reimburse hospitals adequately for the expenses that result from donor care and donor surgery.

Results of the Spanish initiatives show that cadaveric organ donors rose from 550 in 1989 to 1334 in 1999—a 42% increase. This increase was sustained in 2000. The rates of cadaveric organ donation per million inhabitants (31.5) are the highest in the world, and patients on the Spanish waiting list have the best chance of receiving an organ (Fig. 11.8).

The British Medical Association report also lists the following initiatives to increase the numbers of donors:

- increasing the pool of living donation (related and unrelated donors)
- increasing the numbers of non heart beating donors, i.e. patients who die of cardiac arrest, in general wards, accident and emergency or intensive care, who may donate liver and kidneys a short period after death
- introducing presumed consent (opt-out).

Asystolic donation (non-heart-beating)

An initiative at the Leicester General Hospital has suggested that asystolic (non-heart-beating) donation could become an increasingly important source of renal organs. Since 1992, Leicester has identified asystolic donors in the medical wards and the accident and emergency department of the

Table 11.9 International data on organ donation and transplantation in 1998

	France	Greece	Hungary	Italy	Spain	Switzerland	UK and Ireland	USA
Population × 10⁶	60.02	10	10.3	58	39.66	7	62.71	268
Cadaveric donors per million population	16.5	5.7	12.2	12.3	31.5	15.4	13.5	21.6

Statistics taken from data from the Council of Europe (1999).

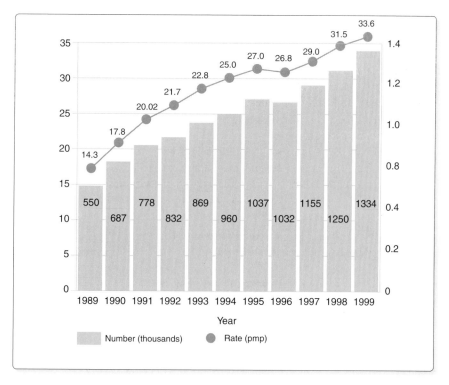

Figure 11.8 Organ donors in Spain: total number and annual rate per million population (pmp). (Statistics supplied by the Spanish National Transplantation Organisation (ONT).)

local hospital. At the time of asystole and following certification of death (providing that there are no medical contraindications to donation), an intraaortic catheter is inserted and ice-cold perfusion of the kidneys commenced. Such perfusion reduces the warm ischaemic damage and allows time for medical/nursing colleagues to approach the family and the coroner for permission to proceed to donation. If permission is granted the kidneys must be removed within 40–45 min of asystole in order to avoid irreversible renal damage.

Ethical concerns about the insertion of the catheter before consent has been given by the family were widely discussed during the planning of this programme and health personnel, the coroner and the general public groups that were consulted gave consent to this initiative. However, following the recent widely reported problems with organ retention after postmortem without family consent that occurred at Alder Hey and other hospitals, it has been decided by the Leicester group that they must now obtain consent before insertion of the intraaortic catheter. This decision will undoubtedly affect the length of time between asystole and cold perfusion of the kidneys.

Interestingly, initial results suggest a marginally higher rate of relative consent in asystolic donation than is usually achieved in brain stem death donation. This may be due to the skill of the staff requesting and also the fact that with asystole the patient appears 'dead' in the conventional sense (cold, pale and cyanosed), thus there may be less psychological denial for the family.

Other centres have introduced asystolic donation programmes and it is hoped that they will provide a useful additional supply of kidneys. However, the limiting factors will be the need for a rapid response time from the retrieval teams and the need for catheter insertion expertise. Such factors may preclude donation from hospitals that are some distance away from the transplant centre.

Opting in/opting out

Within the UK the general public are encouraged to 'opt in' by making the voluntary decision to donate organs. This decision is supported by carrying a donor card and informing relatives of this wish. Thus, donation is a voluntary gift.

Research suggests that approximately 75% of the general public support donation but only 30% carry a donor card. The reluctance to sign and carry a donor card may be due to the fact that death remains a taboo subject within our society and also that many are somewhat superstitious and feel that signing a card may somehow be 'tempting fate'. Furthermore, few of us wish to consider our own mortality.

Additional problems with this system are that in practice, the donor card may not be available at the time of death, or relatives may either be unaware of the donor's wishes or may choose to ignore them. Several groups, mainly patient groups, have pressed for the introduction of an 'opting-out' system, whereby everyone is deemed to wish to donate unless they have registered an objection. The opting-out system has been introduced in Europe (namely Austria and Belgium), and appears to be successful. However, with a true opting-out system the wishes of the family are not considered. At present it is felt by the major health groups in the UK that the denial of the family's wishes is unacceptable practice. Therefore, the government has decided to continue to support opting-in with the introduction of a new national registry, whereby those wishing to donate can register their wishes on to the national computer. The computer can be accessed by critical care staff should death occur. However, relatives will still be asked for consent.

The British Medical Association suggests that by adopting a presumed consent (softer opt-out option), close relatives would not be asked to give permission but rather informed that the individual had not registered an objection. Unless the family object, the donation will proceed and this donation becomes a default position.

Additional areas that the British Medical Association suggests require further consideration include:

- elective ventilation
- paired living kidney exchange.

Elective ventilation

A protocol for increasing organ donation after cerebrovascular death was implemented in the early 1990s (Feest et al 1990), and this protocol stated that 'patients fulfilling the criteria as potential organ donors could be identified on the medical wards; once identified, the relatives could be approached with regard to donation and if permission was given, the patient moved to intensive care for ventilation to facilitate donation'. (This practice became widely known as 'elective ventilation'.) The programme proved successful and in 19 months the hospital reported eight such donations. It was suggested that these results, if replicated throughout the UK, would greatly increase the numbers of donor organs.

However, a legal ruling in 1993 described the act of elective ventilation as 'unlawful' as 'the ventilation was deemed not to have been initiated for the benefit of the patient' (New et al 1994). With the advent of this ruling the elective ventilation programmes were discontinued, but discussions regarding the ethical and legal issues continue in the hope that solutions may be found.

Paired living kidney exchange

Paired living kidney exchange is an exchange system whereby a donor who is incompatible with the intended recipient could donate a kidney to another person whose own donor would provide a kidney in return. Such exchanges have taken place in the USA and south America but to perform these transplants in the UK would require a change in ULTRA guidelines. A special advisory committee has been formed at the Department of Health to prepare recommendations for ministers to seek amendments to the Transplant Act so that paired living kidney exchange could commence in specific designated hospitals.

Conclusions

The British Medical Association recommendations were welcomed by all transplant groups and it is hoped that these innovations will indeed increase donation rates, but it is feared that with the growing waiting lists the demand may always outstrip supply. The solution in the long term may be the introduction of xenotransplantation. (For further reading and to receive a copy of the British Medical Association *Organ Donation Review 2000*, visit www.bma.org.co.uk.)

Xenotransplantation (transplant of animal organs into humans)

To debate all the ethical, moral and practical issues regarding the use of other species for transplantation is beyond the scope of this book. However, from a biological viewpoint, closely related non-human primates such as chimpanzees would be the most preferable for transplantation, since there is no hyperacute rejection problem. However, it has been universally agreed that such species would be ethically unacceptable and impractical since they are endangered species, and dangerous to use because of the possibility of viral transfer or similar disasters. For practicality, the acceptable species would be those in current large-scale usage for food production, such as the pig.

The most obvious and immediate problem confronting the use of xenografts is the problem of hyperacute rejection. Connection of a suitably prepared pig kidney to the blood circulation of a dialysis patient initially results in normal perfusion of the kidney, which becomes pulsatile and pink and may even briefly produce urine. However, within minutes the pulsatility of the kidney lessens, and then ceases, the kidney becoming initially blue and finally almost black as the circulation ceases due to thrombosis. This typical pattern of rapid graft failure was initially described in human kidney allografts and was termed hyperacute rejection. The cause was subsequently shown to be the presence in the recipient of high-titre antibody against the donor tissue, binding the antibody causing complement activation and subsequent activation of the clotting cascade. Blood group ABO incompatibility was a potent source of antidonor antibody that was easily avoided, but some cases of hyperacute rejection still occurred, even after blood group matching. In the case of human allografts it was possible to avoid this fairly rare occurrence by testing for the presence of antidonor antibody and avoiding transplantation when antibody was detected. However, in the case of xenotransplantation between distantly related species, antibody is always detectable despite matching for blood groups, and this antibody came to be known as heterophile or natural antibody.

Two fundamental recent discoveries are the basis for a number of new approaches to prevent xenograft hyperacute rejection, for example by blocking or removing the natural antibody or infusing human complement regulatory proteins. The recent advent of transgenic manipulation has also allowed the concept of developing herds of animals which express high levels of human complement regulatory proteins on their cells. Research is moving so rapidly that already herds of transgenic pigs have been produced and organs from these pigs are undergoing preclinical experimental studies with partially encouraging results.

It now seems likely that combinations of the above approaches will eventually allow transplantation of organs between species such as pigs and humans, avoiding destruction of the graft by hyperacute rejection. However, this is likely to be only the first of several barriers to successful xenograft usage. Other barriers include the processes of cellular rejection that may well be entirely different to those seen in allograft rejection, the problem of species compatibility for crucial molecular and biochemical pathways and, of course, the animal rights movement which promotes heated debate on the moral acceptability of xenotransplantation.

For further information regarding xenotransplantation, refer to Soin & Friend (2001).

PREOPERATIVE MANAGEMENT FOR A RENAL TRANSPLANT RECIPIENT

The transplant call

Transplant recipients report mixed reactions of relief, excitement, anxiety and sadness when they receive the transplant phone call—relief that the waiting time may be over; excitement for the new life ahead; anxiety that the surgery may be difficult or that the transplant may fail; and sadness that a family elsewhere has experienced tragedy in order for the kidney to become available (Dubovsky & Penn 1980).

During the telephone conversation the recipient is informed that a transplant may be possible and to travel to the transplant centre and have nothing further to eat or drink. Brief questions are also asked to clarify current health status and to exclude any infections or other problems that may prevent transplantation.

Some centres contact two recipients for each transplant so that should a positive cross-match occur for one, a second recipient is already prepared, thus minimising the cold ischaemia time. It has been found that contacting two recipients can lead to repeated disappointments, anger and depression, therefore it is preferable to only call one recipient to the transplant centre in the first instance.

Nursing admission

Upon arrival, the recipient and family are welcomed by the nursing team and helped to familiarise themselves with the unit. Brief information is given regarding the forthcoming blood and clinical tests; questions are answered and anxieties explored during the nursing admission procedure (Box 11.7).

Medical assessment

Immediate medical assessment and blood tests are required to assess fluid and electrolyte status (as dialysis may be needed prior to surgery), also to complete the final tissue typing cross-match test, and therefore the medical assessment immediately follows the nursing admission procedure (Box 11.8).

Preoperative dialysis

The results of the medical assessment and blood tests will determine the need for dialysis. Fluid overload and electrolyte imbalance (particularly hyperkalaemia) must be corrected, as they represent an anaesthetic risk and may enhance posttransplantation difficulties.

Haemodialysis with minimal or no heparinisation is often necessary to ensure optimal weight and to reduce fluid overload and serum potassium levels.

■ **BOX 11.7 Nursing admission procedure**

- Blood pressure, pulse, temperature, respirations
- Current weight: dry weight
- Past medical history—renal disease
- Dialysis history—current practice and date and time of last dialysis
- Current health status—recent relevant health events (i.e. blood transfusion/ infections)
- Normal urine output, if any
- Social information
- Allergies
- Name band applied

■ **BOX 11.8 Medical assessment procedure**

- Medical history
- Renal disease history
- Dialysis history
- Current health status—recent relevant events
- Allergies
- Medical examination
- Blood tests:
  - —Urea and electrolytes
  - —Liver function tests
  - —Tissue typing cross-match
  - —Viral screen (as in pretransplant assessment)
  - —Cross-match for 2–4 units of blood available for transplant surgery
- Clinical tests:
  - —Chest X-ray
  - —Electrocardiogram
  - —Midstream specimen of urine, urinalysis

Chronic ambulatory peritoneal dialysis patients may require rapid exchanges to achieve optimal fluid and electrolyte status. The peritoneal catheter exit site should be examined for any signs of infection and a swab taken for culture and sensitivity. Also, following the necessary exchanges the catheter should be drained and a fluid specimen sent for microscopy culture and sensitivity and then the catheter capped, leaving the patient empty of fluid.

Information and emotional support

During the dialysis time, it is often possible to explore individual fears and anxieties and offer emotional support and information regarding postoperative medications and procedures. Recipients are often emotionally labile at this time ('tears and laughter') and require much emotional understanding and support.

Immediate preoperative care

It is usual for the physiotherapist to visit to commence chest physiotherapy and advise regarding postoperative mobility and for the anaesthetist to perform an assessment. Once the tissue typing cross-match has proved negative, the final preoperative preparation begins (Box 11.9).

SURGICAL TECHNIQUE FOR RENAL TRANSPLANTATION

Before transplantation begins, a catheter is placed into the bladder. This allows drainage of the bladder during the transplant operation and also allows the bladder to be filled with solution containing antibiotics to

---

■ **BOX 11.9 Preoperative preparation**

- Skin swabs/nose, throat, axilla and groin swabs—for viral, bacterial and methicillin-resistant *Staphylococcus aureus* screening
- Swabs and dressings to other dialysis lines (i.e. permanent central venous catheters)
- Suppositories (if required)
- Bath/shower/hair wash
- Operation gown
- Marking and dressing (to protect) arteriovenous fistula from inadvertent use of invasive monitoring (e.g. intravenous lines, blood pressure cuffs) and to maintain warmth, thus avoiding clotting
- Anti thrombosis stockings

Preoperative medications
- Ciclosporin
- Azathioprine
- Prednisolone
- Aspirin (unless contraindicated)

Note: Transplant centres may use differing combinations of immunosuppressive medications.

Medications given immediately preoperatively
- Premedication
- Diabetes mellitus: sliding-scale insulin as appropriate

---

facilitate later identification of the bladder for reimplantation of the ureter. The right or left iliac fossa is the normal site for the transplant (Fig. 11.9).

- An incision is made curving from just above the pubic symphysis to just above the iliac crest.
- The inferior epigastric vessels are ligated and divided and an extraperitoneal approach is made down on to the iliac vessels.
- The external iliac artery and vein are freed and small branches or over-lying lymphatics are ligated and divided.
- Clamps are applied to the external iliac vein and the renal vein is anastomosed to the external iliac vein with continuous 5.0 Prolene sutures.
- Clamps are then applied to the external iliac artery and the renal artery on its patch (known as the Carrell patch) is anastomosed with continuous 5.0 Prolene to the external iliac artery (Fig. 11.10). Sometimes the internal iliac artery is used and an end-to-end anastomosis is performed.
- Once the anastomoses are complete, the clamps are released, taking the venous clamps off first. The kidney normally perfuses quickly and one is often able to see immediate urine production.
- The bladder is then filled through the catheter and the ureter put into the bladder and then tunnelled submucosally to prevent urinary ureteric

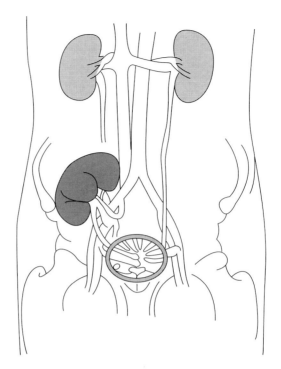

Figure 11.9 Position for the transplant kidney.

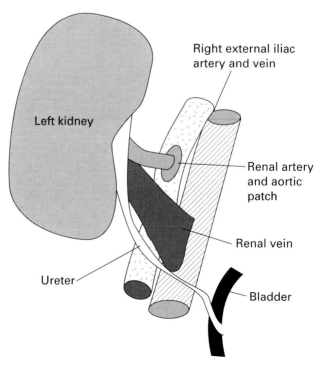

Figure 11.10 The surgical technique for renal transplantation.

reflux (the Leadbetter–Politano technique). Most centres may use an extra vesicle technique which involves splitting the muscle, laying the ureter just above the bladder mucosa and so into the bladder, and closing the muscle over the top. If the bladder has been opened it is closed with two layers of Vicryl. Many units are now using ureteric stents, which are left in situ for 6 weeks. This practice has reduced the incidence of ureteric complications.

• The wound is closed in the usual fashion and the bladder washed out at the end of the procedure.

RENAL TRANSPLANT REJECTION

There are three types of renal transplant rejection:

• hyperacute rejection
• acute rejection
• chronic rejection.

Hyperacute rejection

Hyperacute rejection (Fig. 11.11) occurs rapidly, within minutes or hours of revascularisation of the transplant. It is caused by:

• the presence of preformed cytotoxic antibodies in the recipient's blood (resulting from previous failed transplants, blood transfusions or pregnancies) reacting against the donor's histocompatibility antigens
• ABO incompatibility between the donor and the recipient.

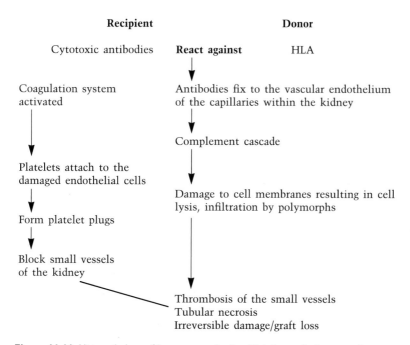

Figure 11.11 Histopathology of hyperacute rejection. HLA, human leukocyte antigen.

The final lymphocytotoxic cross-match prior to transplant should demonstrate that cytotoxic antibodies are present and transplantation should not take place, thus a hyperacute rejection is a very rare phenomenon today.

Hyperacute rejection may be observed during the transplant surgery. Instead of the kidney becoming distended and pink as the arterial and venous clamps are released, as is usual, with hyperacute rejection the kidney will remain flaccid and become blue. Damage is almost always irreversible and the graft is lost.

Acute rejection

Acute rejection (Fig. 11.12) is usually a combination of cellular and antibody-medicated rejection which commonly occurs between 4 days and 2 months after transplantation. The clinical signs of acute rejection may include:

- pyrexia
- renal dysfunction
- weight gain
- fall in urine output
- swelling and tenderness of the transplant
- ankle oedema
- flu-like symptoms.

Acute rejection can usually be controlled by increased immunosuppression; however, a severe rejection may result in some loss of overall graft function.

Chronic rejection

Chronic rejection usually occurs over months or years but may occur much earlier. There is a gradual occlusion of the lumen of the arteries of the kidney with interstitial fibrosis which destroys the graft. The exact mechanisms involved in chronic rejection are still unclear and may be immunological or non-immunological. The first signs of chronic rejection are usually a gradual worsening of renal function with proteinuria.

Immunosuppression regimes

Until 1997, the most commonly used immunosuppression was a 'triple-therapy' regime involving ciclosporin (Sandimmun/Neoral), azathioprine (Imuran) and prednisolone medications. However, the last 4 years have seen the introduction of new immunosuppressive drugs such as tacrolimus (Fk506), mycophenolate mofetil and sirolimus. With the advent of these new drugs many centres now try to use differing combinations of immunosuppression drugs to match the level of risk relating to potential rejection problems (Table 11.10).

Ciclosporin (Sandimmun/Neoral)

Ciclosporin is a natural peptide found in two strains of fungi. It was first introduced into clinical immunosuppression in 1983.

Action

Ciclosporin inhibits interleukin-2 and interferes with the growth and activation of T lymphocytes (Fig. 11.12).

Side-effects

Usually side-effects are dose-dependent and responsive to dose reduction. The commonest side-effects include:

• nephrotoxicity—decreased GFR
• hypertension
• hepatic dysfunction
• hirsutism
• hyperlipidaemia
• hyperkalaemia
• hyperuricaemia
• gum hypertrophy

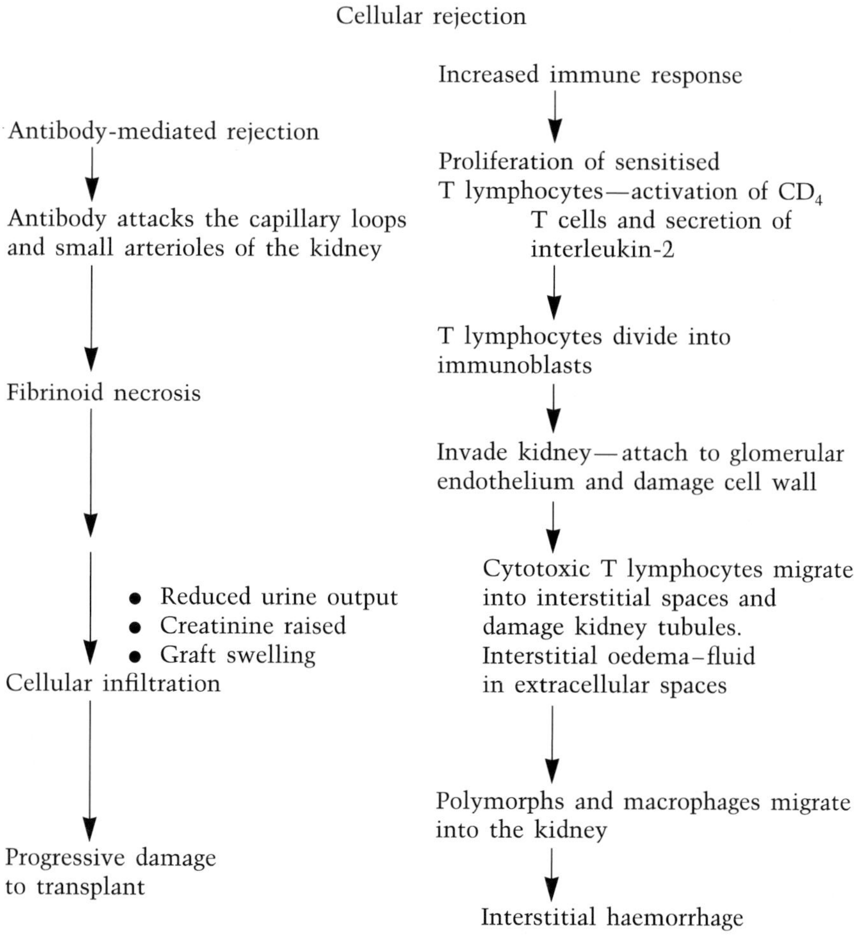

Cellular rejection

Increased immune response
↓

Antibody-mediated rejection
↓

Antibody attacks the capillary loops and small arterioles of the kidney

Proliferation of sensitised
T lymphocytes—activation of CD$_4$
T cells and secretion of
interleukin-2
↓

↓

Fibrinoid necrosis

T lymphocytes divide into
immunoblasts
↓

Invade kidney—attach to glomerular
endothelium and damage cell wall
↓

• Reduced urine output
• Creatinine raised
• Graft swelling

Cytotoxic T lymphocytes migrate
into interstitial spaces and
damage kidney tubules.
Interstitial oedema–fluid
in extracellular spaces
↓

Cellular infiltration
↓

Polymorphs and macrophages migrate
into the kidney
↓

Progressive damage
to transplant

Interstitial haemorrhage

Figure 11.12 Histopathology of acute rejection.

Table 11.10 An example of an immunosuppression protocol

	Immediate function	Delayed graft function	Delayed graft function > 7 days
High-risk PRA> 85% Serious cross-match concern 5–6 HLA mismatches	Basiliximab (Simulect) Tacrolimus Mycophenolate mofetil Prednisolone	½ level tacrolimus	Stop tacrolimus[a] Weekly biopsy
Medium-risk Previously rejected graft 3–4 HLA mismatches or 2 DR mismatches	Ciclosporin (Neoral) Mycophenolate 3–6/12[b] Prednisolone	½ level ciclosporin	Stop CyA[a], start ATG[c] Weekly biopsy
Low-risk All others	Ciclosporin (Neoral) Azathioprine Prednisolone	½ level ciclosporin Stop azathioprine and start mycophenolate 3–6/12[b]	Stop CyA[a], start ATG[c] Weekly biopsy

PRA, panel reactivity; HLA, human leukocyte antigen; CyA, ciclosporin A; ATG, antithymocyte globulin.

[a] Providing renal function is restored and the patient is off dialysis, reintroduce calcineurin inhibitor at full dose (aiming for CyA levels 150–300 ng mL⁻¹ or tacrolimus levels 10–15 ng mL⁻¹, 3 days before stopping ATG. If the patient is still dialysis-dependent at the end of the ATG course, then continue on dual therapy (mycophenolate mofetil (MMF) and steroids). Monitor closely with fine-needle aspiration every 3 days and weekly Tru-cut biopsies. Reintroduce calcineurin inhibitor at full dose (aiming for CyA levels 150–300 ng mL⁻¹ or tacrolimus levels 10–15 ng mL⁻¹ only when renal function is restored and patient is off dialysis.

[b] Continue MMF for 3 months then convert to azathioprine (1.5 mg kg⁻¹ o.d.). However, if the patient has experienced a rejection episode during these first 3 months then the course of MMF must be extended to 6 months before converting to azathioprine.

[c] Start ATG 2 mg kg⁻¹, 10–14-day course (depending on patient response). Give ATG dose when absolute T-cell count >50. See ATG protocol.

- hypomagnesaemia
- hypertrichosis.

Other less common side-effects include:

- muscle weakness
- thrombocytopenia.

Ciclosporin may be started immediately before transplant but because of the known nephrotoxicity it may be withdrawn for the preliminary phase in the presence of primary non-function due to ATN (Table 11.10).

Absorption

Ciclosporin is absorbed with variable efficiency by different individuals; therefore, regular monitoring of whole blood levels must occur. The usual therapeutic range is 200–400 µg mol l⁻¹ during the first 6 months of transplantation, with maintenance doses aimed at levels of 100–200 µg mol l⁻¹. Generally, patients who reject due to inadequate ciclosporin levels usually have levels less than 100 µg mol l⁻¹, while patients with ciclosporin nephrotoxicity usually have levels greater than 500 µg mol l⁻¹ but it is an individual response. Some units are now performing C2 monitoring, i.e. measuring blood concentrations 2 h postdose. C2 is thought to predict more accurately individual patient absorptions than traditional trough monitoring and results in a reduced incidence of acute rejection episodes and acute renal dysfunction.

Tacrolimus (Fk506)

Tacrolimus is a calcineurin inhibitor that, like ciclosporin, works early in T-cell activations. Its action inhibits interleukin-2 and other cytokines that cause early T-cell activation (Fig.11.12)

Side-effects

The commonest side-effects include:

- visual and neurological disturbances
- hypertension
- tremor, headache, insomnia
- raised blood sugar level
- leukopenia.

Sirolimus (Rapamycin)

Sirolimus acts later in the T-cell activation than ciclosporin and tacrolimus. It inhibits interleukin-2-mediated signal transduction pathways (Fig 11.13). Sirolimus is not nephrotoxic, which gives it an advantage over ciclosporin and tacrolimus. It was licensed for use in the UK in 2001.

Side-effects

- hypercholesterolaemia
- hypertriglyceridemia
- thrombocytopenia
- hypertension
- nose bleeds.

Basiliximab (Simulect)

Simulect has recently been licensed in the UK. This monoclonal antibody is given as an infusion before surgery and on the fourth postoperative day.

Action

Basiliximab works by binding specifically to part of the interleukin-2 receptor that is only expressed on activated T lymphocytes. Therefore, it helps to prevent proliferation of antigen-stimulated T cells. It is used in combination with other immunosuppressives to form a baseline therapy (Table 11.10).

Side-effects

None have been reported.

Azathioprine

Azathioprine is a derivative of the anticancer drug 6-mercaptopurine and was introduced into clinical practice in 1962.

Action

Azathioprine inhibits both DNA and RNA synthesis and prevents growth of lymphocytes (Fig. 11.12).

Side-effects

The main side-effect is neutropenia. If the WBC drops to below $3.5 \times 10^9 \, l^{-1}$ the dose should be reduced. If the WBC drops below $3.0 \times 10^9 \, l^{-1}$ the drug should be stopped temporarily.

Other side-effects include:

- alopecia
- general malaise
- muscular pains
- malignancy
- pancreatitis (rare)
- altered liver function
- cholestatic jaundice (rare).

Because of the risk of neutropenia, blood counts must be checked at intervals of not longer than 3 months.

Mycophenolate mofetil

Mycophenolate mofetil was licensed in 1995 and has the same effects as azathioprine.

Action

Mycophenolate mofetil acts by preventing activated lymphocytes from differentiating and proliferating and thereby limiting clonal expansion. In the UK this drug has been used in preference to azathioprine in selected patients who were considered to be at a higher risk of rejection than average (Table 11.10).

Side-effects

Mycophenolate mofetil has significant gastrointestinal adverse effects:

- diarrhoea
- vomiting
- leukopenia.

Prednisolone (corticosteroids)

Action

The action of corticosteroid preparations is complex and involves antiinflammatory responses with blocking of T cells and interleukin-1 (Fig. 11.12).

Side-effects

- cushingoid appearance (facial swelling, swollen abdomen)
- fluid retention
- glaucoma
- increased appetite
- hypertension
- psychosis

- peptic ulceration
- increase in blood sugar levels.

Side-effects with long-term treatment

- subcapsular cataract
- pancreatitis
- skin thinning
- osteoporosis.

Many centres start steroid reduction at 2 months posttransplant and aim to remove steroid therapy at 1 year posttransplant because of the long-term side-effects.

For further information regarding immunosuppression, see Lee & Devaney (2001).

Acute rejection

Rejection treatment consists of an increase in the dose of corticosteroids. Usual practice is to administer daily bolus doses of 500 mg intravenous methylprednisolone over a 3-day period (one bolus each day).

Orthoclone (OKT3) monoclonal antibody

Action

OKT3 is an antibody that reacts with CD-3 molecules on the lymphocytes and depletes them.

Side-effects

- chest pain
- pulmonary oedema
- gastrointestinal disturbances
- fever
- chills
- dyspnoea
- infections.

This drug can cause rapid pulmonary oedema and therefore it is essential that the patient is evaluated for volume overload and given treatment if necessary prior to administration of the drug.

Antilymphocyte globulin—polyclonal antibody

Action

Antilymphocyte globulin inhibits and destroys circulatory lymphocytes through antibody action.

Side-effects

- rash
- fever/chills
- anaphylaxis

- thrombocytopenia/leukopenia
- myalgia.

POSTOPERATIVE CARE AND COMPLICATIONS FOR THE RENAL TRANSPLANT RECIPIENT

In most cases the anaesthetist will insert a triple-lumen central venous line via the internal jugular vein immediately prior to surgery. This line facilitates monitoring of fluid status and central venous pressure (CVP) and allows infusion of fluids and medications during surgery and the early postoperative phase.

Aims of care

The aim of postoperative management is to provide the appropriate care to support primary transplant function and to aid optimal recovery. Initial care involves close monitoring of physical and psychological health, with frequent assessments and adjustments in response to changes in health status.

Immediate postoperative care

Cardiorespiratory status

Immediate baseline observations should be recorded, including blood pressure, pulse, respirations and temperature. Such observations should continue every 30 min until stable and thereafter hourly or as appropriate. Twenty-four-hour ECG monitoring may be routine; however, in some centres such monitoring may only be used for patients in high-risk categories. Close monitoring of respiratory status is essential, as anaesthetic drugs and analgesia may be poorly excreted due to the reduced transplant function, thus depressing respiratory effort and increasing the risk of pulmonary complication. Early chest physiotherapy is essential.

Pain management

The experience of pain is unique to each individual and therefore the use of patient-controlled analgesia is a suitable therapy as it will provide satisfactory pain management, reduce recipient anxiety and facilitate deep breathing and movement. An opiate derivative, such as morphine, is commonly used. Pethidine is avoided because of the possible accumulation of metabolites in the presence of reduced renal function. Recipients often report that the presence of the urinary catheter causes the greatest discomfort.

Hydration: fluid and electrolyte balance

Inadequate hydration may adversely affect transplant function; therefore, the maintenance of an acceptable venous pressure without the complication of fluid overload is an integral element of care. Fluid intake is usually administered through the central venous line. CVP measurements, recorded hourly, and urinary output measurements, recorded hourly, are used as a guide to appropriate fluid intake.

Fluid intake protocol usually involves fluids being administered through an infusion pump with hourly intake equal to the previous hour's output plus 50 mL, with the aim of achieving a CVP level of approximately +10 cm H_2O.

Peripheral line perfusion must also be included in the intake total. Infusion of dopamine may be introduced to help maintain pressure and improve transplant perfusion by reducing vasoconstriction of the smaller renal vessels. Monitoring of serum biochemistry and haemoglobin levels is ongoing and the results will determine the type of intravenous fluid given. Often 5% dextrose is alternated with normal saline. Blood transfusion is rarely required.

Oral fluids are usually introduced within the early postoperative phase (as paralytic ileus is rare) and are gradually increased as appropriate. In uncomplicated cases the CVP line is removed after 48 h and nutrition introduced.

Urine output: catheter care

A urinary catheter will be in situ following the transplant surgery, and the urine may be blood-stained due to the surgical procedures to the bladder and ureter. Clot formation may occur, resulting in pain and anuria. Gentle sterile bladder washouts should be performed to alleviate the problem and re-establish urine flow.

Twenty-four-hour urine output should be recorded and it is, of course, important to note the volume of urine passed from the native kidneys pre-transplantation when assessing urinary totals. Daily urine analysis and biochemistry should be noted and daily catheter specimens obtained for microscopy, culture and sensitivity. The catheter is usually removed on the fifth postoperative day. Some recipients may experience difficulty with voiding and also may have very limited bladder capacity due to pretransplant bladder atrophy. Reassurance and bladder retraining strategies usually help to solve these problems.

Wound management

A wound drain may be present and drainage should be monitored. Observation and aseptic dressing of the wound will be given as appropriate and the sutures removed when healing has occurred. The immunosuppression regime and other contributory factors such as diabetes or malnutrition may impede the healing process.

Infection control

Recipients are immunocompromised and therefore infection control procedures should be strictly followed. Hand-washing should take place before and after each nursing and medical procedure and visitors should be monitored for infections. Medications should include prophylaxis against infection and additional treatments should be commenced if infection is suspected.

The recipient should be helped to achieve personal and oral hygiene of a high standard and aseptic techniques utilised with regard to wound, peritoneal catheter site, urinary catheter and CVP line care. Catheter tips should be cultured for microscopy and sensitivity when removed.

Postoperative medications

- Ciclosporin or tacrolimus: immunosuppression to prevent rejection.
- Azathioprine or mycophenolate mofetil: immunosuppression to prevent rejection.
- Prednisolone: immunosuppression to prevent rejection.
- Co-trimoxazole (Septrin): antibiotic to prevent infection/chest infection, particularly *Pneumocystis*.
- Ranitidine: reduces gastric irritation caused by steroids. Prevents gastric bleeding.
- Nystatin pastilles: prevents oral infection (Candida).
- Aspirin: may be used in some centres to reduce the risk of thrombosis.

Continuing care

Recipients usually recover quickly from the anaesthetic and begin early mobilisation to prevent complications. Diet is introduced on day 1. Constipation may be a problem due to anaesthetic, immobility and analgesia, and gentle laxatives or suppositories may be needed. Self-care is usually achieved by the fifth postoperative day.

Sadness may be linked to thoughts of the donor family and grief and guilt may be expressed that the transplant has resulted from 'another's tragedy'. It is often helpful to give recipients anonymous details such as age, sex and cause of death of the donor, and to offer them the opportunity to write a letter of thanks to the donor family. The expression of thanks usually enables recipients to accept the gift of the organ and to move forward to their new lifestyle.

Anxiety is usually linked to the fear of complications such as rejection, infection and graft loss. Recipients and their families require considerable support, understanding and indepth information during the early postoperative phase, particularly if difficulties occur.

Complications of renal transplantation

Renal dysfunction—acute tubular necrosis

The most common cause of initial non-function after renal transplantation is ATN, which may be due to prolonged hypotension in the donor or difficulties with ischaemia during the donor or recipient surgery. Dialysis support may be required until adequate transplant function is achieved. Haemodialysis, with reduced heparinisation, can be undertaken as necessary (a frequent clotting screen will be required), and peritoneal dialysis recommenced as long as the peritoneum has not been breached by surgery.

Ciclosporin is known to be nephrotoxic and may therefore prolong ATN. Some units may reduce the ciclosporin dosage or withdraw ciclosporin therapy until the ATN is starting to recover. OKT3 or antithymocyte globulin (ATG) may be utilised instead of ciclosporin if ATN is thought to be a potential problem.

Acute rejection

Many transplant recipients will experience at least one episode of acute rejection. Acute rejection is usually a combination of cellular and antibody-

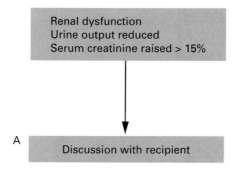

Figure 11.13 Assessment and tests completed in the presence of renal dysfunction during continuing care.

mediated rejection which most usually occurs between 4 days and 2 months following transplantation.

The clinical signs of acute rejection may include:

- pyrexia
- fall in urine output
- rise in serum creatinine
- swelling and tenderness of the transplant

- weight gain
- flu-like symptoms
- ankle oedema.

The diagnosis of acute rejection is usually confirmed by a needle biopsy (see Ch. 6), and treatment is commenced immediately with a daily intravenous bolus of methylprednisolone for 3 days. In severe cases antilymphocyte globulin (horse)/ATG (rabbit) or OKT3 may be commenced. The rejection is usually controlled by the increased immunosuppression; however, a severe rejection episode may result in some loss of overall graft function.

Vascular complications

Transplant renal artery and renal vein thrombosis
Thrombosis of the renal artery or renal vein is a rare complication. Clinical signs of graft thrombosis usually include renal dysfunction, anuria and hypotension. Diagnosis may be confirmed by ultrasound scanning (see Ch. 6). Immediate surgical exploration should be undertaken. In the majority of cases the transplant will be lost.

Transplant renal artery stenosis
Renal artery stenosis usually occurs between 6 and 12 months after transplantation. Signs include graft dysfunction and severe hypertension with a bruit on auscultation over the transplant. Diagnosis is confirmed by angiography. In severe cases intervention may be required either by percutaneous transluminal angioplasty or surgery.

Urological complications
A major urological complication which may occur is avascular necrosis of the distal end of the transplant ureter, resulting in leakage of urine. Surgical reimplantation of the ureter will be required in most cases. This complication has become less common recently due to the use of a ureteric stent.

Infections

Bacterial infections
The clinical signs of infection are similar to those of rejection (pyrexia, tachycardia, flu-like illness), therefore it is important that both possibilities are considered and investigations undertaken to exclude either cause.

Chest infections may result from *Pneumococcus, Haemophilus influenzae, Klebsiella* and *Pneumocystis* (Septrin is often given as prophylaxis for *Pneumocystis* during the first 6 months posttransplant). Infection may develop rapidly, resulting in the need for ventilation. Early treatment with appropriate antibiotic therapies is essential.

Fungal infections
Oral *Candida* is common and many centres use nystatin as prophylaxis for the first 2 months following transplant. Oral hygiene of a high standard should be encouraged.

Vaginal *Candida* may also occur and recipients may be reluctant to report this problem, particularly to a male clinician in an outpatient setting. Recipients should be informed that *Candida* is a potential problem and that treatment will be required.

Viral infections

Cytomegalovirus

Cytomegalovirus (CMV) infection is usually acquired during childhood and early adulthood and is a minor flu-like illness. However, this minor illness can cause major complications in the immunosuppressed transplant recipient. CMV disease, after transplantation, may occur because of:

- reactivation of latent disease in a CMV-positive recipient. Such reactivation is generally classed as 'secondary CMV'
- transmission of CMV from a CMV-positive donor to a CMV-negative recipient through the transplanted organ. This is classed as 'primary CMV'.

CMV may also be transmitted through whole blood transfusions, hence many centres require that all renal patients receive CMV-negative blood.

CMV vaccinations for all transplant recipients in the pretransplant phase would be an ideal solution to this problem but, as yet, no clinically acceptable vaccines have been formulated. Also matching so that CMV-negative recipients receive CMV-negative grafts would help to minimise the difficulties experienced, but such matching is not always possible in practice. Therefore, primary CMV disease does occur and can cause morbidity and mortality.

The usual time for manifestation of CMV disease is 4–8 weeks posttransplantation. Clinical signs include swinging pyrexia, rigors, malaise and, in extreme cases, pneumonitis, retinitis, gastroenteritis and encephalitis.

Some centres use aciclovir as prophylaxis in all high-risk recipients (such as CMV-negative recipients receiving CMV-positive grafts). Other centres monitor serological progress and treat as appropriate. With primary disease, admission to hospital and treatment with ganciclovir is often necessary.

Herpes simplex and varicella zoster virus

Herpes simplex (type I and type II) commonly cause problems in the first months following transplantation. Oral and anogenital lesions may occur. Recipients may be reluctant to report such problems due to anxiety and embarrassment. Therefore, recipients should be aware that these lesions may arise and that they occur because of reduced immunity, not because of other social issues. Sympathetic and understanding care should be offered and treatment with aciclovir may be required.

Reactivation of the latent varicella zoster virus may also occur and present as classical 'shingle' lesions. Treatment with aciclovir is often necessary to prevent systemic complications. Disseminated varicella zoster (chickenpox) can be dangerous in immunosuppressed patients, resulting in some cases of severe illness with encephalitis, pneumonitis and meningitis. The recipients must be aware of the problems associated with such viral infections and should be encouraged to report signs and symptoms or contact with infected others.

RECIPIENT DISCHARGE FROM HOSPITAL AND CONTINUING CARE

If recovery has been uncomplicated the transplant recipient may be discharged home on the 7th to 10th postoperative day.

The educative and developmental intervention is very important for transplant recipients. They must have sufficient knowledge to monitor their health status, be understanding of medication regimes and report problems if they arise. Assessment of learning difficulties should be completed soon after transplant so that relevant interventions may be implemented to aid learning, knowledge and eventual independence. Physical barriers such as impaired sight and hearing can be aided by electronic blood pressure monitoring equipment. Language and literacy difficulties can be resolved with diagrammatic information, translations and medication presented in daily dosette boxes, all promoting personal independence, although family members may be included in teaching sessions as appropriate.

The 'named nurse' may assess learning abilities (with an informal, non-threatening discussion) posttransplant and plan a teaching information programme, implement this programme and evaluate progress. Written information is given as appropriate both verbally and in the form of a written information booklet. At the time of discharge the recipient should have the following knowledge (Box 11.10).

■ **BOX 11.10 Recipient predischarge knowledge**

- Record and report changes in:
  - Pulse
  - Temperature
  - Respirations
  - Weight
  - Blood pressure
  - And understand the relevance of such changes
- Measure and record 24-h urine output
- Understand the action, dosage and side-effects of medication and the need for compliance
- Recognise the signs of rejection
- Recognise the signs of infection
- Have telephone numbers of the transplant centre and know how to contact staff
- Recognise the need to alert transplant personnel in the light of any of these changes

Drug charts and monitoring booklets should be utilised as part of a self-medication programme introduced as recovery allows or on the second postoperative day.

Immediately after discharge, recipients will be seen very frequently in the outpatient clinic and it is important that nursing intervention identifies developmental needs so that the recipient's knowledge base continues to expand and psychosocial care is offered. Reports suggest that some recipients feel that only the renal function and transplant progress is monitored, not the rehabilitation of the 'whole person'. Therefore, holistic care is essential, addressing psychosocial needs with physical needs; such care may be most appropriately offered by a transplant nurse practitioner who can offer continuity of care as well as understanding and support.

The aim of ongoing care is to empower the recipient to achieve optimal individual rehabilitation. It is essential to help the recipient achieve a balance between monitoring health and gaining normality. One of the most important posttransplant psychosocial tasks that the recipient needs to accomplish is the gradual relinquishing of the sick role and the eventual return to non-patient status (Christopherson 1987). Medical and nursing staff can give a confusing message by referring to recipients as patients and demanding strict adherence to rigid health protocols, whilst at the same time insisting that transplantation offers a return to 'normality'.

Flexibility of care, understanding and encouragement are required to enable recipients to take control of their lives and achieve the highest quality of life possible. Ongoing health monitoring will continue and problems may occur, but advice and support should be available throughout the complete transplant experience.

Ongoing care: information and support for transplant recipients

- Peritoneal dialysis catheter: if transplant function is satisfactory, the peritoneal dialysis catheter is removed at 3 months posttransplant. The ureteric stent is usually removed at 6 weeks after transplant.

- Diet: follow a normal diet, but taking care with weight gain due to increased appetite and freedom from the renal diet. If cholesterol or lipid levels are raised, dietary restrictions may be necessary.

- Vaccinations and travel: transplant recipients should not receive live vaccines. Therefore, it is important to consult the transplant centre before travel immunisations are given. Foreign travel is encouraged but recognition of possible infection sources is necessary so that suitable precautions may be taken.

- Skin care: immunosuppression predisposes recipients to skin damage from trauma and sun and increases the risk of skin malignancies. Therefore, dermatological monitoring and advice should be given and recipients should use factor 25–30 sun block during sun exposure and report any skin lesions.

- Fertility: female patients should be aware of fertility issues and be given advice with regard to birth control measures. Intrauterine devices are not recommended because of the risk of infection. Condoms or the mini-pill are the most appropriate therapies. Recipients should, ideally, wait at least 1 year before considering pregnancy. Advice should be available with regard to pregnancy risks in individual cases. Recipients cannot breast feed after delivery as the immunosuppression may transfer to the baby.

• Employment: recipients may return to work as soon as they feel able as long as graft function and health are satisfactory and employment does not put either at risk. Help should be available for those recipients seeking employment.

• Health education: smoking is discouraged due to the risk of enhanced cardiorespiratory and vascular complications. Exercise and activity are encouraged, although contact sports such as rugby or karate may put the graft at risk. Female patients should have regular cervical smears and breast examinations because of the increased risk of malignancy. Male patients should be monitored for potential malignancies and encouraged to perform testicular self-examination.

• Psychological health: psychological support should be available to help with sexual problems, body image problems and marital problems.

• Social needs: help and advice should be available for social needs such as benefits, housing and return to work.

SUMMARY

A successful renal transplant can provide the best quality of life for those with ESRF. As one patient, who received a transplant in 1972 when aged 9 years, has said: 'It is amazing that the special gift from the donor has enabled me to achieve my career and personal goals and has resulted in the creation of a new family – a gift for generations to come'.

REFERENCES

British Medical Association. Organ donation in the 21st century—a review. June 2000. Available at: www.bma.org.uk 9 Nov 2001.

Buckley PE. The delicate question of the donor family. Transplant Proc 1989; 21:1411–1412.

Carlisle D. Life-giving FATWA. Nurs Times 1995; 91:2.

Christopherson LK. Cardiac transplantation: a psychological perspective. Circulation 1987; 75:57.

Committee on Microbiological Safety of Blood and Tissue Transplantation. Guidance on the microbiological safety of human tissues and organs used in transplantation. NHS Executive 1996 HSG (96) 26 Revised 2000.

Conference of Medical Royal Colleges and their faculties in the United Kingdom. Br Med J 1976; ii:1187–1188.

Conference of Medical Royal Colleges and their faculties in the United Kingdom. Lancet 1979; ii:1069–1070.

Conference of Medical Royal Colleges and their faculties in the United Kingdom. Br Med J 1991; i:32.

Conference of Medical Royal Colleges and their faculties in the United Kingdom. Lancet 1998; i:261–262.

Connerney I, Bartlett S. Depression, readmissions and quality of life in kidney transplant patients. Psychosom Med 2001; 63:91–190.

Coulter M. The needs of family members in ICUs. Intens Care Nurs 1989; 3:4–10.

Council of Europe. European consensus document. Meeting the organ shortage—current status and strategies for improvement of organ donation. International figures on organ donation and transplantation activities 1998. Recommendations of the select committee of experts on the organisational aspects of co-operation in organ and tissue transplantation. Transplant Newslett 1999; 4:1.

Department of Health. Guidance on the microbiological safety of human tissues and organs used in transplantation. HSG (96) 26. London: NHS Executive, 1996.

Didlake RH, Dreyfus K, Kerman RH, Van Buren CT, Kahan BD. Patient non-compliance: a major cause of late graft failure in cycylosporin-treated renal transplant. Transplant Proc 1988; 20: 63.

Dubovsky SL, Penn I. Psychiatric considerations in renal transplant surgery. Psychosomatics 1980; 21:481.

Evans RW, Manninen DL, Garrison LP Jr et al. The quality of life for patients with end stage renal disease. N Engl J Med 1985; 312:553.

Feest TG, Riad HN, Collins CH et al. Protocol for increasing organ donation after cerebrovascular deaths in a district general hospital. Lancet 1990; 335:1133.

Fellner CH, Marshall JR. Twelve kidney donors. JAMA 1968; 206:2703.

Flowers JL, Jacobs S, Cho E et al. Comparison of open and laparoscopic live donor nephrectomy. Ann Surg 1997; 226:483.

Fuggle SV, Belger MA, Johnson RJ et al. A new national allocation scheme for adult kidney transplantation in the UK. Clin Transplant 1998; 107–113.

Galpin C. Body image in end stage renal failure. Br J Nurs 1992; 1:21.

Garrison RN, Bentley FR, Rague GH et al. There is an answer to the shortage of organ donors. Surg Gynaecol Obstet 1991; 173:391–396.

Gilks WR, Bradley BA, Gore SM, Klanda PT. Substantial benefits of tissue matching in renal transplantation. Transplantation 1987; 43:669–674.

Gore SM, Hinds CJ, Rutherford AJ. Organ donation from intensive care units in England. Br Med J 1989; 299:1193–1197.

Harvard Medical School. Report of the ad hoc committee of Harvard Medical School to examine the definition of brain death. Definition of irreversible coma. JAMA 1968; 205:337.

Hilton BA, Starzomski RC. Families decision making about living related kidney donation. Am Nephrol Nurs Assoc J 1994; 21:346.

Human Tissue Act 1961. HSC (IS) 156. London: Department of Health and Social Security, 1975.

Jacobs C, Johnson E, Anderson K et al. Kidney transplants from living donors: how donation affects family dynamics. Adv Renal Ther 1998; 5:89.

Jain N. Evolution and development of a renal transplant co-ordinator for the Asian community. EDTNA/ERCA J 1999; xx:5.

Jofre R, Lopez-Gomez JM, Moreno F et al. Changes in quality of life after renal transplantation. Am Kidney Dis 1998; 32:93.

Kemph JP. Renal failure, artifical kidney and kidney transplant. Am J Psychiatr 1966; 122:1270.

Klein J. Natural history of the major histocompatibility complex. New York: John Wiley, 1986.

Levey AS, Hon S, Bush HL Jr. Kidney transplantation from unrelated living donors: time to reclaim a discarded opportunity. N Engl J Med 1986; 314:914.

Mathew TH. Recurrent disease after renal transplantation. Transplant Rev 1991; 31.

Molter NC. Needs of relatives of critically ill patients. A descriptive study. Heart Lung 1979; 8:332.

Montgomery RA, Ratner LE. The laparoscopic donor nephrectomy. In: Morris PJ, ed. Kidney transplantation principles and practice. 5th ed. New York: Saunders, 2001.

Mori/UKTCA/BACCN. Report of a 2 year study into the reasons for relatives' refusal of organ donation. Obtained from UKTCA secretariat. Newcastle Upon Tyne: Royal Victoria Infirmary, 1995.

Morris PJ. (ed.) Kidney transplantation principles and practice. London: Saunders, 2001.

Morris PLP, Jones B. Transplantation versus dialysis—a study of quality of life. Transplant Proc 1988; 20:23.

Morris PJ, Johnson RJ, Belger MA et al. Analysis of factors that affect outcome of primary cadaveric renal transplantation in the UK. Lancet 1999; 345:1147–1152.

Najarian JS, Chavers BM, McHugh LE et al. Twenty years or more of follow up living donors. Lancet 1992; 340:807.

New W, Solomon M, Dingwall R et al. A question of give and take. Research report no. 18. London: Kings Fund Institute, 1994.

Novitzky D. Selection and management of cardiac allograft donors. Curr Opin Organ Transplant,1998; 3:51–61.

Pallis C. Brain stem death: the evolution of a concept. In: Morris PJ, ed. Kidney transplantation, principles and practice. 4th edn. London: Saunders, 1994: 71–85.

Rovelli M, Palmeri D, Vossler E et al. Non-compliance in renal transplantation recipients: evaluation by socio-economic groups. Transplant Proc 1989; 21:3979.

Russell S, Jacob R G. Living related organ dontation: the donor's dilemma. Patient Education Counselling 1994; 21:89.

Simmons RG, Hickley K, Kjellstrand CM et al. Donors and non donors: the role of the family and the physician in kidney transplantation. Semin Psychiatr 1971; 3:102.

Simmons RC, Klein SD, Simmons RL. The gift of life: the social and psychological impact of organ transplantation. New York: John Wiley, 1977.

Smith MD, Kappell DF, Province MA et al. Living related kidney donors: a multicentre study of donor education, socioeconomic adjustment and rehabilitation. Am J Kidney Dis 1986; 8:223.

Soin R, Friend PJ. Renal xenotransplantation. In Morris PJ, ed. Kidney transplantation principles and practice. 5th edn. New York: Saunders, 2001.

Surman OS. Psychiatric aspects of organ transplantation. Am J Psychiatry, 1989; 146:972.

Terasaki PI, Cecka JM, Gjertson DW et al. High survival rates in kidney transplants from spousal and living unrelated donors. N Engl J Med 1995; 333:333.

UK code of practice. A code of practice for the diagnosis of brain stem death prepared by a working party established through the Royal College of Physicians on behalf of the Academy of Medical Royal Colleges at the Health Department (Department of Health) London: 1998.

Wakeford RE, Stepney R. Obstacles to organ donation. Br J Surg 1989; 76:35–39.

Wilkinson P. A qualitative study to establish the self perceived needs of family members of patients in a general intensive care unit. Intens Crit Care Nurs 1995; 11:77–86.

Community nursing in renal care

Victoria Warmington

12

■ CONTENTS

■ LEARNING OUTCOMES FOR THIS CHAPTER

- To understand the need for increased community care for those with renal failure
- To review the aims and roles and responsibilities of the community renal nurse
- To describe the factors involved in successful home dialysis
- To evaluate the needs of patients on home dialysis.

INTRODUCTION

In this chapter the reader gains an understanding of the complex nature of community nursing and the breadth of role the community renal nurse has in the care and management of the dialysis patient and family at home.

The many factors involved in the success of home-based dialysis therapy in reducing patient morbidity are discussed, and central to this is the role of the nurse. The family and other carers are acknowledged as playing a vital role in caring for patients on home dialysis. The need to include other members of the primary healthcare team is recognised as an essential component to safe, effective dialysis in the community.

THE NATURE OF COMMUNITY AND COMMUNITY CARE

Many authors have sought to define the terms 'community' and 'community care'. Walshe (1997) and Hennessy & Swain (1997) argue that community is resistant to a satisfactory definition. 'Community' implies a group of people, all of whom share something in common, which could be race, work, religion, a social activity or simply the area in which they live. In respect of planned resources and services, a community is usually defined geographically (Hennessy & Swain 1997). All societies have a notion of community that is recognised and realised in many different ways (Walshe 1997). A community gives care and support to those within it (Skidmore 1997). This liaison with family and friends means that they are relied upon to give support and often assume the role of care provider for extended periods (Newby 1996). In the case of those needing dialysis this means lifelong comfort and help. This traditional support is continued through the length of the illness.

It has been argued that planners and providers of healthcare need to understand the nature and function of a community in order to ensure that the particular needs of those people living within it are met appropriately and sensitively. Nurses working in community settings must understand and have knowledge of the community in order to plan and implement effective nursing care (Hennessy & Swain 1997).

THE MOVE TO THE COMMUNITY

The provision of care in the community underpins one of the main philosophies of the National Health Service (NHS), namely enabling patients to live longer, as independently as possible, and to enjoy a better quality of life (Department of Health, 1990).

In the latter half of the 20th century there has been a rapid medical technological expansion. Alongside this, there has been a return to care in the community. The increased sophistication of and demand for primary care, community nursing and outreach services mean that patients with a chronic illness and using a life-saving treatment can be cared for and be self-caring at home.

As the number of patients reaching end-stage renal failure rises, so does the requirement for dialysis services. The increased demand for haemodialysis (HD) has led to a crisis in renal replacement. The development of home programmes during the 1960s and 1970s and increase in use of continuous ambulatory peritoneal dialysis (CAPD) in the late 1970s further changed the emphasis of home dialysis, and with this came an introduction of community dialysis nurses working within renal units. Marks (1991) argued that providing care at home for dialysis patients is an excellent example of a clinically safe, organisationally feasible and financially viable alternative to hospital-based care: this remains true today. Lunts (1999) argues that home HD can be a viable, indeed an optimal treatment for many patients. Technological advances alongside economic constraints of publicly funded healthcare systems are often cited as the reasons for the increase in home-based and self-care treatments (Wellard & Street 1999). The provision of community renal care is recognised as an effective means of minimising hospital admission for preventable dialysis-related problems

(Fawcett-Henesy 1999, Warmington & Baxter 1996). Above all, what must remain paramount is the preference the patient has for the location of the treatment and nursing care.

It is not until the patient is discharged home from the training programme that the unsupervised self-administration therapy commences. Until this point, the patient will have been closely supervised during the learning process and will always have had a renal nurse available to ask and assist in problem-solving situations and to answer any questions. After this level of input from the renal team, going home to be in charge of the dialysis treatment can be a worrying and frightening time for the patient and the family or carers. This is where the community renal nurse has such a vital role.

THE AIM OF THE COMMUNITY RENAL NURSE

Many patients requiring dialysis are elderly and have comorbid conditions. As such they will need long-term community nursing care if they are to remain at home and well on their treatment. A comprehensive approach, taking into account socioeconomic, cultural, psychological and environmental factors and their effect on the patient and family is the cornerstone of holistic community nursing practice. As well as this broad view, community renal nurses will have very specific aims relating to reducing the risk of dialysis-associated problems. Keogh (1999) has outlined the core aims of a community renal nurse as follows:

- to prevent peritonitis and exit-site infections
- to preserve vascular access in home HD patients
- to provide health education
- to assist with ordering supplies
- to promote open lines of communication.

These will be discussed in more detail later in this chapter.

THE ROLE OF THE COMMUNITY RENAL NURSE

Community nursing has been established by the United Kingdom Central Council for Nursing, Midwifery and Health Visiting (UKCC) at specialist practice level (UKCC 1994) and was identified as making a significant contribution to the care of individuals, families and the community as a whole. Specialist care is linked to specific types of intervention for particular patient groups (McGee 1998). In order to function as a specialist community practitioner nurses need to undergo preparation that equips them with specific skills to meet the needs of patients. McGee (1998) highlights that specialist practitioners are expert care-givers and need to be directly involved in patient care.

In the current climate of financial restraint and providing value for money, any service needs to have clearly defined aims as to what it hopes to achieve. With the broad aims outlined above, it can be seen that the community renal nurse has a complex role not simply directed at physical tasks.

It could be argued that community nurses have a different relationship with patients and the family compared with hospital nurses. In the community, the patients' homes are their territory and the nurse is a guest. The nurse should abide by the 'rules of the house', showing due respect and consideration for the patient's customs, creed and culture.

The community renal nurse must accept the patient's norms and values and continue to nurse the patient in a non-judgemental manner, regardless of the home conditions. A patient's home environment may not always be suitable for peritoneal dialysis (PD) or HD. By approaching the patient sensitively the nurse could encourage the patient to keep a clean area for carrying out exchanges. Reinforcing the importance of cleanliness on subsequent visits is an important part of the community renal nurse's role. Working within these values, the community renal nurse can be an effective provider of care and assist in preventing some of the infectious complications of PD and HD.

By the nature of the illness and treatment needed, it is acknowledged that patients receiving HD and PD need long-term follow-up care. The spectrum of potential complications associated with dialysis therapy and the need for ongoing education and training require expert nursing care and this is best provided where the patient carries out the treatment. As such, the role of the community renal nurse is an exciting and challenging one. It can be the cornerstone of the team by occupying the privileged position of knowing the patient, family, home life and other factors involved in the patient's day-to-day lifestyle.

Renal nurses can facilitate this supportive and educational network by bringing together the patient, family, community and other members of the multidisciplinary team to maintain optimum health and independence of the patient. Enthusiasm and commitment to this approach are essential for the success of any renal replacement programme (Uttley & Prowant, 1994).

Brindle & Brown (1991) outline the five aims of a nurse specialist, which can be applied to the role of the community renal nurse and the holistic role in the care and management of home dialysis patients:

- Control symptoms.
- Support and advise.
- Coordinate care.
- Meet practical needs.
- Supply education and training.

CONTROL OF SYMPTOMS

Patients dialysing at home are in charge of the therapy and it is therefore essential that the patient and carer have the knowledge and ability to ensure that the patient remains asymptomatic of uraemia, fluid overload and dehydration.

After the initiation of treatment, patients usually feel significantly better and can be convinced that the renal replacement therapy is necessary and of great benefit. However, those involved in the care of renal patients would not deny that the treatment is monotonous and time-consuming and, as such, technique and skills can become slack. The community dialysis nurse, with other members of the renal team, must try to maintain the patient's enthusiasm and motivation to continue the treatment as prescribed in order to ensure the patient stays well and symptom-free for as long as dialysis continues.

On the first home visit following initiation of dialysis it is important that the nurse establishes some baseline observations with the patient, including the patient's target weight, state of hydration, peripheral oedema, blood pressure (BP) and urine output as well as exercise tolerance level. Patients should always be aware of their target weight and the ensuing symptoms and any potential complications should this vary. Some patients may not feel confident enough to change their CAPD regime by using different-strength bags or increasing or decreasing their fluid intake without first consulting their nurse. As such, patients should be encouraged to understand the importance of BP recordings and the pattern of their weight so that over time they may feel confident and thus more in charge of the treatment. Keogh (1999) argues that giving care needs to be balanced with ways that help patients assume control of their dialysis and their life. The community renal nurse must take on the responsibility of empowering patients to do this. Empowerment can promote choice and control for patients by enhancing skills and independence. Involving patients and their families in decision-making can be a very positive practice for both the patient and the nurses involved in the care.

On subsequent home visits, baseline targets previously set with the patient should be checked and revised as required. As a patient begins to feel better, appetite may improve and the taste sensations return. A weight increase is expected and in this situation an accurate fluid and weight assessment will be carried out on each home visit and a new target weight agreed. Patients can often become dehydrated as their flesh weight increases as they try to maintain a target weight by using extra hypertonic exchanges or take off too much fluid during HD. It is important to reinforce the difference between flesh and fluid weight on subsequent home visits to prevent an unnecessary admission to hospital for rehydration.

Advice previously given is reinforced and can be further explained. A practical example of this could be if a patient experiences itching. In this situation the nurse may think it appropriate to take a blood sample to check the patient's serum phosphate and calcium levels. Advice regarding the importance of taking phosphate binders with meals should be offered. Feedback can then be given to the dietitian, highlighting problems encountered and re-referring patients back to the dietetic service as necessary (Case Study 12.1).

It is the community nurse's responsibility to reinforce the awareness of when and how to take the prescribed medication. By providing information about the indication for medication the patient is more likely to be aware that drug therapy is an integral part of dialysis success.

Another vital aspect of symptom control is the management of the patient's anaemia. The anaemia of chronic renal failure is a well-documented

---

■ CASE STUDY 12.1

Mr Clark is a 72-year-old man who has been using continous ambulatory peritoneal dialysis (CAPD) for 4 months. He uses 4 × 2000-mL exchanges a day (1 × 3.86% and 3 × 1.36%). He has no difficulty adhering to his 1500-mL fluid allowance and his wife takes charge of his dietary management.

Mr Clark called the community renal nurse requesting a visit, since he had been experiencing itching for the previous week, which had been worsening in the last 2 days. Prior to the visit the nurse checked his most recent biochemical results which had been taken at a routine clinic visit 3 weeks previously:

Urea 23.1 mmol L^{-1} Creatinine 745 μmol L^{-1} Potassium 4.8 mmol L^{-1}
Phosphate 1.8 mmol L^{-1} Corrected calcium 2.30 mmol L^{-1}

During the visit the community renal nurse established that Mr Clark was doing his four prescribed exchanges a day and was taking his phosphate binders (calcium carbonate 1 tablet tds) with meals. Mr and Mrs Clark discussed aspects of his diet with the nurse. He was eating according to his diet sheet given to him by the renal dietitian at his last outpatient appointment and was managing to eat within his allowances of phosphate-rich foods. From observation and closer questioning about anything else Mr Clark may have been eating, the nurse established that he had been consuming toffees and fudge that he had been given for his birthday. Mr Clark confessed to eating rather too many of them! He was advised that these are high in phosphate and might be contributing to his symptoms.

The community renal nurse took a blood sample from Mr Clark and arranged to ring him later that day with the results and any course of action deemed necessary by the medical staff. The results showed that Mr Clark's serum phosphate was indeed high, at 2.15 mmol L^{-1} and his calcium remained within normal limits. After discussion with the medical staff it was decided to increase Mr Clark's calcium carbonate to 2 tablets tds for a week and then recheck his blood. Mr Clark was informed of this decision, and he agreed with it. Three days later Mr Clark felt back to normal and his blood results 1 week later confirmed this.

---

occurrence and imposes many restrictions on a person's activity level and way of life. Active involvement in coordinating the prescribed erythropoietin (EPO) administration will ensure the correct dose and route and potential side-effects will be minimised, therefore keeping the patient's safety paramount (UKCC 1992). The community renal nurse may need to involve district and practice nurses in the administration of the EPO in situations where the patient or carer does not wish to or when it has been assessed as inappropriate. Teaching community nurses about EPO ensures safe and effective patient care as well as promoting optimum health and well-being for the patient. The provision of up-to-date literature for nurses and patients is an important aspect of care.

Collection of blood samples will be required to monitor the patient's haemoglobin levels. Any adjustments in the EPO dose need to be discussed with the renal team and fed back to the patient and the community nurse involved. Periodically, blood sampling for control of uraemia may be necessary. Discussion of test results must first take place with the medical staff before any action deemed necessary is followed through. The patient should be informed of results to encourage involvement in care and also to avoid unnecessary worry.

SUPPORT AND ADVICE

Nurses are at the forefront of providing care and support to patients suffering from a chronic illness and this is undoubtedly the key role of the community renal nurse (Lok 1996). Patients and the family will require frequent help, guidance, information and support before commencing, and for as long as PD or HD is used. Good-quality home support, prevention and early detection of problems that a patient may encounter can reduce the number of hospital inpatient episodes or attendances in the outpatient clinic (Fawcett-Henesy 1999, Uttley & Prowant 1994). It is argued that patients with chronic illnesses may well have increased mortality and morbidity if care and supervision in the community are denied to them, although there appears to be no hard evidence to support this theory. Preventing patients from being admitted to hospital for a dialysis-related problem should be one of the key objectives of providing a home visit service (Keogh 1999, Warmington & Baxter 1996). The community team should audit this aspect of the role in order to prove its effectiveness.

Ideally, any prospective patient and family should have met the hospital and community renal nursing team prior to commencing therapy, especially as dialysis is now viewed as a lifelong long-term option (Lunts 1999). Seeing the patient and family at home before dialysis commences can gain the patient's trust and provide information and support in a non-threatening environment. Keogh (1999) argues that patients should be offered a predialysis assessment at home. In this way, the patient and family can begin to establish a relationship before dialysis is required. Support and advice to the patient and family should begin at the first point of referral. There is often only a short amount of time available for nurses and other team members to prepare the patient and family for what could be lifelong and life-altering treatment (Uttley & Prowant 1994).

Although Jaffe & Skidmore-Roth (1993) highlighted 'ineffective family coping' as one of the major problems for carers, these difficulties are still experienced today. A patient's chronic illness can often exhaust the supportive capacity of the carer. Family members have been expected to be involved with home dialysis since the mid-1960s and, although patients are taught to dialyse themselves, the spouse or other carer will become involved in the treatment and can experience considerable stress (Brunier & McKeever 1993). Keogh (1999) has identified that patients will need continuing support from those providing informal care, who are often family members. Various studies have shown that women carers have recalled feelings of depression before the onset of home dialysis and that the pattern of communication and dynamics of the relationship had changed.

Stressors of chronic dialysis affect whole families, not just patients (Wagner 1996). Depression and anxiety are well-recognised phenomena in patients with end-stage renal failure (White & Greyner 1999). Depression has been associated with a higher rate of dialysis complications and a lower survival rate. Anger and hostility are both factors which hinder adaptation to home dialysis. An awareness of psychological and emotional factors is required alongside good assessment skills so that the effects of these problems are minimised. Patients' abilities to adapt to their new lives can be hastened and enhanced by support and advice from the community renal nurse. Indeed, McClure (2001) argues that with this support patients have the opportunity to become 'expert paltients'. Nurses need to recognise and respond to the tremendous emotional impact that chronic illness and its treatment can have on families and the patient's life (Hyde 1998, White & Grenyer 1999). The family's ability to adapt to the dialysis is influenced by many factors such as cultural values, quality of the family relationship and communication. Nurses need to understand the impact renal failure can have on the family, thus ensuring care is focused on the individual patient and family needs. Various studies (Brunier & McKeever 1993, White & Grenyer 1999) have shown that carers complain of fatigue from the extra work dialysis imposes, social isolation, role changes within the family and financial uncertainty. The community renal nurse is well placed to refer patients to appropriate services for further help either within health or social services, provided centrally from the hospital or more locally where the patient lives. The well-being of any carer is paramount to the patient as well as to the health service as a whole.

A variety of strategies to avoid crisis scenarios within a family can be initiated:

- assessing the family's need for help in the home and referring any identified needs on to the appropriate service
- encouraging and referring families to use home care and other community resources instead of relying solely on relatives and friends
- advocating the use of respite services to lessen the workload on care-givers
- any communication with patients and carers needs to be in understandable language, avoiding jargon and unfamiliar words.

Caring at home puts a strain on family relationships. The burden of the care may fall on one family member, imposing physical, mental and emotional strain. Acknowledging that renal failure has periods of stable health interspersed with unexpected acute episodes such as peritonitis, as 'normal'—may allieviate some fears and anxieties the patient and family may have. Many restrictions are imposed on partners of patients using HD at home, as they have to be present throughout the dialysis session. The nurse can then introduce a range of interventions, primarily by providing accurate information about the treatment regime, the likely progress and outcome, thus alleviating any fears and anxieties. It is essential to allow time for questions, answers and clarifications on each visit. In the non-threatening environment of the home, the family, carers and the patient should be encouraged to discuss the options available for change should they be unhappy with the treatment. More sensitive subjects can be more easily discussed (Uttley & Prowant 1994). There is no pressure on the patient to hurry and the nurse will not be called away to another task.

Some of the perceived benefits to the patient and family from provision of support in the community were identified (Stewart 1991) and are still relevant today. Deficits in knowledge and skill in dialysis technique can be identified and corrected by the nurse, which may help with the prevention of infections and the 'knock-on' complication of ill health and hospital admission. The patient and family's ability to adjust to the demands of dialysis can be monitored and referrals made to appropriate services as necessary.

Family members and the patient have an opportunity to air problems and seek answers to physical, psychological, sexual and emotional needs away from the hospital environment. As a result, patients and families will feel supported and less isolated.

Patients may benefit from support from each other. The community renal nurse can facilitate this by introducing people in similar circumstances by encouraging membership of the local kidney patients' association attached to the renal unit. As supportive as renal staff are, they are no substitute for direct experience of life on dialysis that other patients and carers can offer.

An area where the community renal nurse can offer expertise and skill is in the terminal care of patients who withdraw from treatment. The decision to withdraw from or to terminate dialysis involves the patient, family and all members of the team. Psychological aspects of treatment withdrawal are discussed in Chapter 3.

Once a decision has been made to cease dialysis, the patient needs to be reassured that staff will continue to provide appropriate comfort and care until death, and to the family and carers afterwards (Oreopoulos 1994). At this stage it is the duty of the nursing staff to provide terminal care to the dying patient with pain relief, advice on fluid control, support and reassurance. When a patient chooses to die at home, support from district nurses and other services for care and terminal support at home can be arranged. A link to the hospital can be maintained by the continuation of home visits. It is important to maintain a level of contact with the family after the patient has died. The community renal nurse can offer emotional support to the family as well as practical help and advice. The family may need help to organise removal of supplies. Partners of patients have often described a double loss when a patient on dialysis dies—loss of their family member as well as their role of carer, which has been described as their 'job'.

COORDINATING CARE

Nurses working in community settings frequently use the role of coordinator. The community renal nurse is likely to be the patient's named nurse for home treatment. As many agencies, both health and social, are often involved in supporting patients at home, a care coordinator requires a familiar knowledge of the community in which the patient lives. The primary benefit of well coordinated community services is good-quality healthcare delivered to patients. Coordinated services between hospital and community teams avoid unnecessary duplication and foster patient-focused sensitive care.

The coordination of home- care services has become increasingly important and complex as new technology and treatment methods are developed. Older people who may not have been offered dialysis 10 years ago are now being offered renal replacement therapy, most commonly PD. Older adults will often require more nursing and social care input as the dependencies increase. With the complex and inseparable nature of health and social care, it is important that a referral network has been established. This ensures that patients receive appropriate services with the minimum of delay.

COMPLEX HOME-CARE REGIMEN

For patients who have many professionals involved in their care, confusion can arise if roles and responsibilities are not clearly defined. Well-coordinated community services will avoid this.

A home visit shortly following discharge will support the patient whilst adjusting to dialysis at home. Ideally, the nurse should be present for the first CAPD exchange or HD session. Sensible planning is needed to ensure that a patient is not discharged from the training programme until all parties involved, including the patient, are ready and any community care requirements are in place. Examples of problems and their solutions that a patient may experience are:

- lack of knowledge of any part of the treatment regimen
- unavailability of the community nurse for initial support
- significant alteration in customary lifestyle.

Starting home PD and HD has a major impact on family life. Others involved should be made aware of the patient's new treatment and aspects of care involved. Any additions to the existing package of care need to be made explicit to the person responsible and added to the care plan. This may include the home carer breaking up the empty boxes from the CAPD fluid or putting out the patient's clinical waste for collection. Although these tasks may seem trivial, they are vital to a patient who is not able to do them.

Meeting any carers involved together with the patient is an excellent opportunity for the professionals to meet and discuss the individual roles and agree on a common aim—well coordinated seamless care to meet the patient's individual needs.

As a coordinator, the community renal nurse is in an ideal position to keep all members of the renal team informed of the patient's progress and ability to continue with the demands that dialysis imposes. Feedback is vital to the hospital team as well as to the patient's general practitioner (GP). The community renal nurses liaise with GPs regarding the patient's ongoing condition and ability to continue the dialysis and any alterations in treatment (Wilkie & Brown 1994). Informing all professionals involved with the patient fosters a cohesive team approach, which is so vital in the care and management of patients on dialysis.

CARE PLANNING

Under the present Patient's Charter (Department of Health 1995), patients are entitled to a needs assessment carried out to a high standard. The community care plan should include the following:

- the patients' own description of their needs and how they can best be met
- the opportunity to have an advocate present—this could be a friend or relative
- assistance for people whose first language is not English
- listening to carers' views and ideas
- taking account of carers' ability and willingness to participate in care
- coordinating the involvement of different agencies to provide the most comprehensive assessment
- giving accurate information (Department of Health, 1995).

The document *A Framework for Local Community Care Charters in England* (Department of Health 1994) sets out the entitlements a patient can expect from a care plan:

- It is in writing.
- It is shared with users and their carers.
- It covers all services when more than one agency is involved.
- It gives contact points.
- It gives a statement of when the assessment and care plan will be reviewed to ensure they are still appropriate.

When formulating a care plan, the community renal nurse must take the above points into account. It is important that prescribed nursing care is evaluated at agreed intervals to ensure that the care plan remains pertinent to the patient's current needs.

Nursing care plans and notes need to be accessible to all members of the renal nursing staff, especially for the out-of-hours service when a patient may require treatment. This ensures that patients receive individualised nursing care according to the prescribed plan.

MEETING PRACTICAL NEEDS

Although patients at home using dialysis are self-caring, the nurse has a practical role in maintaining the patient's health with effective dialysis therapy. During routine visiting the community renal nurse may encounter problems that require prompt nursing action. The patient, however, may not be forthcoming with information. With experience and sensitive questioning, the nurse can discover any difficulties patients could be having with the dialysis.

With PD the importance of exit-site care must be reinforced to the patient and carer and this should be discussed on each home visit. It may be necessary to take a swab from the exit site for culture if it has become inflamed and is discharging. According to the individual unit policy, oral antibiotic therapy can be initiated. Should the patient have an exit-site infection, it may be possible to discover the likely cause so this can be avoided in future. A demonstration of the correct exit-site care and catheter immobilisation technique can be given to the patient. Observation of carrying out the procedure and an explanation of modifications to technique are necessary.

Peritonitis remains the most common and challenging problem to patients using PD. Apart from the preventive role, practical skills are required in its diagnosis and nursing management. In many units the standard policy for the diagnosis and treatment of PD peritonitis is nurse-led. Having established that a patient has peritonitis, an experienced renal nurse can decide whether the patient is unwell and requires medical attention and possible hospital admission. If the patient remains clinically well, the community nurse may take specimens of dialysis effluent and administer antibiotic therapy according to the renal unit's protocol. It may be necessary to teach the patient or carer to inject the PD bags with antibiotics or involve the district nurses, depending on the treatment protocol and the patient's needs.

Follow-up visits during episodes of peritonitis may be necessary to ensure the fluid is clearing and that the patient remains well.

In conjunction with the renal dietitian it may be appropriate to give the patient protein supplementation in the form of sip feeds to counteract protein loss during the peritonitis episode.

Patients using HD at home have different needs requiring practical help. The community renal nurse needs to be present for the first home dialysis session, gradually withdrawing, thus promoting the patient's independence and confidence. Difficulties with cannulation may be encountered, and the patient will require assistance and education regarding inserting needles correctly and identifying new sites to use. Visiting during a dialysis session is an excellent opportunity to observe the patient and carer's technique of setting up and commencing treatment or completing dialysis. Reiterating parts of the training programme, in particular trouble shooting, ie. when to give saline, what to do if there is a power failure, is important and reassuring for the patient and the dialysis partner. Reinforcing fistula care is a necessary part of continuing education for the patient (see Ch. 7).

In the predialysis period the patient will have been given information about the changes to the home that will need to be made. Other members of the renal team will be involved, such as the social worker and the renal technician. Patients will have the benefit of practical advice and experience of the nurse who can demonstrate the amount and suitability of an area in which to store PD fluid. Suggestions as to the most appropriate place for exchanges may be helpful. For patients using PD any adjustments required in the home can be discussed and planned prior to the initial fluid delivery. Storage of large amounts of fluid can cause anxiety to the patient and their family. These can be relieved by practical interventions by the community renal nurse (Keogh 1999).

Although covered in the training programme, patients may need information reinforced and help to adjust dialysis to their home conditions. A flat, cleanable surface for CAPD exchanges and a sink nearby for hand-washing are desirable. A hook to hang the bag up to drain fluid in will be needed as well as a suitable device for warming the fluid and a set of scales for monitoring the daily weight. These are often supplied by the hospital.

As already discussed, it is agreed that dialysis significantly alters patients' lifestyles and that of their families. Part of the community dialysis nurse's role is to help patients to adjust to the rigours of dialysis and to advise and encourage them to fit the treatment into their life with the minimum disruption. At the same time it is important to acknowledge that commencing dialysis can be stressful and a difficult time for the patient and family.

Encouraging a normal life for the patient includes taking holidays. Indeed, some patients may not have realised that this was possible. The community renal nurse will explain to patients the procedure involved in taking a holiday and how the correct supplies reach the destination, and reassuring patients that they will be given a contact name, address and the telephone number of the nearest renal unit may allay any fears.

Putting patients in touch with others who have had a positive experience of a holiday whilst on dialysis could be a deciding factor for others to have much needed respite from some daily routines.

SAFE DISPOSAL OF CLINICAL WASTE IN THE COMMUNITY

PD and HD generate large amounts of clinical waste and patients need to be aware of the correct disposal methods of the waste in the community. Waste disposal from dialysis treatment at home raises different problems from those in the hospital environment.

Liaison with the patient's local authority environmental services department to reinforce the nature and risks which can arise from unsafe disposal of clinical waste is essential, as it can be hazardous to health or the environment if dealt with incorrectly (Department of the Environment 1990).

In the UK, all dialysis waste must be disposed of in a yellow clinical waste bag, sealed with a tie to avoid leakage. Arrangements should be made with the local authority for collection of the waste on a specific day. Until the collection, the waste should be kept inside the patient's home. All waste containers should be left outside for the minimum amount of time possible to reduce any risks of infection to others (Department of the Environment 1990). Local authorities have a duty to collect clinical waste, and there should be no need for nursing staff to transport health care waste.

EDUCATION AND TRAINING

Much of the professional nurse's time spent in a patient's home involves teaching both implicitly and explicitly (Zastocki & Rovinski-Wagner 2000) and even more has been documented regarding patients' needs for information concerning treatment or condition. Patient education depends on sound clinical knowledge and the ability to transfer pertinent and useful information to patients (McGee 1998).

Dialysis is undoubtedly monotonous and demanding and has along with it a spectrum of complications, some potentially life-threatening. The period of training a patient undergoes should not be viewed as an isolated event. The need for ongoing education for patients and family is essential, as dialysis is for life if the patient is unsuitable for transplantation. As such, the community renal nurse as a specialist practitioner has a vital role in continuing education, updating practical skills, knowledge and technique for dialysis patients, carers and healthcare professionals. With an indepth nursing knowledge of the specialty, the community renal nurse needs to be involved in teaching other nurses (McGee 1998).

As previously mentioned, two vital aims of any community renal nursing service are to prevent infectious complications of PD and to preserve vascular access. A home visit provides an excellent opportunity to observe these practical skills and confirm the patient or carer's competence at carrying them out (Keogh 1999).

Accurate nursing assessment is required to establish the patient's current level of knowledge before building on this to increase the understanding of the treatment (Thomas 1998). Dialysis patients already have to invest much time in treatment and self-care and therefore may not wish to spend 'free time' focusing on the illness and making additional visits to hospital. In this situation, a home visit will update the patient and family education and training in patient's home, using familiar equipment to update dialysis skills, knowledge and technique.

In order to learn, patients need to be actively involved in the process to ensure the best is gained from the experience (Ewles & Simnett 1999). When teaching, it must be relevant and interesting to the patient (Webb 1994). In this situation a variety of approaches are required but the main theme of education and retraining will be the promotion of self-care. Motivation is an essential ingredient for the teaching and learning experience. Zastocki & Rovinski-Wagner (2000) argue that this can be more important in successful learning than the patient's level of intelligence or the amount of formal education received.

District nurses often require more formal training, such as attendance at renal study days, although the district nurse can gain much knowledge and practical skills during a joint home visit with the community renal nurse and the value of these interactions should not be underestimated. In this scenario, patients have an opportunity to voice their needs, and a plan of care can be formulated that is acceptable to the patient and family. The success of taking dialysis into the community has been highlighted by many authors (Keogh 1999, Simoyi 1993, Warmington & Baxter 1996). Specialist nurses working in the community should use their expert knowledge and skills to care for patients and to pass on that skill to other nurses by teaching and demonstration. By disseminating such knowledge and skills to members of the primary healthcare team, the provision of a seamless service is more likely.

CULTURAL CONSIDERATIONS IN COMMUNITY CARE

Culture and background have an important influence on many aspects of people's lives (Helman 2000). This includes beliefs, behaviour, emotions, language, religion, rituals, family structure, diet, dress, body image as well as attitudes to illness and pain. All of these have important implications for health and nursing care. That the UK is a multicultural society made up of a range of racial groups is no longer disputed. Within each racial group will be a further division of social classes, language, religious beliefs, education, attitudes, beliefs and values (Elliott 1994). Although there are broad cultural values shared by those who live in the UK, there is a wealth of subcultures in each society. It is critically important to be sensitive to the needs of each culture.

Understanding those cultural influences that affect a person's behaviour is part of the planning of care. The challenge to nursing presented by a multiethnic society impacts upon individual practitioners (Gerrish et al 1996). Gerrish et al (1996) further argue that there is little evidence of a comprehensive response in preparing nurses to meet the needs of multiethnic clients.

Commencing dialysis requires a change in or modification of behaviour. Patients from minority ethnic groups can never achieve this unless healthcare professionals are aware of factors such as family, religion, health and illness and how these shape behaviour.

In order to achieve effective community care the particular needs of patients and families have to be addressed (Elliott 1994). Coordinated information about the people and geographical area served is important. Building up a profile will aid in providing data on population, causes of renal failure, key health problems and local available services for referral. Roderick et al, (1994) argue that ethnic composition is a vital determinant of a population's need. From this study it was concluded that the ethnic composition of a population has an appreciable impact on an area's requirement for renal replacement therapy.

Difficulties with communication and language may be experienced. A family member is often used to help with translation. This situation may not be appropriate, since it cannot be assumed that a patient is willing to discuss personal details through family members. Nor can it be assumed that the correct interpretation is given. Accordingly, a local interpreting or link-worker service may be a preferred option. The latter acts as more of an advocate to the patient. Fuller & Toon (1988) state that the following are desirable attributes when using a link-worker or interpreter:

- is fluent in both languages
- has some training in interpretation

- has some medical knowledge
- has a good knowledge of how the health service works
- is available every time the patient is seen
- is accepted and trusted by the patient and health worker
- is sensitive to the patient's and health worker's needs
- will not allow his or her own beliefs to override those of the patient
- puts the patient at ease
- has a good memory and pays attention to detail
- can translate fine shades of meaning
- is able to tell the health worker when the patient has problems and why
- is aware of the cultural expectations of both patients and health workers and can explain them to both
- is the same sex as the patient
- is able to carry the responsibility.

Although these attributes are highly desirable, they are not necessarily achievable simultaneously. With our multiethnic population, minority ethnic health should not be an added extra but a part of mainstream funding (David 1998).

CLINICAL EFFECTIVENESS IN COMMUNITY CARE

There is an ever-growing pressure on all healthcare professionals across all specialties to demonstrate the value and effectiveness of the service they provide (Walshe 1997). In the current climate of economic constraint and demanding value for money, all publicly funded employees need to prove their worth. Gough (1995) argues that determining the impact and value of care provided by community nurses is particularly difficult. This is, according to Gough (1995), because the work of community nurses is highly private, hidden behind closed doors and with a traditionally unvocal patient group.

The nature of community renal nursing is concerned with aspects of health promotion, prevention of infection, support, advice and teaching, all of which can be difficult to measure in terms of health gain for the patient and the impact the service has on the patient's life. Walshe (1997) argues that those working in the community have remarkably little evidence with which to justify certain patterns of clinical practice.

There appears to be no published evidence as to the clinical effectiveness of community renal nurses. The assumption is that they provide an essential, valuable and needed service caring for an ever-increasing home dialysis patient population. It is vitally important that community renal nurses articulate their worth by demonstrating that their service can, for example, reduce admission rates for dialysis-related problems if this type of service is to continue.

As community nurses are major providers of healthcare, they must assume a key role in measuring the quality of services, effectiveness of care and documenting costs (Gough 1995). A major challenge is to prove the value of the expert contribution community renal nurses can make.

SUMMARY

With the recognised shift of more technical treatments into the community, patients using home PD and HD can be safely cared for and managed by community renal nurses together with district nurses and visits to the hospital multidisciplinary team.

The community is a complex mixture of health and social care and the nurse needs to have a sound knowledge of available treatments as well as the needs of the patients on dialysis at home. This enables a comprehensive and sensitive service to be available to renal patients, wherever the treatment is carried out.

REFERENCES

Brindle C, Brown K. Community health care. New York: Macmillan Magazines, 1991.

Brunier GM, McKeever PT. The impact of home dialysis on the family: literature review. ANNA J 1993; 20:653–658.

David M. Cultural awareness and customer care. In: Castledine G, McGee P, eds. Advanced and specialist nursing practice. Oxford: Blackwell Science. 1998: 158–162.

Department of Health. The Health Service. The NHS reforms and you. London: HMSO, 1990.

Department of Health. A framework for local community care charters in England. London: DOH, 1994.

Department of Health. The patient's charter and you. Raising the standard. London: HMSO, 1995.

Department of the Environment. Environmental protection act 1990. Waste management. The duty of care. A code of practice. London: HMSO, 1990.

Elliott O. Working with black and minority ethnic groups. In: Webb P, ed. Health Promotion and patient education. A professional's guide. London: Chapman & Hall, 1994:195–213.

Ewles L, Simnett I. Promoting health. A practical guide to health education. 4th ed. London: Baillière Tindall, 1999.

Fawcett-Henesy A. Chronic disease: the challenge for nursing and midwifery. EDTNA/ERCA J 1999; XXV:45–48.

Fuller FHS, Toon PD. Medical practice in a multicultural society. Oxford: Heinemann Medical Press, 1998.

Gerrish K, Husband C, Mackenzie J. Nursing for a multi-ethnic society. Buckingham, Philadelphia: OUP, 1996.

Gough P. Measuring the effectiveness of community health nursing. In: Sines D, ed. Community health care nursing. Oxford: Blackwell Science, 1995:356–373.

Helman CG. Culture, health and illness. 4th ed. Oxford: Butterworth-Heinemann, 2000.

Hennessy D, Swain G. Developing community health care. In: Hennesy D, ed. Community health care development. Basingstoke: Macmillan, 1997:1–36.

Hyde C. Quality of life and coping in home haemodialysis patients. EDTNA/ERCA 1998; 24:10–12.

Jaffe M, Skidmore-Roth L. Home health nursing care plans. 2nd edn. St Louis: Mosby, 1993.

Keogh AM. Dialysis at home; the role of the renal community nurse. Br J Homecare. 1999; 1:50–56.

Lok P. Stressors, coping mechanisms and quality of life among dialysis patients in Australia. J Adv Nurs 1996; 23: 873–881.

Lunts P. Rediscovering home haemodialysis. Returning choice to patients. EDTNA/ERCA J 1999; 25:40–42.

Marks L. Home and hospital care: redrawing the boundaries. Research report no. 9. London: Kings Fund Institute, 1991.

McClure L. Caregivers and community nurses: co-experts in care? In: Hyde V, ed. Community nursing and health care. Insights and innovations. London: Arnold, 2001: 95–118.

McGee P. Specialist practice in the UK. In: Castledine G, McGee P, eds. Advanced and specialist nursing practice. Oxford: Blackwell Science, 1998:135–145.

Newby N. Chronic illness and the family life-cycle. J Adv Nurs 1996; 23:786–791.

Oreopoulos DG. Is there a right time to say no to life? Editorial. Int Soc Peritoneal Dialysis 1994; 14:205–208.

Roderick PJ, Jones I, Raleigh VS et al. Population need for renal replacement therapy in Thames regions: ethnic dimension. Br Med J 1994; 309:1111–1114.

Simoyi P. Taking dialysis to the community. Commun Outlook 1993; 3:37–38.

Skidmore D. Community care. Initial training and beyond. London: Arnold, 1997.

Stewart G. The renal nurse consultant: perspectives on a new role. Approaches to cost effective, quality care for the renal patient. EDTNA/ ERCA J 1991; 16:2–4.

Thomas N. Patient education. In: Challinor P, Sedgewick J, eds. Principles and practice of renal nursing. Cheltenham: Stanley Thornes, 1998.

United Kingdom Central Council for Nursing, Midwifery and Health Visiting. Code of professional conduct. London: UKCC, 1992.

United Kingdom Central Council for Nursing, Midwifery and Health Visiting. The future of profesional practice—the Council's standards for education and practice following registration. London: UKCC, 1994.

Uttley L, Prowant B. Organization of the peritoneal dialysis program—the nurses' role. In: Gokal R, Khanna R, eds. The textbook of peritoneal dialysis. Dordrecht: Kluwer Academic Publishers, 1994:335–355.

Wagner C. Family needs of chronic hemodialysis patients: a comparison of perceptions of nurses and families. ANNA J 1996; 23:19–26.

Walshe K. Clinical effectiveness: the challenge for community nursing. In: Hennessy D, ed. Community health care development. Basingstoke: Macmillan Press, 1997.

Warmington V, Baxter E. A supportive partnership for CAPD patients. Professional Nurse 1996; 11; 767–768.

Webb P. (ed.) Health promotion and patient education. A professional's guide. London: Chapman & Hall, 1994.

Wellard SJ, Street AF. Family issues in home based care. Int J Nurs Practice 1999; 5:132–136.

White Y, Grenyer BFS. The biopsychosocial impact of end-stage renal disease: the experience of dialysis patients and their partners. J Adv Nurs 1999; 30:1312–1320.

Wilkie M, Brown C. Sharing the management of patients on CAPD. Prescriber 1994; 5:61–65.

Zastocki DK, Rovinski-Wagner C. Homecare: Patient and family instructions. 2nd Ed. Philadelphia, PA: WB Saunders, 2000.

Clinical standards and nursing audit

Nicola Thomas

13

CONTENTS

LEARNING OUTCOMES FOR THIS CHAPTER

- To understand the process of setting, delivering and monitoring standards
- To identify the four elements of clinical governance
- To evaluate the different national and international clinical guidelines that are available to the renal nurse
- To plan and evaluate the components of a clinical nursing audit of dialysis care.

INTRODUCTION

In 1998, the Secretary of State announced specific measures to ensure that 'all patients should receive a first class service' (Department of Health 1998). This document highlighted that there are unacceptable variations in performance and practice, and in clinical outcomes. The previous chapters in this book have to some extent highlighted the inequalities in renal care (lack of autonomous renal services in some parts of the country; low acceptance rates for renal replacement therapy, particularly for older people; and poor numbers of specialist nurses) across the UK.

This chapter will explore the ways in which renal nurses can promote a high-quality service, through understanding of the clinical governance framework, knowledge of clinical standards, and evaluation of best practice guidelines. Nurses have a vital role to play in the promotion of quality care in the renal specialty and are in a key position to understand the needs of individual patients and their carers.

SETTING, DELIVERING AND MONITORING STANDARDS

Over the past 10 years, the renal specialty has seen the emergence of a number of national and international standards for renal care and these clinical guidelines will be discussed in more detail later in the chapter.

When the government's way of setting clear national standards was announced in 1998, the main strategy for this was through National Service Frameworks (NSF) and through a National Institute for Clinical Excellence (NICE). In July 2001, the work commenced on the NSF for kidney disease with the announcement of the co-chairs of the external reference group.

National service frameworks

As outlined in the Department of Health (1997) paper 'The new NHS', the government will work with the professions and representatives of users and carers to establish clearer, evidence-based NSFs for major care areas and disease groups. That way, patients will get greater consistency in the availability and quality of services, right across the National Heath Service (NHS). The government will use them as a way of being clearer with patients about what they can expect from the NHS.

So, the NSFs will:

- set national standards and define service models
- put in place programmes to support implementation
- establish performance measures against which progress within an agreed timescale will be measured.

Although it may be some time before the Renal Service Framework is published, the Kidney Alliance in 2001 produced some service standards and recommended the structures that are necessary to deliver them in the new NHS. These are discussed later in the chapter.

National institute for clinical excellence

NICE produces and disseminates clinical guidelines based on relevant evidence, associated clinical audit methods and information on good practice. The Institute will identify new and existing health interventions, collect evidence, consider the implications for clinical practice, disseminate the findings, implement at a local level and monitor the impact. To date, the only guidelines produced by NICE that are specifically relevant to renal practice are those that are written on Renal Care in type 2 diabetes mellitus. These were out for consultation at the end of 2000 and the final version is expected in 2002. For further details look on the NICE website: www.nice.org.uk.

DELIVERING QUALITY STANDARDS

Once the Renal NSF has been published, the Department of Health (1998) has stated that 'we need consistent action locally to ensure that national standards and guidance are reflected in the delivery of services'. That action will be guided by a single, robust framework—a new system of clinical governance—to monitor healthcare at a local level.

Clinical governance

Clinical governance can be defined as a framework through which NHS organizations are accountable for continuously improving the quality of

---

■ **BOX 13.1 Main components of clinical governance (NHS Trusts)**

- Clear lines of responsibility and accountability for the overall quality of clinical care
- A comprehensive programme of quality improvement activities, e.g. audit, evidence-based practice, continuing professional development, effective monitoring of clinical care
- Clear policies aimed at managing risks
- Procedures for all professional groups to identify and remedy poor performance, e.g. critical incident reporting, complaints procedures, staff supported to report any concerns about colleagues' professional conduct

---

Source: Department of Health (1998). Crown copyright material is reproduced with the permission of the Controller of HMSO and the Queen's Printer for Scotland.

their services and safeguarding high standards of care by creating an environment in which excellence in clinical care will flourish. Central to this initiative is the understanding that everyone in clinical care is responsible for delivering a high-quality service (Middleton & O'Donaghue 2001). The main components of clinical governance are shown in Box 13.1.

So what does all this mean for renal nurses? It could be argued that many of these suggested systems are already in place, but they do not necessarily work within an integrated and cohesive framework. This chapter will now go on to explore the ways in which renal nurses can contribute to improving the quality of patient care and work within a true partnership with patients, doctors and other members of the interprofessional team. As the Royal College of Nursing (2000) has recognized, nurses have a key role in implementing clinical governance and maximum use should be made of their skills and expertise to improve quality.

CLINICAL EFFECTIVENESS

Clinical effectiveness is about doing the right thing in the right way and at the right time for the right patient (Royal College of Nursing, 1996). The NHS Executive (1998) described several key activities needed to support clinically effective practice and these include:

- selecting a particular aspect of practice to question or examine
- finding out from the literature and professional networks and other sources what is best practice and critically appraising the available literature and sources
- implementing and/or learning how to provide best known clinical practice
- confirming that you are providing best practice on a day-to-day basis
- changing practice to make improvements if necessary.

In renal nursing practice we are fortunate to have a variety of clinical standards and guidelines to help us achieve clinically effective practice. In other words, many of the clinical guidelines that are available have been based on research evidence or expert opinion, so we do not have to examine all aspects of our care as it has already been done for us. There now follows a review of the most important clinical standards and guideline documents available for renal nurses.

CLINICAL STANDARDS AND BEST PRACTICE GUIDELINES

In 1990, the European Dialysis and Transplant Nurses' Association/European Renal Care Association (EDTNA/ERCA) commenced work on writing European clinical standards and in 1995 published European Standards for Nephrology Nursing Practice (Van Waeleghem & Edwards 1995). This document was published alongside the European core curriculum for a postbasic course in nephrology nursing (Kuentzle & Thomas 1995), as part of the Association's strategy for the development of quality care in Europe (Kuentzle et al 1997). These standards were one of the first publications that recommended specific guidelines for renal clinical practice. An outline of the key components is shown in Box 13.2.

Box 13.3 shows an example of one of the standards—discontinuation of treatment (dialysis). As can be seen from the example, these standards are based on the Dynamic Standard Setting System as first described by Kitson for the Royal College of Nursing in 1990. These standards are broad to allow for differing renal care practices across Europe and have been made more specific for local use. They were based on opinion, as a group of experienced healthcare professionals came together in a working group to define specific levels of practice.

Since 1995, the EDTNA/ERCA has developed a Research Board and each year carries out a collaborative research project. In past years, topics for the collaborative research project have been vascular access (Van Waeleghem

---

■ BOX 13.2 EDTNA/ERCA European standards for nephrology nursing practice (Van Waeleghem & Edwards 1995, with permission)

Fundamental aspects of care
- Conservative management
- Education of staff
- Psychological support
- Discontinuation of treatment

Specific treatment modalities
- Haemodialysis
- Peritoneal dialysis
- Paediatric renal replacement
- Acute renal failure
- Transplantation

■ **BOX 13.3 Discontinuation of treatment**

Standard statement

Nephrology patients and their families will be positively supported when decisions to discontinue treatment are made, whether by themselves, members of the family, or by the multidisciplinary team, in order that the patient may die with dignity.

Structure criteria

1. The multidisciplinary team will provide appropriate bereavement and counselling support for patients and their families.
2. The nephrology nurse will have access to courses on bereavement and counselling skills.

Process criteria

1. The nephrology nurse will assess, plan and implement the most appropriate care to meet the needs of patients and their families during the dying and grieving process.
2. The nephrology nurse will refer patients and their families for bereavement counselling, as necessary.
3. The nephrology nurse will give patients and their families information about external agencies which provide bereavement counselling.
4. The nephrology nurse will ensure that the care environment is relaxing, non-judgemental, and provides patients and their families with maximum privacy.
5. The nephrology nurse will document all planned care and support, identifying the patients and/or families with special needs.

Outcome criteria

1. Patients and/or their families state that they were supported and encouraged to discuss their fears about, and adjustment to, impending death, and the processes of grieving and bereavement.
2. There is evidence that patients and their families have had access to bereavement counsellors and/or external agencies, as necessary.
3. The nephrology nurse has documented and evaluated the ongoing support for and interactions with the patient in the care plans.
4. Liaison between bereavement counsellors and/or external agencies and the nephrology team is documented as effective and appropriate.

---

et al 2000), dietary advice (Nevett et al 2000) and water treatment (Lindley et al 2000). It is hoped that as a result of these European surveys into clinical practice, evidence-based clinical guidelines will result, and work is commencing on haemodialysis and water treatment guidelines at present. For further information visit the EDTNA/ERCA website at www.edtna-erca.org.

Nutritional guidelines have been developed by EDTNA/ERCA in 2001 and there are other guidelines for nutrition, as described in Chapter 9.

So, some guidelines have been developed on consultation with expert groups whilst others have been developed on opinion and evidence. An example of these is the K/DOQI guidelines (Kidney Disease Outcome Quality Initiative, originally called DOQI or Dialysis Outcome Quality Initiative).

The core principles of the K/DOQI guideline development process are:

* scientific and methodologic rigour using an evidence-based approach
* an interdisciplinary approach
* independence of work groups to facilitate an unbiased approach to guideline development, without influence of organizations or industry
* openness of the guideline development process. Draft guideline statements are subjected to a three-stage review process that invites comment from groups that the guidelines will affect.

Since the original development of the DOQI guidelines in haemodialysis and peritoneal dialysis, there have been developments in certain areas of care, such as anaemia management. For this reason the K/DOQI guidelines are being redeveloped at present and they should be ready for publication in 2002. An example of part of the original DOQI guideline on haemodialysis dose is shown for information in Box 13.4. Each guideline is supported by a rationale based on evidence and opinion. For further information, visit www.kidney.org/professionals/doqi.

Within the UK, the Renal Association published the second edition of *Treatment of Adult Patients with Renal Failure—Recommended Standards and Audit Measures* in 1997. A third edition is expected and consultation on some modality-specific guidelines, such as peritoneal dialysis, are taking place during 2001. This important document is being used as a framework for clinical audit throughout many renal units in the UK, and Box 13.5 shows the main content. For further information, visit the website: www.renal.org/

As discussed in Chapter 1, the Kidney Alliance (2001) has published seven National Service Standards which constitute the core objectives of a strategic plan for renal services for the next decade. In most cases, the evidence base for the recommendations is described. Box 13.6 shows a summary of the National Service Standards and Box 13.7 an example of a Service Standard.

■ **BOX 13.4 DOQI guideline 4: minimum delivered dose of haemodialysis (adults—evidence, children—opinion)**

The dialysis care team should deliver a *Kt/V* of at least 1.2 (single-pool, variable-volume) for both adult and paediatric haemodialysis patients. For those using the urea reduction ratio (URR), the delivered dose should be equivalent to a *Kt/V* of 1.2, i.e. an average URR of 65%. URR can vary substantially as a function of fluid removal, however.

■ BOX 13.5 Renal Association standards 1997

- Practical aspects of comparative audit—definition of standard, medium- and high-risk patients
- Haemodialysis standards
- Peritoneal dialysis standards
- Transplantation standards
- Acute potentially reversible renal failure
- Chronic renal failure (predialysis)
- General nephrology
- Blood-borne viruses and microbiology
- Quality of life

For further information visit the website: www.renal.org.

■ BOX 13.6 Kidney Alliance National Service Standards

- Predialysis: retarding progression and reducing the comorbid burden in renal disease
- Preparation for renal replacement therapy
- Vascular and peritoneal dialysis
- Effective delivery: Renal Association Standards and continuous quality improvement
- Patient/carer experience
- Conservative management of end-stage renal failure, palliative care and withdrawal from dialysis
- Equity of provision

EVALUATION OF GUIDELINES

There are numerous other local, national and international guidelines that renal nurses can access for achieving clinically effective practice, although Mead (2000) questions how useful these guidelines can actually be in promoting good practice. She summarises her debate with the following recommendations—guidelines are guides, not rules; practitioners must critically appraise the included evidence; national guidelines must be adapted to local circumstances; and it is vital to ensure judicious and selective guideline development.

It is helpful to have a checklist to evaluate how useful guidelines are to a local renal nursing team. The following questions could be used for evaluation:

- Are the guidelines based on evidence, expert opinion or both?
- What is the quality of the evidence? (well-conducted clinical studies, reports, opinions, clinical experience of respected professionals)
- Are the guidelines specific enough?

■ BOX 13.7 National Service Standard 5

Patient/carer experience
- ESRF patients should receive care and support which encourage inclusion of therapy into their overall lifestyle. Treatment should be in comfortable and convenient surroundings and delivered at times consistent with regaining or maintaining employment and maximising rehabilitation into society.
- ESRF patients should expect to access regular HD, CAPD and outpatient review as close to their homes as possible. Access to consultant time, nursing, dietetic, social work, counselling advice and pharmacy support should be equitable irrespective of place of residence or treatment. For the majority, one-way travel time for these services should be less than 30 min.
- HD centres should have parking, waiting and changing areas appropriate for 'lifelong' attendance.
- RRT patients with intercurrent problems requiring hospitalisation should expect to be admitted to single-sex areas in dedicated nephrology wards staffed by nurses trained in renal medicine and dialysis. Nephrology beds should be expanded in line with the expansion of dialysis stock so that the admission of a RRT patient to an 'outlying' ward is exceptional.
- Each patient should have a named nurse responsible for assessment and planning of care.
- Patients and carers, through their local KPAs and the NKF, should expect to be involved in local planning and the setting of Service Level Agreements and to be co-opted on to provider planning committees, on to renal subgroups of RSCGs and on to national initiatives, including the setting of clinical standards.
- Dialysis patients should be free to holiday in the UK or overseas. This will require investment in the health economies of popular UK destinations. It will require the creation of facilities in all HD units for temporary 'isolation' of patients returning from areas overseas which are high-risk for blood-borne virus infections.

ESRF, end-stage renal failure; HD, haemodialysis; CAPD, continuous ambulatory peritoneal dialysis; RRT, renal replacement therapy; KPA, Kidney Patients' Association; NKF, National Kidney Foundation; RSCG, Renal Specialised Commissioning Group.

- Are the guidelines local, national or international?
- Have patients been involved in the development?
- Do the guidelines measure nursing?

The last point is difficult to evaluate, as of course nurses do not work in isolation and therefore all members of the multiprofessional team contribute to patient outcome. But it is important that nurses recognise that it is nursing that they have to measure, and not necessarily the easier-to-measure variables such as blood pressure, potassium level, Kt/V and haemoglobin levels. What matters to patients is the depth of the communication, the skill of the teaching and the quality of their life, and although it is recognized that all of these are very difficult to measure, surely nurses must strive to evaluate these as part of the audit process.

NURSING AUDIT

The NHS Executive (1998) described how to design and carry out a clinical audit. See Figure 13.1 for an overview of this process.

For renal nurses, it has been shown that, although there are many national and international guidelines available, one of the difficulties is how to select topics for audit that really matter to patient care. It is recognized that quality-of-life instruments may be one way of measuring more qualitative outcomes, but that in itself is challenging as 'there are no agreed methods of assessment

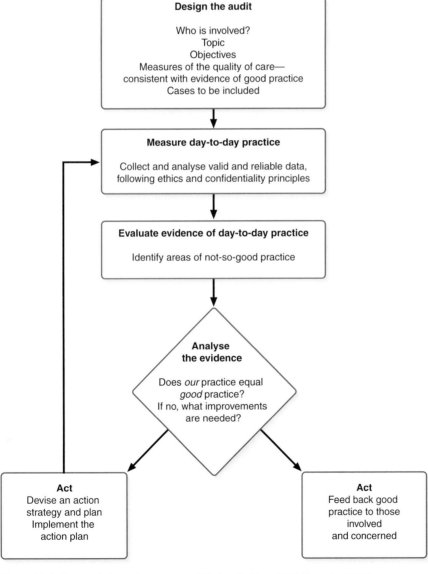

Figure 13.1 How to design and carry out a clinical audit. (From NHS Executive 1998.)

upon which audit of this aspect of renal care can be based' (Renal Association 1997). There has been some ongoing work by the Renal Nurse Advisory Group on this issue and results are awaited with interest.

SUMMARY

Increasingly, renal nurses are being asked to present clinical audit findings on behalf of the multiprofessional team, and it is important to remember that patients are also to be included in the audit cycle. There are international (European Kidney Patients' Foundation: CEAPIR), national (National Kidney Foundation: NKF) and local patients' associations which are ready to participate. Renal nurses are contributing to the culture of continuous quality improvement in patient care and have a very important role to play in implementation of clinical governance.

REFERENCES

Department of Health. The new NHS. London: HMSO, 1997.

Department of Health. A first class service. Quality in the new NHS. London: HMSO, 1998.

Kidney Alliance. End-stage renal failure. A framework for planning and service delivery. Kidney Alliance, 2001.

Kitson A. The dynamic standard setting system. RCN standards of care paper. London: RCN, 1990.

Kuentzle W, Thomas N (eds). European core curriculum for a post-basic course in nephrology nursing. Ghent, Belgium: European Dialysis and Transplant Nurses Association/European Renal Care Association, 1995.

Kuentzle W, Thomas N, Hartley-Jones J. Developing a strategy for the quality of renal care in Europe. Jpn J Clin Dialysis 1997; 13:21–25.

Lindley L, Lopot F, Harrington M et al. Treatment of water for dialysis: a European survey. EDTNA/ERCA J 2000; XXVI:22–27.

Mead P. Clinical guidelines: promoting clinical effectiveness or a professional minefield? J Adv Nurs 2000; 31:110–116.

Middleton R, O'Donaghue D. Clinical governance in the field of renal medicine. Br J Renal Med 2001; Vol 6:17–20.

Nevett G, Nagel C, Elseviers M et al. Provision of dietary advice in selected centers across Europe. EDTNA/ERCA J 2000; XXVI:34–40.

NHS Executive. Achieving effective practice. A clinical effectiveness and research information pack for nurses, midwives and health visitors. London: HMSO, 1998.

Renal Association. Treatment of adult patients with renal failure. Recommended standards and audit measures. Bristol: Renal Association, 1997.

Royal College of Nursing. Clinical effectiveness. A Royal College of Nursing guide. London: Royal College of Nursing, 1996.

Royal College of Nursing. Improving quality of care—RCN guidance for nurses on clinical governance. Available: www.rcn.org.uk/services 11 Oct 2001.

Van Waeleghem JP, Edwards P. European standards for nephrology nursing practice. Ghent, Belgium: European Dialysis and Transplant Nurses Association/European Renal Care Association, 1995.

Van Waeleghem JP, Elseviers M, Lindley L. Management of vascular access in Europe Part 1. EDTNA/ERCA J 2000; XXVI:28-33.

Future trends in renal nursing

14

Jean Yves De Vos

■ LEARNING OUTCOMES FOR THIS CHAPTER

- To identify the challenges that renal nurses may face in the future
- To find solutions to cope with the healthcare needs of tomorrow
- To evaluate the ways in which renal replacement therapies will look in the future
- To analyse the challenges facing renal nurses in the 21st century.

INTRODUCTION

Forty years ago, patients with kidney failure faced a brief future. Now, renal failure can often be treated successfully for several decades with dialysis techniques or transplantation. Although the technology existing to date is simple and on the whole well supported, dialysis treatments may last for hours and often involve additional hours of travel to and from dialysis centres, 3 or more days a week for the rest of an individual's life.

For the year 2000, the global number of dialysis patients treated worldwide is estimated at over 1 million people (Editorial Spotlight 2000).

Advances in immunosuppressive therapy, better surgical and medical insight and management of transplanted renal failure patients together with important steps towards successful xenotransplantation programmes have led and will continue to lead towards improved survival of patients with renal failure. In addition the improved care of patients who are dependent and will stay dependent on dialysis techniques, together with structural, molecular and pharmacological developments, continues to enhance the efficacy and safety of dialysis.

Recent successes in harvesting and expanding renal cells in vitro and the development of biologically active synthetic materials allow for the creation of three-dimensional functioning renal units, which in the future may be applied ex vivo or in vivo for partial or full replacement of kidney function—the bioartificial kidney.

Even the generation of human tissues and organs through genetic engineering in specialised labs will become reality in this century.

However, despite all these promising future initiatives, in view of the ever-increasing number of patients with renal failure and the increasing costs related to this, all these new innovations will not necessarily solve everything.

As discussed in Chapter 1, there will not be enough facilities to meet the demand for care due to funding and staff shortages. This has led to a possibly arbitrary selection of patients with renal failure needing treatment.

Even for those who will get treatment, satisfactory results will be diminished as a consequence of overutilisation of existing facilities and staff. This includes potentially dangerous and indiscriminate reduction of session lengths and limitation on the use of advanced and sophisticated materials and techniques.

Under such frightening perspectives, dialysis treatments that are widely available and give excellent patient outcomes at a reasonably low cost will be essential (Amiel & Atala 1999, Shapiro 1979, Zickler 1998).

WHO WILL NEED RENAL REPLACEMENT IN THE FUTURE?

Worldwide there is about a 7–10% yearly increase in the numbers of patients with renal failure (Editorial Spotlight 2000).

Approximately 760 000 patients received dialysis worldwide in 1996. Of these, 19.7% were in Europe; 28.3% in the USA; 1.4% in Canada; 11.2% in the Far East; 9.5% in Latin America; 21.8% in Japan and 8.1% in the rest of the world. For the year 2000 it was projected that over 1 million people would be treated for renal failure (US Renal Data System 1996).

Reasons for this increase are multiple, e.g. patients are often treated for decades because of better insight into treatment opportunities and improved development of treatment modalities.

Also, as a consequence of these medical and technical improvements, patients with larger and multiple pathologies are treated. This includes older patients and those with diabetes. The number of older patients has increased constantly over time as people live longer than in the past due to better healthcare provision and better working conditions, at least in industrialised countries. The number of people over 65 years is increasing by 7–8% per year.

As people grow older, one consequence is that they are more prone to having multiorgan failure, and caring for these complex needs is one of the many challenges facing renal nursing today.

Demographic profiles of those in Europe on chronic dialysis at present are as follows: about 10% are 15–45 years; about 30% are 46–65 years; and about 58% are over 65 years. About 10% of the 58% group are over 80 years (European Renal Association/European Dialysis and Transplant Association (ERA/EDTA) Registry 1999). In the UK, the second national Renal Registry Report showed that at the start of renal replacement therapy, 46% of patients were aged 65 or more and 33% were aged 70 or more in England and Wales in 1998 (Ansell & Feest 1999).

Another increasing group of patients are those with diabetes. At present these make up around 20–25% of the dialysis patients in Europe, and over 50% in the USA (ERA/EDTA Registry1999, Organisatie van Paramedici der Dialyse en Transplantie afdelingen (ORPADT) Questionaire 1997, US Renal Data System (USRDS 1999)).

These special groups of patients need very different and often more complicated care than those who are younger. More complex care means advanced caring skills, increased care time and higher costs.

WHO WILL CARE FOR THOSE WITH RENAL FAILURE?

It is clear that the need for broader care skills and time per patient will be the major challenge when treating constantly increasing numbers of patients with more complicated renal failure due to age and multiple organ failure.

At present there is projected to be a shortage of nurses and doctors within the industrialised countries worldwide, a time when numbers of patients are increasing yearly and pathology is demanding extra care. It has been estimated that there is a 16–20% shortfall in the number of nurses required in acute hospitals in the UK (Millar 2000). A survey of renal units carried out for the Kidney Alliance in 1999/2000 showed that, of the 55 renal units surveyed, only four stated that recruitment and retention of nurses was not a problem (Kidney Alliance 2001).

An increase of 7–10% per year of those on dialysis means that in 10–15 years' time we will treat double the number of patients that are treated today.

What can be done about the shortage of nurses? There has been much recent publicity concerning the lack of nurses in the UK and in Europe (Kennedy 1999). Strategies include recruitment overseas, although this in itself is not without problems (Mahoney 2001), continuing education for those who are new to renal care and the overall challenge of improving working conditions and the social–financial recognition of the profession.

Another route might be to employ more healthcare support workers into the renal specialty, although specialist in-service education is essential for this group of healthcare workers. There has been much debate in the UK about the employment of healthcare support workers and many renal units are now using non-registered practitioners to take on specialist nursing skills (Kidney Alliance 2001), such as cannulation of fistulae. Many clinical nurse managers are having to evaluate the effects of a changing nursing skill-mix and are re-evaluating the roles of the healthcare assistant (Thornley 2000).

A renal nurse working in today's healthcare environment needs additional skills due to the changed profile of the patients to be cared for—older people and those with comorbid conditions such as diabetes, heart disease and cancer.

At present, staff/patient ratios within Europe are about one nurse per four patients in the best situation and up to one nurse per six patients in chronic haemodialysis programmes. Staff/patient ratios for chronic peritoneal dialysis programmes and home haemodialysis programmes are much more widely spread within Europe, even within one single country (EDTNA/ERCA 1999–2000, ORPADT Questionnaire 1997, UK Renal Registry Data 1999).

This staff/patient ratio has not really changed over the years, whilst patient care has differed enormously. Technical advances, such as controlled ultrafiltration, fully automatically controlled dialysis equipment and automated peritoneal dialysis devices have facilitated easier control of the treated patient but this still does not balance with the more complicated care need of patients.

At present and in the future, renal care centres will be needed to train or employ multispecialised renal care nurses to deal with this new patient profile. There will be a need for nurses with extra skills in addition to renal care skills which are already essential. This includes knowledge and regular updating on care and treatment of diabetes mellitus, older adults, wound care, infection control, psychosocial support and other pertinent issues.

There will be a need to invest in allowing renal care workers to follow specific courses and conferences nationally and internationally. Renal care nurses will become more multidisciplinary in future. At the least they should cover knowledge of the total care needed for the new renal care patient, but importantly, they should work closely together with skilled and educated specific care workers such as dietitians, social workers, technicians, medical doctors, psychologists and podiatrists.

SOCIOECONOMIC CHALLENGES

Renal failure patients represent fewer than 1% of the population needing medical care while at present they consume over 5% of total medical expenditure (Editorial Spotlight 2000).

There is no doubt that caring for more patients will open debate on what all this will cost in future, and if society will still be able to afford this.

Healthcare resources all over the world are restricted in relation to economic welfare. Each society will have to define how much can be spent for what purpose.

There might be a lack of resources, not only because of the higher number of renal care patients with often more complex pathologies to be treated in the next decades, but also because of ever-increasing costs when using newer but more expensive techniques and equipment.

Renal care workers will play an important role, in collaboration with authorities, private insurance companies and renal care industries, in planning for the best use of available resources.

There will be a need for multidisciplinary leadership of nephrologists, nurses, social workers, dietitians and patients. We will have to decide together which patient requires which renal replacement according to the individual profile of each patient.

ADVANCES IN RENAL REPLACEMENT THERAPIES

This section explores challenging future perspectives that could help the next generation to cope with the socioeconomic difficulties encountered when treating those with renal failure.

Extracorporeal treatments

There have been improvements in recent years in technical advances such as ultrafiltration control, blood volume control, blood temperature monitoring, electrolyte profiling, ultrafiltration profiling, online efficiency measurements and individualised treatments.

Over the next decades the evolution of effective use of biofeedback systems, in which biosensor technology will enable automatic steering of an individuals' treatment according to biological needs, is anticipated. Further reading can be found in Grassmann et al (2000). However, it is believed that those often costly new innovations will not solve all the challenges of renal healthcare (Parker 2000).

Costs of in-centre dialysis have risen progressively during the last 20 years due to a series of improvements in dialysate composition (better but more expensive water treatment and concentrate production), newer but more expensive membranes, more sophisticated equipment, increased use of more expensive techniques such as haemofiltration and haemodiafiltration, staffing, transportation and other issues. As well as cost, there are the pressures of increased numbers of patients and, in the UK, dialysis services are under intense pressure. In a recent survey of provider trusts (Kidney Alliance 2001), 31 out of 56 autonomous centres reported their dialysis programmes as 'tight, bordering on clinical compromise'.

Although home haemodialysis has declined dramatically over the last 20 years, from 41% in 1983 to 3.2% in 1998 in the UK (UK Renal Registry Data, 1999), many studies (Kenley et al, 1995) have suggested that it offers the optimum dialysis in terms of outcome. Improvement in quality of life of some selected groups of patients, such as younger people in employment, is attested to by the revival of home haemodialysis, more specifically, short daily dialysis or long nocturnal dialysis, in which treatment frequency can be increased (Hombrouckx et al 1989, Kenley et al 1995, Kjellstrand & Ing 2000). Renewed interest is being generated by the development of a small wearable dialysis device offering slow continuous therapy during the day time and eventually in combination with nocturnal dialysis (Hombrouckx et al, Unpublished work, 2000).

One of the reasons for the superior cost-effectiveness of home therapy is the reduced need for staffing and lower overhead costs in general. Studies have shown that treatment costs for a home dialysis patient are about half of the treatment cost for an in-centre patient. In some cases the reported savings are even greater (Kenley et al 1995).

To date, however, only 3% of European dialysis patients younger than 65 years perform home haemodialysis and this is predominantly in the UK and in France (ERA/EDTA Registry 1999).

Daily dialysis

The present commonly used haemodialysis schedules of 3–6 h three times a week is only a pragmatic compromise between the observation that it sustains patients reasonably well for long periods of time while twice a week did not (Kjellstrand & Ing 2000).

Studies have shown that if frequency of dialysis is increased, while total dialysis time per week is kept stable, this may lead to improved haematocrit, blood pressure control and general patient well-being, as well as the possibility of reducing or stopping some medication, such as antihypertensive therapy (Case Study 14.1).

There is no doubt about the medical superiority of daily dialysis when compared to thrice-weekly dialysis schedule.

At present there are no more obstacles for a wider application of this superior dialysis mode since some dialysis industries now offer basic but reliable dialysis machines for use at home (Kjellstrand & Ing 2000). For many, home therapy means improved quality of life, independence and flexibility, personalised dialysis and an active professional and social lifestyle.

Peritoneal dialysis

Another home therapy modality is peritoneal dialysis (see Ch. 8). Some promising future aspects are now explored.

Peritoneal dialysis is currently the dialytic treatment with the best cost/benefit ratio. However it is used worldwide in fewer than 20% (10–70%, varying from country to country) of end-stage renal disease treatments in the vast majority of countries (ERA/EDTA Registry 1999). The main factors for limiting a wider dispersion and a longer duration of peritoneal dialysis treatment are the fear of infection complication and the progressive reduction of the purifying efficiency and ability to maintain fluid balance and acceptable clearance over time. In future, better prevention of infection will be developed through newer and better techniques, and the possible use of vaccines against microorganisms which are frequently implicated in peritonitis (Amiel 1999, Atala Shapiro 1979, Zickler 1998).

Genetic engineering

Within the domain of transplantation, tissue engineering following genetic engineering sounds like science fiction, but it is not any more. Much is expected from this domain (Williams 1997).

The aim is to produce cells (such as kidney beta cells) which could be used in specific applications ex vivo and in vivo in the near future (Aebisher et al 1999, Roberts 2000). It is believed that by the year 2020 some diseases could be eradicated by replacing the defective genes. Bioengineers are already able to generate specific cells in specialised biolaboratories. The principle

■ CASE STUDY 14.1: Daily dialysis

This case study highlights the experience with ultra-short daily home haemodialysis in patients with end-stage renal failure in a dialysis unit in Belgium. The unit's nephrologist is a strong believer in increasing the dialysis frequency for haemodialysis patients in order to achieve better quality of life and improved long-term outcome.

The first patient was a 66-year-old woman who had been on chronic dialysis for 15 years because of polycystic kidney disease. As a result of increasing problems of general well-being and polyneuritis she accepted a change from 3 × 4 h a week to 5 × 2 h a week.

The ultrafiltration rate decreased from 875 mL h^{-1} to 750 mL h^{-1}. Cramps, hypotensive episodes, nausea and vomiting disappeared. Her blood pressure decreased from 150/90 mmHg to 120/80 mmHg without the need of antihypertensive therapy. Haematocrit rose from 28% to 36% without erythropoietin. Phosphate binders decreased from 6g day^{-1} calcium carbonate to zero. Nerve conductivity improved from 33 m s^{-1} to 40 m s^{-1} after 6 months. Mean weekly Kt/V increased from 3.6 to 6.4.

The second patient was a 57-year-old woman suffering from polycystic kidney. She was treated 6 × 1 h 45 min a week from the beginning while awaiting kidney transplantation. Daily home haemodialysis was her first choice as she was still an active teacher and she lived with her husband, who was blind and needed her help. The ultrafiltration rate on dialysis was 660 mL h^{-1}. No cramps, hypotensive episodes or nausea were experienced. Blood pressure was kept at 120/70 mmHg without any antihypertensive therapy. Haematocrit was kept at 33% without the need for erythropoietin. No phosphate binders were needed. Nerve conductivity stayed at 47m s^{-1}. Mean weekly Kt/V was 7.8.

Note: Be careful when comparing Kt/V values when different treatment frequencies are used. Weekly Kt/V values are not simply to be divided by the number of sessions a week to get comparable values of objective dialysis dose.

Results

In the first patient, general well-being improved significantly, as did the biological parameters and nerve conductivity. Ultrafiltration needs per dialysis session were significantly lower than before, resulting in better dialysis tolerance and significantly lower dry body weight. Antihypertensive drugs were no longer needed.

In the second patient, general well-being was good from the beginning. There was no polyneuritis, good blood pressure control, low ultrafiltration needs and, good biological parameters. She was able to continue teaching and supporting her blind husband.

In both patients no problems with vascular access (both native fistulae) were encountered despite increased number of weekly punctures.

■ **CASE STUDY 14.1:** *(Continued)*

Conclusions

- Fewer dialytic complications (cramps, hypotensive episodes, nausea)
- Less need for medication: no or little erythropoietin, no phosphate binders, no antihypertensive drugs; only vitamins (D, B and folic acid) and some iron were needed
- Increased dialysis dose
- Increased or stable nerve conductivity (electromyogram)
- Better dialysis tolerance due to low ultrafiltration rates
- Better control of hydration status
- More physiological therapy due to daily elimination of solutes
- More stable and better metabolic condition.

---

would be to inject or transplant a biodegradable framework with human stem cells in the sick patient. After administering the growth factors, specific functioning cells or tissues or organs will develop within the human body, restoring normal function. This will definitely cause a revolution, as a limited number of people would then need chronic dialysis treatment, for a limited time before and during the process of regeneration.

Already there is a new trend among parents to save their newborn baby's umbilical cord blood as a potential source of stem cells for use within the family. These stem cells can then be used in the future by the bioengineer to generate desired specific cells, tissue or organs. What is important is that no immunosuppressive drugs would be required as cells and tissues would be recognised as the patient's own (Editorial Transplantation 2000).

At present an implantable bioartificial kidney, consisting of a haemofilter and hollow fibre dialyser wherein human proximal tubular renal cells have been grown on the outside of the fibres, has been constructed and clinically applied (Cutler 1997). Also pancreatic islet cells (beta cells) have been grown successfully but are still rapidly lost due to hypoxia. Isolation of the beta cells from pigs is another possibility. Isolation of human cadaver pancreas is possible, but due to the large numbers of pancreas (at least five) needed to isolate sufficient cells to treat one adult with diabetes for only a limited time, this is not the first choice (Editorial Spotlight 2000). Grafting a whole pancreas together with a renal graft offers a good alternative for those with diabetes mellitus and renal failure.

SUMMARY

The future of renal care will initiate heated debate and raise many ethical questions. For the moment, the most pressing issues in the UK have been highlighted by the Kidney Alliance (2001). There is congestion in many renal units and some areas of the country are without autonomous renal services or even satellite units. There are also huge difficulties in the recruitment and retention of nurses.

The way forward needs to support continuous quality improvement through interprofessional working, where nurses are seen to contribute on an equal footing within the healthcare team. Evidence-based practice and clinical audit are moving the renal nursing profession forward, together with recent appointments of nurse consultants within the nephrology specialty.

Finally, all the associations involved in renal care must work together with those who have experienced the service to ensure that renal care is truly patient-centred.

REFERENCES

Aebisher P, Lysaght MJ, Parenteau N et al. Special report on the promise of tissue engineering. Sci Am 1999; April:37–65.

Amiel GE, Atala A. Current and future modalities for functional renal replacement. Urol Clin North Am 1999; Feb:235–246.

Ansell D, Feest T. Second annual report of the UK Renal Registry. Available: www.renalreg.com/report99 3 Oct 2001.

Cutler DS. A look at potential ESRD treatment alternatives for the future. The bio-artificial kidney. Nephrol News Issues 1997; 11:14–15.

Editorial. Spotlight. Dialysis Transplant 2000; 29:514–518.

Editorial. Transplantation. Nephrol News Issues 2000; 14:66.

EDTNA/ERCA. Research board projects 1999–2000 data. Available: RB.office@pandora.be 3 Oct 2001.

European Renal Association/European Dialysis and Transplant Association (ERA/EDTA) Registry. (1999) Report on management of renal failure in Europe. Available: erareg@amc.uva.nl 3 Oct 2001.

Grassmann A, Uhlenbusch-Körwer I, Bonnie-Schorn E et al. Recent advances in dialysis fluid management and outlook—dialysis fluid of the future. In: Composition and management of hemodialysis fluids. Germany: Pabst Science, 2000:244–287, 306–307.

Hombrouckx R, Bogaert AM, Leroy F et al. Limitations of short dialysis are the indications for ultrashort daily auto dialysis. Trans Am Soc Artifi Intern Organs 1989; 35:503–505.

Kenley RS, Twardowski Z, Depner T et al. Will daily home hemodialysis be an important future therapy for ESRD? Semin Dialysis 1995; 8:261–274.

Kennedy A. A problem shared: a Europe wide approach to the chronic nursing shortage. World Irish Nurs 1999; 7:14–15.

Kidney Alliance. End-stage renal failure—a framework for planning and service delivery. Kidney Alliance, 2001.

Kjellstrand CM, Ing T. Daily hemodialysis: history and revival of a superior dialysis method. Available: http://www.aksys.com/SuperiorMethod.htm Nov 2000.

Mahoney C. NHS foreign recruitment sparks attack by WHO. Nurs Times 2001; 97:5.

Millar B. Situations vacant. Nurs Times 2000; 96:24–25.

Organisatie van Paramedici der Dialyse en Transplantie afdelingen (ORPADT) Questionnaire 1997. A survey of nephrology nursing care and treatments in Belgium. Nephrol News Issues 1998;11:53–56.

Parker TF. Technical advances in hemodialysis therapy. Semin Dialysis 2000; 13:372.

Roberts M. Conference report on the American Society for Artificial Internal Organs (ASAIO) meeting. Dialysis Transplant 2000; 29:663–692.

Shapiro FL. Hemodialysis and alternative treatments. A look into the near future. Nephron 1979; 24:2–6.

Thornley C. A question of competence? Re-evaluating the roles of the nursing auxiliary and health care assistant in the NHS. J Clin Nurs 2000; 9:451–458.

UK Renal Registry Data 1999. Available: www.renalreg.com 3 Oct 2001.

US Renal Data System (USRDS). Annual report. 1996 Available: www.usrds.org 11 Oct 2001.

Williams D. Engineering a concept: the creation of tissue engineering. Med Devices Technol 1997; 8:8–9.

Zickler P. Perspectives on dialysis therapy. Biomed Instrument Technol 1998; 36:627–630.

Index

Note: References to figures are indicated by 'f' and references to tables are indicated by 't' when they fall on a page not covered by the text reference.